European status report on road safety

Towards safer roads and healthier transport choices

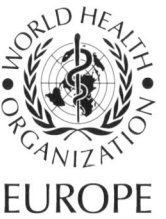

Abstract

This report presents the status of road safety in the WHO European Region and provides a baseline assessment of how far 49 countries have come in implementing the recommendations of the *World report on road traffic injury prevention*. In the Region, road crashes result annually in 120 000 deaths, 2.4 million injuries and a great economic burden, which may be up to 3% of a country's gross domestic product. Road traffic injuries are the leading cause of death among people 5–29 years old. Vulnerable road users such as pedestrians, cyclists and users of motorized two-wheelers constitute 39% of all road traffic injury fatalities, with pedestrians being more at risk in the eastern part of the Region. Countries differ greatly in mortality rates for road traffic injuries; the average in low- and middle-income countries is twice that in high-income countries. Countries' policy responses in providing road safety for their citizens have differed. This report proposes the following areas of action: narrow the gap between countries with the lowest and highest mortality rates; provide better protection for vulnerable road users; develop a well-resourced multisectoral road safety strategy in each country; design and enforce comprehensive legislation; and develop and implement healthier transport policies. In addition, country profiles on the current status of road safety are presented for the 49 participating countries.

Keywords

Accidents, traffic – statistics and numerical data
Accidents, traffic – economics
Safety management – organization and administration
Wounds and injuries – prevention and control
Europe

ISBN 978 92 890 4176 8

Suggested citation: *European status report on road safety: towards safer roads and healthier transport choices*. Copenhagen, WHO Regional Office for Europe, 2009.

Address requests about publications of the WHO Regional Office for Europe to:
Publications
WHO Regional Office for Europe
Scherfigsvej 8
DK-2100 Copenhagen Ø, Denmark
Alternatively, complete an online request form for documentation, health information, or for permission to quote or translate, on the Regional Office web site (http://www.euro.who.int/pubrequest).

© World Health Organization 2009

All rights reserved. The Regional Office for Europe of the World Health Organization welcomes requests for permission to reproduce or translate its publications, in part or in full.
The designations employed and the presentation of the material in this publication do not imply the expression of any opinion whatsoever on the part of the World Health Organization concerning the legal status of any country, territory, city or area or of its authorities, or concerning the delimitation of its frontiers or boundaries. Dotted lines on maps represent approximate border lines for which there may not yet be full agreement.
The mention of specific companies or of certain manufacturers' products does not imply that they are endorsed or recommended by the World Health Organization in preference to others of a similar nature that are not mentioned. Errors and omissions excepted, the names of proprietary products are distinguished by initial capital letters.
All reasonable precautions have been taken by the World Health Organization to verify the information contained in this publication. However, the published material is being distributed without warranty of any kind, either express or implied. The responsibility for the interpretation and use of the material lies with the reader. In no event shall the World Health Organization be liable for damages arising from its use.

Text editing: David Breuer
Design and layout: L'IV Com Sàrl, Le-Mont-sur-Lausanne, Switzerland
Cover mural: ©Artist, John Sakars; photography of mural: ©Claudia Aubertin-Vedova/Studio Southwest
Printed by Servizi Tipografici Carlo Colombo, Rome, Italy
Made possible through funding from Bloomberg Philanthropies

Contents

Acknowledgements — v

Foreword — vi

Executive summary — vii

1. Introduction — 1
    1.1 Road traffic injuries: a health priority — 1
    1.2 Rising inequality in the Region — 3
    1.3 Road traffic injuries and other transport-related health effects — 4
    1.4 International institutional response — 5
    1.5 Why this survey? — 6
    1.6 Objectives — 7
    1.7 Structure of the report — 7

2. Methods — 9

3. Findings — 11
    3.1 Great inequality in fatal and non-fatal road traffic injuries in the Region — 11
    3.2 Very many non-fatal injuries — 13
    3.3 Vulnerable road users are at risk — 13
    3.4 Health information systems need to be improved — 15
    3.5 The economic costs of road traffic injuries — 16
    3.6 Lead agency and national strategy on road safety — 17
        3.6.1 More countries need a national strategy for road safety — 17
        3.6.2 Expenditure on road safety varies greatly, and this expenditure is far less than the costs of road traffic injuries — 19
    3.7 Legislation on and enforcement of risk factors — 20
        3.7.1 Speed control needs to be improved and more widespread — 21
        3.7.2 Controlling drink–driving is a priority — 21
        3.7.3 Wearing helmets — 22
        3.7.4 There is much room for improvement in wearing seat-belts and using child car restraints — 22
        3.7.5 Better legislation and enforcement are needed — 23
    3.8 Road safety management — 24
        3.8.1 Better transport and urban policy to improve mobility and road safety — 24
        3.8.2 Other aspects of road safety management — 28

4. Conclusions — 29
    4.1 Key findings — 29
    4.2 Key actions — 31

5. References — 33

6. Country profiles — 35

Annexes 137

Annex 1.	Explanatory notes for Annexes 2–13	138
Annex 2.	Indicators explored in the questionnaire developed for the *Global status report on road safety*	142
Annex 3.	General information, vehicles, road traffic deaths and proportions of road user deaths by type and road traffic injuries for countries in the WHO European Region	144
Annex 4.	Mortality rates for road traffic injuries per 100 000 population by gross national income per person in the WHO European Region, 2008	146
Annex 5.	Sample objectives from national strategies implemented in countries in the WHO European Region	147
Annex 6.	Estimated economic costs of one death in selected countries in the WHO European Region	149
Annex 7.	Drinking and driving laws, enforcement and road traffic deaths attributed to alcohol in countries in the WHO European Region, 2008	150
Annex 8.	Seat-belt and child restraint laws, enforcement and wearing rates in countries in the WHO European Region, 2008	152
Annex 9.	Speed limit laws and enforcement in countries in the WHO European Region, 2008	153
Annex 10.	Helmet laws, enforcement and wearing rates in countries in the WHO European Region, 2008	154
Annex 11.	Road safety management, strategies and policies in countries in the WHO European Region	156
Annex 12.	Prehospital post-crash care systems in countries in the WHO European Region, 2008	160
Annex 13.	National data coordinators and survey respondents in countries in the WHO European Region	161

Acknowledgements

Many international experts and WHO staff have contributed to developing this report. WHO gratefully acknowledges the contributions made to this report by the following people.

Francesco Zambon, Dinesh Sethi and Francesca Racioppi wrote the report. Dinesh Sethi and Francesco Zambon provided coordination for developing it. Francesco Zambon conducted the statistical analysis and compiled country profiles. Francesco Mitis provided comments on drafts and contributed to sections of the report. Manuela Gallitto provided administrative support. Rimma Kuznetsova provided administrative support, contributed to compiling country profiles and statistical annexes and helped in obtaining photographs. Nicoletta Di Tanno helped in obtaining photographs. Maria Charnaya helped with editing drafts and contributed to sections. Luigi Migliorini and Tatiana Kolpakova provided support and commented on drafts.

Tamitza Toroyan, Margie Peden and Etienne Krug provided support for the coordination of the project and commented on drafts. Kidist Bartholomeos helped with data processing. Alison Harvey contributed to the country profiles. Meleckidzedeck Khayesi and Matts-Ake Belin commented on drafts. Steven Lauwers helped to obtain photographs.

The following external peer reviewers provided very helpful comments: Dinesh Mohan, Indian Institute of Technology, Delhi, India; María Seguí-Gómez, University of Navarra, Pamplona, Spain; Elizabeth Towner, University of the West of England, Bristol, United Kingdom; and Heather Ward, University College London, United Kingdom.

Country-level data could not have been obtained without the invaluable support of: the heads and staff of WHO country offices; the national data coordinators (Annex 13); all respondents and attendees of the consensus meetings in countries (Annex 13); and government officials who cleared the information for inclusion in the report.

The report also benefited from the contributions of the following people: David Breuer, who edited the report; graphic designers from L'IV Com Sàrl, who produced the design and layout; Tatiana Alekseeva, for information used in Box 9 on *The happy road of childhood*; John Sakars, artist for the mural reproduced on the cover and graciously on loan from Welland Centennial Secondary School, Ontario, Canada; and Claudia Aubertin-Vedova/Studio Southwest for the photograph of the mural.

Finally, the World Health Organization wishes to thank Bloomberg Philanthropies for its generous financial support for the development and publication of this report.

Foreword

Road traffic injuries are a major public health problem in the WHO European Region and cause the premature deaths of some 120 000 people every year. They are the leading cause of death in children and young adults aged 5 to 29 years. In addition to these deaths, about 2.4 million people are estimated to be so seriously injured as to require hospital admission each year. This is a strain on the resources of health systems as they strive to provide quality emergency trauma services while faced with other competing priorities. In addition to the pain and suffering experienced by the families of loved ones, road traffic injuries cause a substantial economic loss to society: up to 3% of the gross domestic product of any given country.

The evidence that road traffic injuries can be prevented is compelling, which makes the current situation all the more unacceptable. Countries that have invested in road safety for many decades have shown that effective strategies can reduce the size of the loss. Much of the evidence for effective prevention is summarized in the *World report on road traffic injury prevention* and the accompanying *Preventing road traffic injury: a public health perspective for Europe*, which were launched on World Health Day 2004. These reports and the accompanying advocacy activities helped to raise global awareness of the problem and called on policy-makers and practitioners to take evidence-based action against this leading cause of death and disability. Further, the contents of these reports informed the methodology used in a WHO global assessment of road safety.

The present publication uses a standard survey methodology, allowing policy-makers for the first time to make a thorough assessment of the road safety situation in 49 participating countries. It provides an important baseline for the progress made in implementing the actions proposed in the *World report on road traffic injury prevention*. It provides both a regional overview and detailed country profiles. It shows that many countries in the European Region use multisectoral strategies that have consistently lowered the mortality from road traffic injuries. Yet this achievement is uneven across the Region and the higher mortality rates suggest that many low- and middle-income countries need to make a stronger effort to make roads safer for their citizens. The publication also highlights the plight of vulnerable road users, especially pedestrians in the east of the Region and motorized two-wheelers in the south.

By providing a baseline assessment of what has been done in countries, this publication aims to mobilize efforts in the whole Region and highlights future actions to fill the gaps. These actions consist of both healthier transport policies and multisectoral evidence-based strategies to prevent this leading cause of death and disability. Tackling road safety is an investment in a healthier and more equitable future for our citizens.

Marc Danzon
WHO Regional Director for Europe

Executive summary

Key findings

In 2004, the World Health Organization (WHO) and the World Bank jointly launched the *World report on road traffic injury prevention*. The report provided evidence on the magnitude of the burden of road traffic injuries and on how to tackle road safety and recommended several actions for countries to implement. In 2008, WHO undertook a project to assess the status of road safety globally and to determine whether countries are implementing the recommendations of the *World report on road traffic injury prevention*. The survey used a standardized method with a questionnaire administered to representatives of the health, transport, justice and education sectors, academia and nongovernmental organizations. The project has led to the publication of the *Global status report on road safety*, which provides global results and regional reports from each of the six WHO regions. This publication reports in detail on the results from 49 participating countries in the WHO European Region. The survey has provided numerous key findings for the Region.

Large-scale problem

Annually, road crashes result in almost 120 000 fatalities and 2.4 million injuries in the Region. Road traffic injuries represent the leading cause of death among adolescents and young adults.

Great inequality in fatal and non-fatal road traffic injuries in the Region

Mortality rates for road traffic injuries differ widely between countries in the Region, with rates being twice as high in low- and middle-income countries as in high-income countries. Mortality rates in the Commonwealth of Independent States (CIS) are up to four times higher than those of the Nordic countries. Trends have been falling in many high-income countries but not in low- and middle-income countries, many of which are in the CIS.

Vulnerable road users are at risk

Pedestrians, cyclists and users of motorized two-wheelers constitute 39% of all deaths in road crashes. They are more likely to be more seriously injured. The proportion of pedestrians involved in road crashes is highest in CIS countries. High vehicle speeds and urban design place these road users at increased risk.

Costs of road traffic injuries severely burden countries' economies

The health service costs of treating the people injured and disabled by road crashes are very high as are the costs borne by families, communities and society at large due to forgone production. The economic burden of road crashes is as much as 3% of gross domestic product.

National strategies on road safety often fail to set measurable targets

About one third of the countries surveyed do not have a national, multisectoral strategy on road safety. Even the countries that do are not always able to set measurable targets that can be properly monitored and evaluated.

Enforcement of laws on vehicle speed, drink–driving and use of seat-belts, child car restraints and helmets is unsatisfactory in many countries

Many countries have inadequate legislation to control speed in urban areas, drink–driving and the use of helmets (for riders of motorized two-wheelers), seat-belts and child car restraints. Even well-designed legislation has no effect if it is not properly enforced. In most countries in the Region, the current enforcement of speed control, drink–driving and use of helmets, seat-belts and child car restraints is reported as not being effective enough.

Policies on walking and cycling and public transport services are not always factored into strategies on road safety and on transport systems

Only one third of the countries are implementing national policies on both public transport and walking and cycling. Even fewer countries have introduced measures to better manage private car use. This is of concern given the potential ill health associated with physical inactivity and environmental harm.

Recommendations for action

Based on these findings, the following areas of action are proposed, built on those proposed in the *World report on road traffic injury prevention*.

Inequality in road traffic injury deaths should be narrowed

More attention needs to be given to road safety throughout the Region. Some high-income countries have shown sustained political commitment and developed innovative strategies and technologies for reducing road traffic deaths and serious injuries. Countries with poorer road safety records need to take up this experience.

Vulnerable road users need better protection

Governments need to protect all road users and not neglect the needs of pedestrians, cyclists and riders of motorized two-wheelers. Road safety stakeholders need to work together to implement evidence-based action to guarantee better protection, especially in low- and middle-income countries.

More countries need a well-resourced multisectoral road safety body to take forward a strategy for safety

Such a body should involve all stakeholders in developing a multisectoral strategy that clearly designates responsibilities and authority as to who should do what, where and when.

Better enactment and enforcement of legislation on road safety could save lives

Governments need to ensure that comprehensive laws cover the main risk factors of speed, drink–driving and use of helmets (for riders of motorized two-wheelers), seat-belts and child car restraints. Enforcement of such legislation needs to be improved. This requires well-publicized enforcement campaigns, perceived certainty of being apprehended and severity and promptness of punishment for violations. Many countries need to put this winning combination in place.

Sustainable transport policies present a large untapped opportunity for health and environmental gains

Sustainable transport policies represent an important opportunity for contributing to achieving other public health and environmental goals. More countries could reap the multiple benefits of investing in policies that promote public transport, cycling and walking. Land-use and transport policies that encourage such modes of transport will provide multiple health gains by reducing injuries, decreasing respiratory illness, preventing noncommunicable disease through physical activity and mitigating the negative effects of climate change. Making roads safer for vulnerable road users will help to encourage greater mobility with walking and cycling. One way of achieving this is by implementing transport policies that integrate road safety with environmental and health concerns.

The report provides 49 country profiles on road safety that include data collected in the survey and can serve as a tool for assessing the road safety situation and stimulating debate and action nationally and can act as a baseline for future reference, assessment and monitoring.

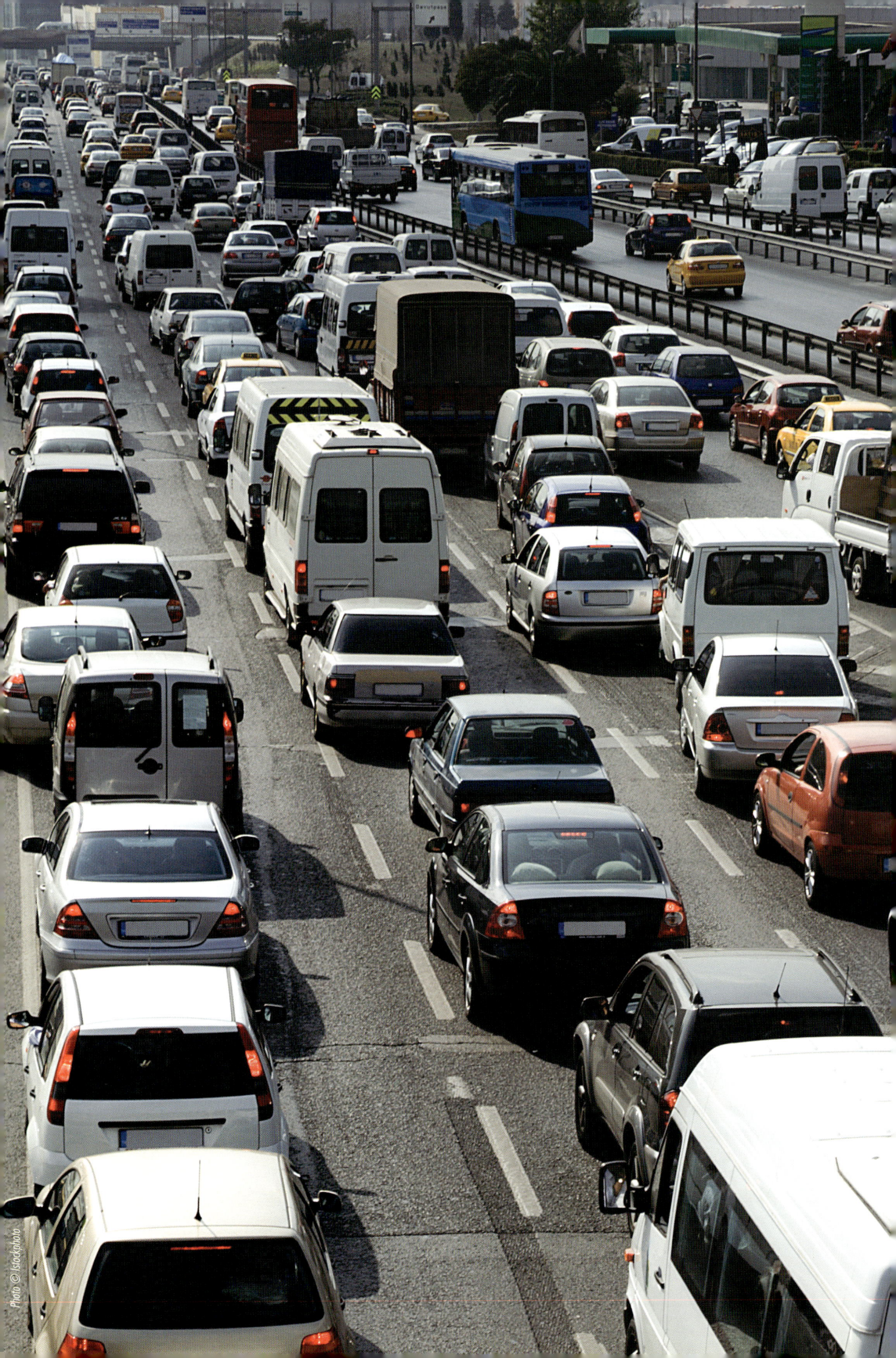

1 Introduction

1.1 Road traffic injuries: a health priority

Road traffic injuries are a major public health problem in the 53 countries of the WHO European Region. The annual death toll from road traffic injury is estimated to be 129 000 according to WHO's Global Burden of Disease project for 2004 (Table 1) *(1)*. In addition, road crashes injure more than 2.4 million people each year *(2)*. The problem is especially severe for people aged 5–29 years, for whom road traffic injuries are the leading cause of death (Table 1). Males are more likely to die than females from road traffic injury; they make up three fourths of road traffic deaths *(3–5)*. Underlying these stark statistics but less well described are the many more who suffer a temporary or permanent disability from their injury and the families emotionally devastated by the loss of loved ones. Many people may be driven into poverty by the loss of a family breadwinner or by the prolonged health and social care required for people with disabilities *(6)*. The costs of care and rehabilitation are considerable, and societal costs have been estimated at up to 3% of gross domestic product (GDP) *(7,8)*.

Nevertheless, many effective preventive strategies exist, and many European countries are among the safest in the world *(2)*. There is therefore potential to take up the challenge and reduce the burden of road traffic injuries by applying lessons of good practice. A good starting-point for this is to understand the baseline situation, which is one purpose of this report.

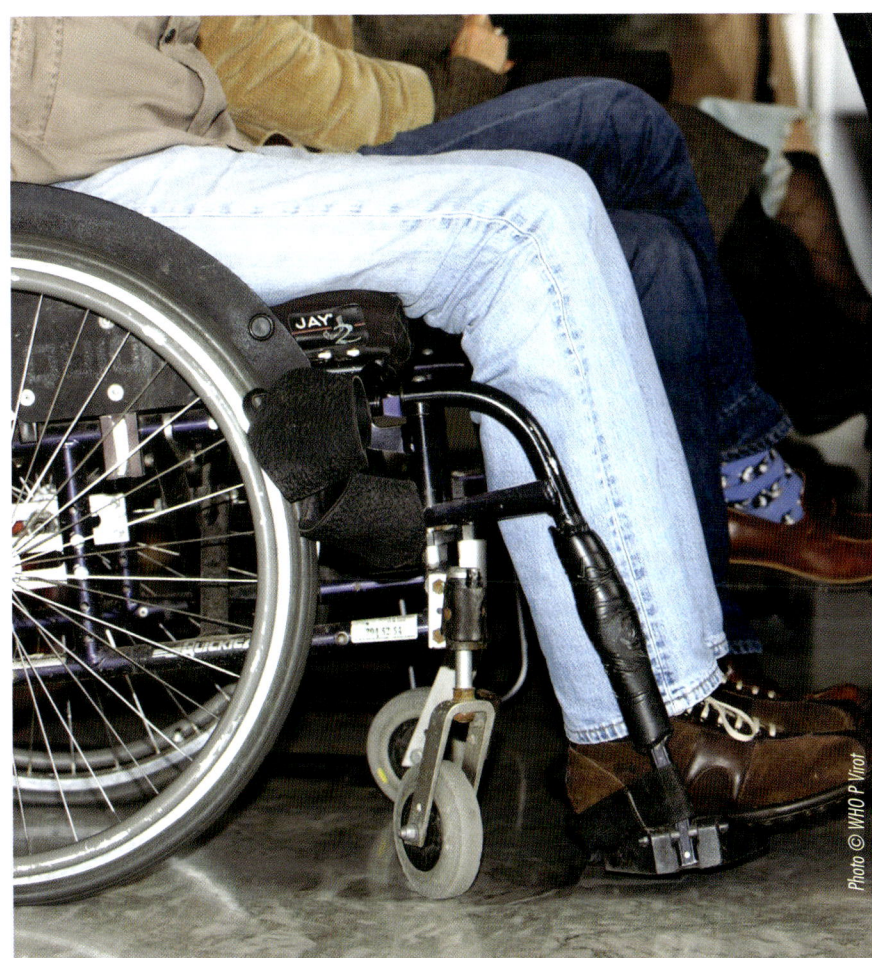

Table 1. Number of deaths for leading causes by age group in the WHO European Region, 2004

Rank	0–4 years	5–14 years	15–29 years	30–44 years	45–69 years	70+ years	Total
1	Perinatal causes 87 500	Road traffic injuries 4180	Road traffic injuries 39 300	Ischaemic heart disease 56 900	Ischaemic heart disease 679 400	Ischaemic heart disease 1 554 600	Ischaemic heart disease 2 295 600
2	Lower respiratory infections 34 500	Drowning 2430	Self-inflicted injuries 29 500	Self-inflicted injuries 41 000	Cerebrovascular disease 314 900	Cerebrovascular disease 1 020 200	Cerebrovascular disease 1 363 600
3	Diarrhoeal diseases 32 400	Lower respiratory infections 1930	Violence 14 900	Poisoning 33 600	Trachea, bronchus, lung cancer 190 900	Chronic obstructive pulmonary disease 176 300	Trachea, bronchus, lung cancer 370 700
4	Congenital anomalies 25 800	Leukaemia 1680	Poisoning 14 100	Road traffic injuries 33 200	Cirrhosis of the liver 112 400	Trachea, bronchus, lung cancer 168 900	Colon and rectum cancer 238 100
5	Meningitis 5360	Congenital anomalies 1390	HIV/AIDS 7010	Tuberculosis 28 900	Colon and rectum cancer 83 500	Colon and rectum cancer 148 300	Lower respiratory infections 234 700
6	Upper respiratory infections 3000	Self-inflicted injuries 1280	Tuberculosis 7000	Cirrhosis of the liver 27 400	Breast cancer 75 200	Lower respiratory infections 139 300	Chronic obstructive pulmonary disease 233 800
7	Drowning 2470	Lymphomas, multiple myeloma 700	Drowning 6570	Cerebrovascular disease 23 000	Stomach cancer 65 400	Hypertensive heart disease 130 700	Cirrhosis of the liver 184 900
8	Road traffic injuries 1740	Epilepsy 650	Ischaemic heart disease 4610	Violence 22 600	Self-inflicted injuries 57 500	Alzheimer and other types of dementia 128 400	Hypertensive heart disease 179 000
9	HIV/AIDS 1660	Violence 640	Cerebrovascular disease 4380	HIV/AIDS 13 700	Chronic obstructive pulmonary disease 54 600	Diabetes mellitus 106 700	Breast cancer 158 400
10	Endocrine disorders 1650	Cerebrovascular disease 590	Leukaemia 4250	Inflammatory heart diseases 10 700	Poisoning 52 300	Stomach cancer 82 000	Diabetes mellitus 155 400
11	Poisoning 1140	Endocrine disorders 590	Cirrhosis of the liver 3800	Breast cancer 10 300	Lower respiratory infections 46 800	Prostate cancer 77 100	Stomach cancer 155 100
12	Fire 1080	Poisoning 560	War and conflict 3700	Trachea, bronchus, lung cancer 10 200	Hypertensive heart disease 45 100	Breast cancer 72 500	Self-inflicted injuries 150 500
13	Leukaemia 970	Falls 530	Falls 3590	Lower respiratory infections 9400	Diabetes mellitus 42 800	Inflammatory heart diseases 68 600	Alzheimer and other types of dementia 137 400
14	Hepatitis B 950	War and conflict 470	Drug use disorders 3010	Drowning 9000	Inflammatory heart diseases 39 800	Nephritis and nephrosis 53 100	Road traffic injuries 129 100
15	Inflammatory heart diseases 780	Upper respiratory infections 430	Inflammatory heart diseases 2740	Falls 7900	Pancreas cancer 39 100	Pancreas cancer 51 600	Inflammatory heart diseases 122 900
16	Epilepsy 730	Fire 430	Lower respiratory infections 2730	Drug use disorders 7500	Road traffic injuries 36 500	Lymphomas, multiple myeloma 44 700	Poisoning 107 000
17	Violence 690	Meningitis 390	Epilepsy 2310	Stomach cancer 6800	Tuberculosis 33 600	Falls 44 600	Prostate cancer 97 300
18	Iron-deficiency anaemia 680	Nephritis and nephrosis 350	Nephritis and nephrosis 2200	Colon and rectum cancer 5500	Mouth and oropharynx cancer 33 300	Bladder cancer 43 100	Pancreas cancer 93 300
19	Falls 660	Inflammatory heart diseases 270	Congenital anomalies 2120	Fires 5300	Lymphomas, multiple myeloma 27 300	Cirrhosis of the liver 41 100	Perinatal causes 87 600
20	Hepatitis C 560	Diarrhoeal diseases 260	Lymphomas, multiple myeloma 2090	Alcohol use disorders 5200	Liver cancer 27 100	Liver cancer 35 500	Nephritis and nephrosis 80 300

Source: The global burden of disease: 2004 update *(1)*.

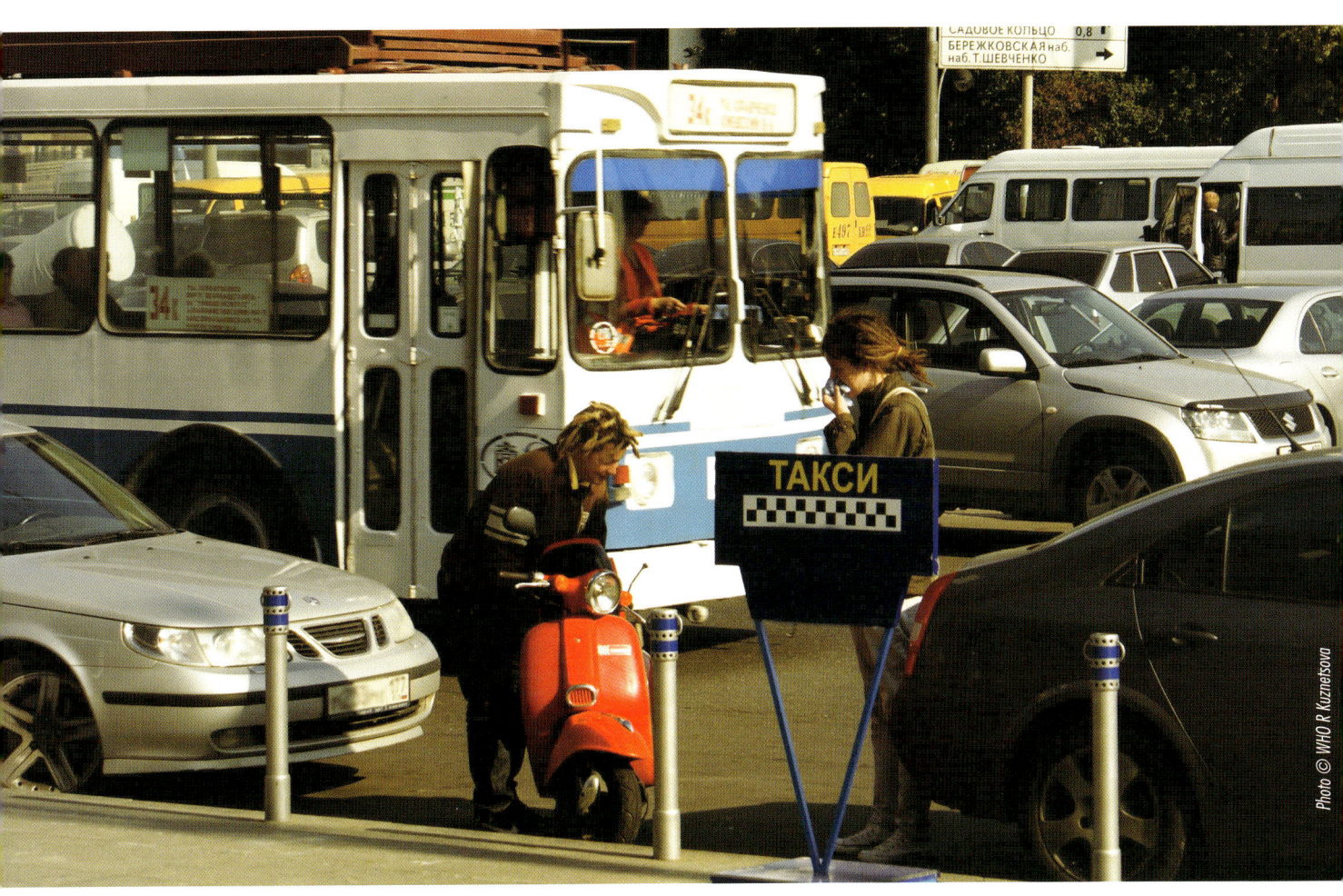

1.2 Rising inequality in the Region

The burden of road traffic injuries is unequal in the Region. Whereas mortality rates from road traffic injuries have declined overall in the Region, this is in stark contrast to the Commonwealth of Independent States (CIS[1]), which have the highest rates (Fig. 1). In the CIS, mortality rates peaked in the early 1990s and, after an initial fall, are climbing again. This differs from the European Union (EU), where rates are falling, making the gap even wider (9,10). Even the EU has great inequality, with the Nordic countries (Denmark, Finland, Iceland, Norway and Sweden) having far lower death rates than the Baltic countries (Estonia, Latvia and Lithuania) and those of southern Europe. In the Region, the age groups most at risk as pedestrians are children and older people, and young males are most at risk as car occupants or riders of motorized two-wheelers (2,7,11). Socioeconomic determinants are important, and even high-income countries in Europe have described a widening gap, with the children of deprived families at much greater risk than the children of affluent families (12,13). Exposure to hazardous traffic situations in unsafe environments and unsafe vehicles and less access to safety equipment and emergency trauma services are some of the factors that put lower-income people at greater risk. Further, many countries in Europe have undergone political and economic transition, and road infrastructure, vehicle safety and regulatory practices have not kept up with motorization (14). In addition, risk factors such as alcohol and speed need to be taken into account (4).

---

[1] CIS countries consisted of Armenia, Azerbaijan, Belarus, Georgia, Kazakhstan, Kyrgyzstan, Republic of Moldova, Russian Federation, Tajikistan, Turkmenistan, Ukraine and Uzbekistan at the time the data were collected.

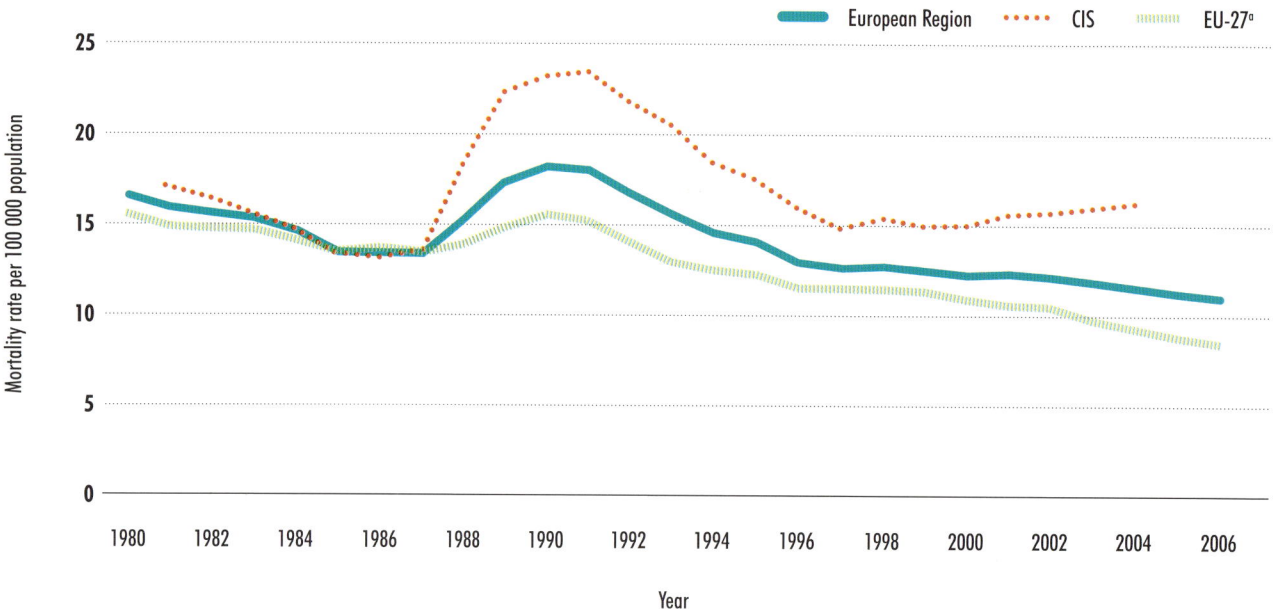

Fig. 1. Mortality rates from road traffic injuries per 100 000 population, WHO European Region, CIS and EU, 1980–2006

[a] Those 27 countries that now make up the EU.

Source: European Health for All database (10).

1.3 Road traffic injuries and other transport-related health effects

Road transport is essential to human and societal development because people and goods need to move and access needs to be provided to jobs, education, health care and other services and amenities. However, it also exposes people to the risk of road traffic injuries, and the number of deaths due to road traffic injuries would continue to increase if left unchecked (15). This would add to the burden of other transport-related health effects such as respiratory illness and the ill health related to physical inactivity and climate change.

For example, the level of transport-related air pollution is a major public health concern in most countries in the Region, where air pollution contributes to a similar number of deaths to those arising from road traffic injuries (16). In addition, transport-related emissions of gases that cause climate change may contribute to extreme weather events with harmful effects on human health (17). There are other effects on health, including pervasive annoyance induced by road traffic noise and constraints on the development of neighbourhood support networks. By discouraging the use of safe cycling and walking for transport, this contributes to cardiovascular disease, diabetes and obesity. These disproportionately affect urban poor people, living in areas with higher levels of pollution and fewer options for safe physical activity (18–20).

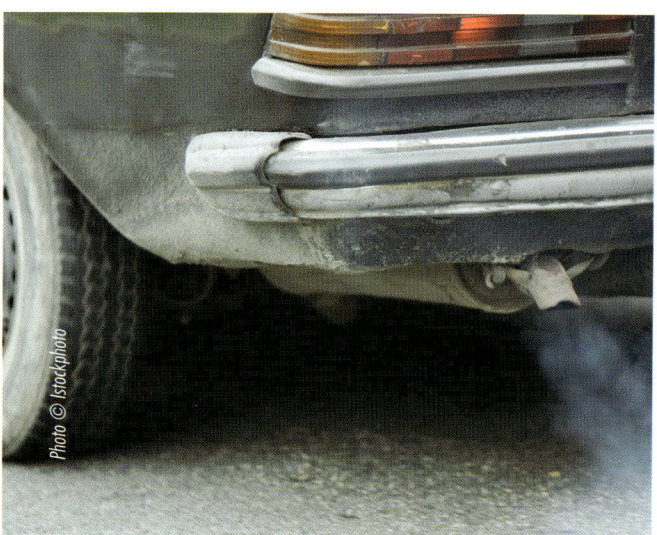

Taken together, these transport-related health effects add to the high burden and cost of road traffic injuries, strengthening the case for implementing sustainable transport strategies to reduce such illnesses and costs. Arguments for addressing road safety should therefore take into account the additional non-injury health benefits such actions would bring (Box 1). Conversely, more sustainable transport strategies that promote walking and cycling need to address the issue of safety for these vulnerable road users *(2)*. As a response to the concern about the environmental and health threats of climate change, speed-reduction policies that aim to reduce greenhouse gases will also make roads safer (Box 2).

1.4 International institutional response

Road safety has moved up the political agenda in recent years, and intergovernmental bodies have launched several policy initiatives *(23,24)*. The launch of the *World report on road traffic injury prevention* by WHO and the World Bank on World Health Day 2004 *(4)* refocused attention on the plight of victims of road crashes and proposed a multisectoral and evidence-based approach to preventing road traffic injury (see below). A companion publication *Preventing road traffic injury: a public health perspective for Europe (2)* was also released that describes the burden of road traffic injuries and urges action in the context of transport policies in the WHO European Region. World Health Assembly resolution WHA57.10 on road safety and health calls upon Member States to mobilize public health action to reduce the burden of road traffic injuries. These actions require a multisectoral response from transport, justice, health, industry and civil society.

Box 1. Addressing road safety as part of sustainable transport policy

The Transport, Health and Environment Pan-European Programme (THE PEP) addresses road safety as a key factor in overall policies on sustainable transport systems. In terms of health effects, this has the additional contribution of promoting transport policies that, in addition to road safety, also work towards reducing emissions of noise and air pollutants and providing conditions that promote walking and cycling. THE PEP promotes strategies developed to improve road safety that also take into account these other health effects to deliver multiple health benefits. Such broader approaches are more cost-effective investments than those focusing on a single health outcome. For example, maintaining speeds below 30 km/h to reduce death or serious injury saves on both the costs of avoided injuries and also on the costs resulting from ill health due to air pollution, noise and the barrier effect of fear of unsafe roads, which prevents walking and cycling.

Source: THE PEP – Transport, Health and Environment Pan-European Programme *(21)*.

Box 2. Speed reduction and transport demand management beyond road safety: opportunities for multiple benefits

The EU energy and climate package targets a 20% overall reduction in greenhouse gases by 2020 and highlights the need for the transport sector to contribute actively. In the EU, growing transport volumes have raised emissions by 27% between 1990 and 2006 (excluding the international aviation and marine sectors) *(22)*.

Reducing speed by enforcing speed limits and using intelligent speed assistance devices can contribute to reducing CO_2 emissions and saving lives. The same applies to policies to manage the demand for transport. Interestingly, these measures are increasingly featured in the portfolio of policies considered as part of the strategy to reduce emissions of greenhouse gases, noise and air pollutants *(22)*.

The United Nations General Assembly has passed several resolutions calling on governments to address the global road safety issue (Box 3).

WHO Regional Committee for Europe resolution RC55/R9 on the prevention of injuries provides a public health framework for prevention in the European Region. Further, the United Nations Economic Commission for Europe, the International Transport Forum and the

Organisation for Economic Co-operation and Development all undertake work on road safety. The EU European Road Safety Action Programme *(25)* urges the EU countries to halve road crash fatalities by 2010 compared with 2000 through a combination of measures, including better vehicle safety with both active and passive measures, improving road infrastructure and safer road user behaviour through licensing, regulations and enforcement. At the national level, there have been innovative approaches such as the Zero Vision approach in Sweden (Box 4).

1.5 Why this survey?

To address the state of global road safety and to evaluate whether Member States have implemented the recommendations of the *World report on road traffic injury prevention (4)* (Box 5), WHO undertook a project on a global status report on road safety. This survey assesses whether actions proposed in the *World report on road traffic injury prevention* are being implemented in 178 countries. The *Global status report on road safety (5)* was launched on 15 June 2009 in New York. Six regional reports have also

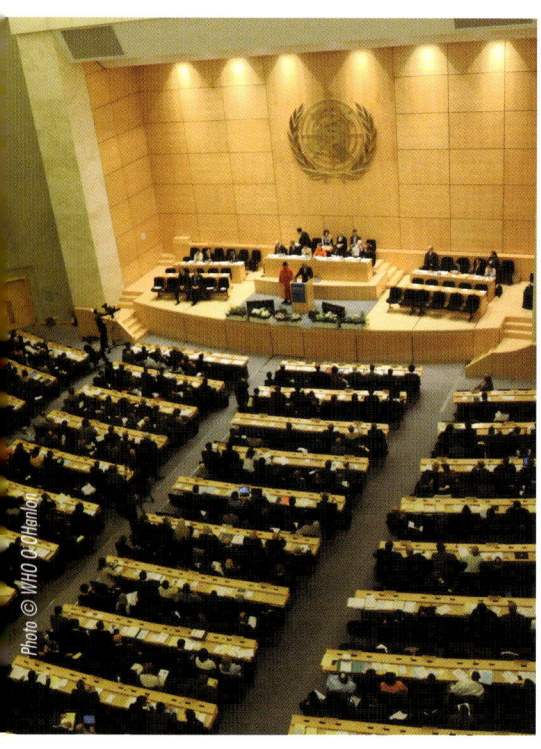

Box 3. United Nations General Assembly resolution A/Res/62/244 on improving global road safety

The United Nations resolution on improving global road safety in March 2008 reaffirms the importance of addressing global road safety and invites Member States to participate in developing the *Global status report on road safety (5)*. It also welcomes the offer by the Government of the Russian Federation to host the United Nations Ministerial Summit on Road Safety in Moscow in 2009. The Summit aims to bring together delegations of ministers and representatives working on transport, health, education, safety and traffic-related law enforcement issues *(23)*. Ministers from all Member States will have an opportunity to discuss progress in implementing the recommendations developed by the *World report on road traffic injury prevention (4)* and the United Nations General Assembly resolutions on improving global road safety. The Summit will be an opportunity for Member States to exchange information and best practices. Further, if the delegates adopt the proposed Decade of Action, this will prove to be a further catalyst for change.

Box 4. The Zero Vision approach

The Zero Vision envisages a future in which no one is killed or seriously injured on the roads and originated in Sweden. The main tenet of the Zero Vision policy is the belief that human failure is inevitable. It emphasizes the principle that speed and safety are not tradable. This means that policy-makers must do everything within their control to ensure that road crashes do not result in fatality or serious injury. The policy has thus focused on developing road infrastructure design to mitigate the consequences of road crashes and on measures to reduce the transfer of energy on impact, mainly by limiting speed. The approach now has a strong foothold in Sweden's national road safety system and has been adopted by other European countries. The new design of some of the roads allows for greater safety and mobility. Finally, although Zero Vision does place great responsibility on road builders and managers, it still recognizes the importance of other approaches and, among other things, works to improve vehicle safety and legislation.

Source: Racioppi et al. *(2)*.

been developed, and this publication describes the survey and its results in the WHO European Region. This report is primarily intended for European policy-makers and practitioners concerned with road safety and mobility from diverse sectors such as health, transport, justice and land use.

1.6 Objectives

This publication describes the state of road safety in European Member States by using standardized methods. The objectives of the project were:
- to assess the status of road safety in European Member States as measured against a core set of road safety indicators;
- to define the gaps in road safety nationally and in the WHO European Region;
- to help countries identify the key priorities for intervention;
- to stimulate road safety activities at a national level; and
- to provide a baseline to monitor progress in the future.

1.7 Structure of the report

This report has two main parts. The first part briefly describes the key findings in the European Region and their implications. After discussing the methods, key findings of the main report are presented as follows:
- data on fatal and non-fatal injuries;
- economic costs of road traffic injuries;
- lead agency and national strategy on road safety;

> **Box 5. Recommendations of the *World report on road traffic injury prevention***
>
> The *World report on road traffic injury prevention* (4) calls for a "systems approach" to road safety that examines the component parts of the system (infrastructure, vehicle and road user) in developing strategies for prevention. To help countries achieve progress in road safety, the report provides six universal recommendations.
> 1. Identify a lead agency in government to guide the national road traffic safety effort.
> 2. Assess the problem, policies and institutional settings relating to road traffic injury and the capacity for road traffic injury prevention in each country.
> 3. Prepare a national road safety strategy and plan of action.
> 4. Allocate financial and human resources to address the problem.
> 5. Implement specific actions to prevent road crashes, minimize injuries and their consequences and evaluate the impact of these actions.
> 6. Support the development of national capacity and international cooperation.

- legislation on and enforcement of risk factors; and
- road safety management.

These are followed by conclusions and key actions.

This publication includes detailed country profiles of road safety for each of the 49 participating countries with some explanatory notes on methods. Each two-page country profile tabulates data obtained in the survey assessing road safety nationally and sets a baseline for future follow-up. National experts, researchers and policy-makers can use the profiles as a resource for country-specific action and studies. Country profiles can be used for international comparison, but there are limitations due to differences in definitions, surveillance, costing and other methods between countries. Annexes 3–12 provide results for each country for most of the variables.

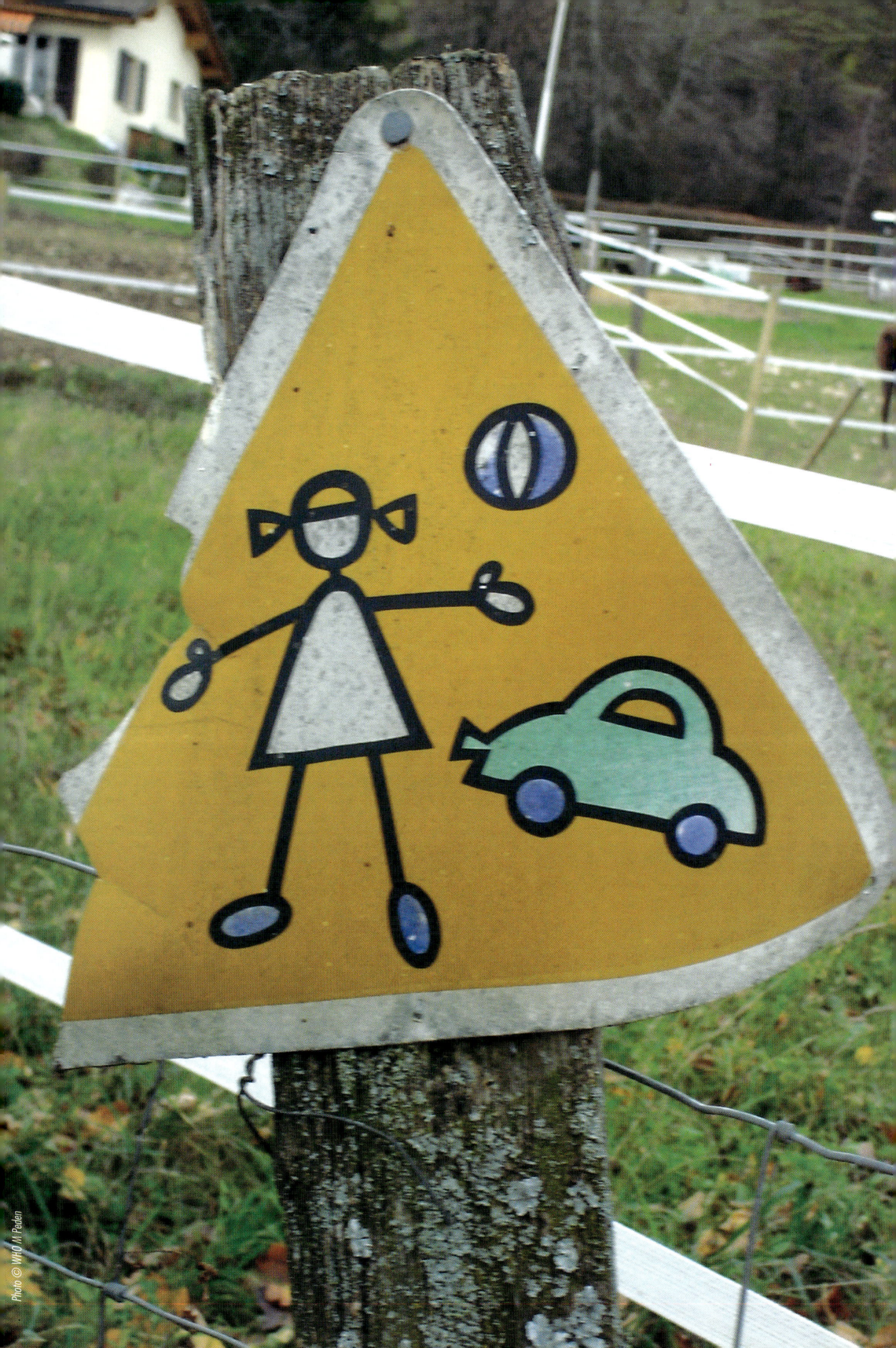

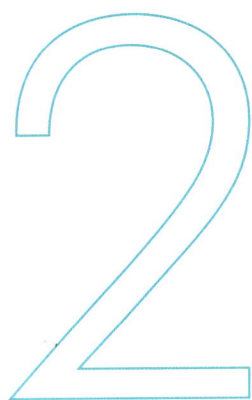

2 Methods

A self-administered questionnaire was developed using the content of the *World report on road traffic injury prevention (4)* as a basis for selecting items. An international panel of experts advised on the questionnaire design for the survey and the data collection methods. The questionnaire was used:

- to collect data on the burden of injuries, exposure to risk and vehicle and infrastructure standards;
- to define the institutional framework for road safety;
- to gather information on the economic costs of road traffic injuries;
- to record legislation and the enforcement of measures to control some of the main risk factors such as speed, alcohol and safety equipment;
- to identify road safety management; and
- to describe pre-hospital care.

Annex 2 describes the indicators in more detail.

Fig. 2 shows the methods for data processing. The health or transport ministries nominated national data coordinators in the 49 responding Member States (92% of the Region's Member States). Each national data coordinator was trained in the standard methods and facilitated a consensus meeting of a multisectoral group of up to eight road safety experts. The methods stipulated that experts be selected from the health, transport and enforcement sectors, and membership by academia and nongovernmental organizations was encouraged. Each respondent was asked to fill in the questionnaire before the meeting and then discuss each answer at the consensus meeting so that each country would have one official response. Data collection commenced in March 2008 and was completed in September 2008. The Regional Data Coordinator validated the data in consultation with the national data coordinator, and a final completed questionnaire was agreed on. These data were then used for processing and inclusion in the report. Annex 13 lists the national data coordinators and expert panels. Annex 3 lists the participating countries, together with relevant demographic, economic and development indicators.

Fig. 2. Methods of the survey

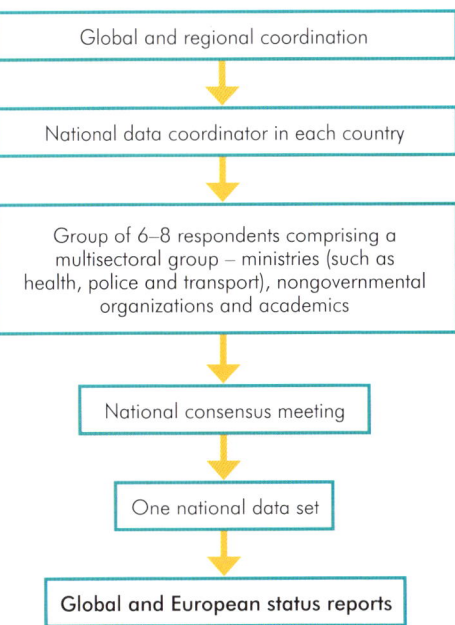

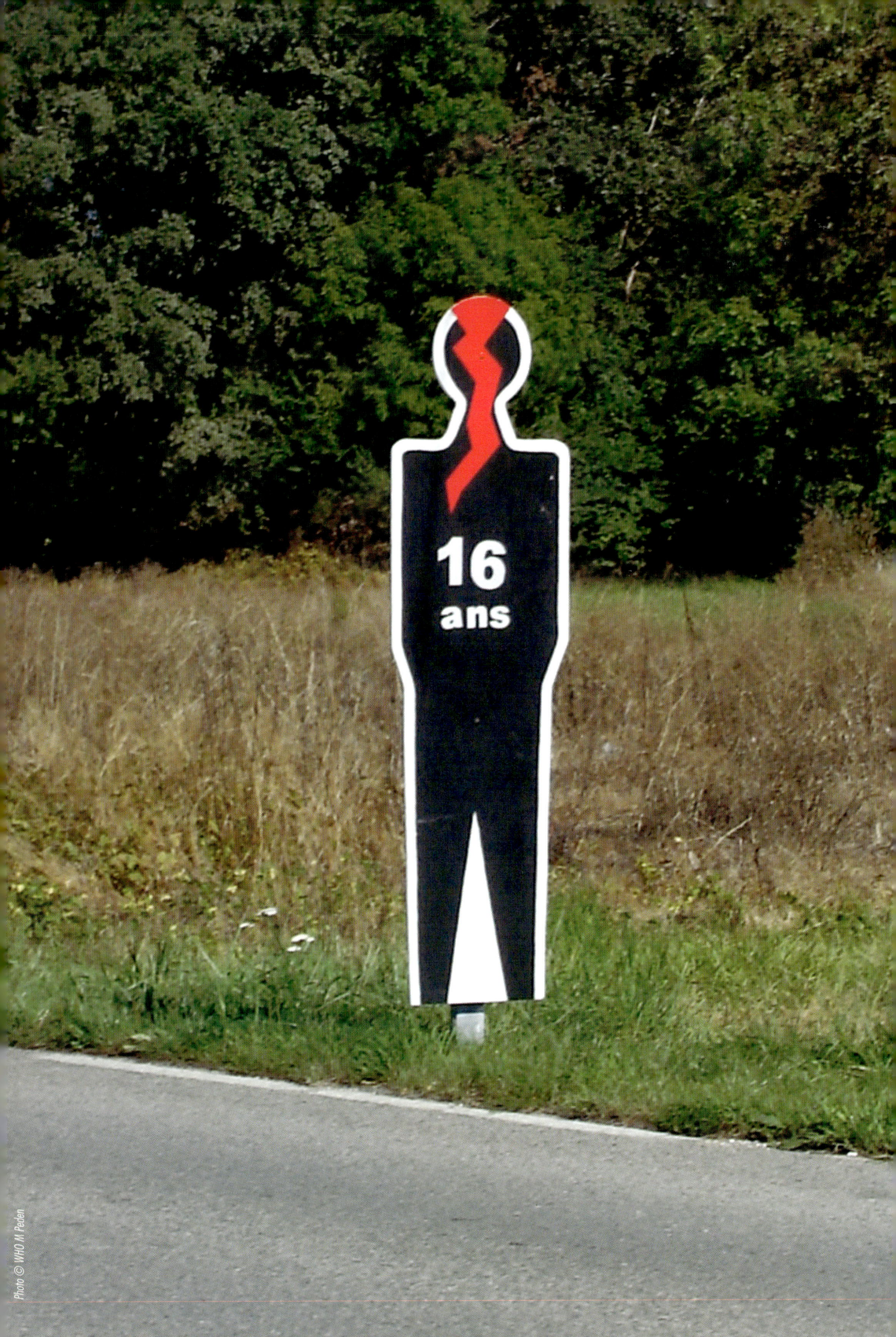

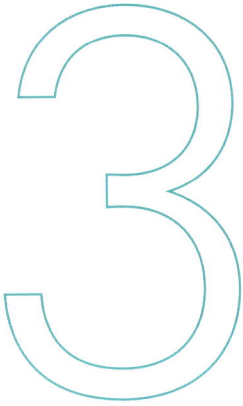

Findings

3.1 Great inequality in fatal and non-fatal road traffic injuries in the Region

The study shows that 120 000 people die annually in road crashes in the Region, confirming other estimates (1). The mortality rate from road traffic injuries in the Region is 13.4 per 100 000 population, lower than the global rate of 18.8 per 100 000 population (4). However, there is great inequality in the Region, as shown by the mortality rates in Fig. 3[1] (these data have been modelled for some countries to correct for differences in definition and completeness). The rate in low- and middle-income countries is 18.7 per 100 000 population, twice as high as that in high-income countries (7.9 per 100 000 population). The Nordic countries have some of the lowest mortality rates in the Region and in the world (average 5.7 per 100 000 population). In contrast, the average mortality rate in CIS countries (21.8 per 100 000 population) is nearly four times higher. Kazakhstan has by far the highest mortality rate in the Region (30.6 per 100 000 population), followed by other CIS countries such as the Russian Federation (25.2 per 100 000 population) and Kyrgyzstan (22.8 per 100 000 population). Among the EU countries, Lithuania and Latvia have the highest mortality rates (22.4 and 17.9 per 100 000 population respectively). Most countries in the western part of the Region have downward trends, as the graphs presenting trend data in the country profiles show. However, such decreasing trends are not consistent among countries in the eastern part of the Region, where mortality rates are increasing or remain unchanged.

Men account for 80% of young adult fatalities. The risk among young adults aged 20–24 years is five times greater in Estonia and Lithuania than in Norway. Similarly high mortality rates among young adults are reported in the southern part of the Region, in such countries as Croatia, Greece, Montenegro and Slovenia.

The Russian Federation, Ukraine and Kazakhstan make up 23% of the population of the Region but account for 43% of the regional burden of road traffic fatalities. With its 36 000 victims,[2] the Russian Federation has the highest death toll in numbers in the Region.

---

[1] Annex 3 presents the number of fatalities adjusted for the 30-day definition of road traffic death and the modelled mortality rates. Annex 1 presents detailed information on the modelled data.

[2] The Russian Federation reported 33 308 victims dying within 7 days of the crash; 35 972 is the adjusted number of victims dying within 30 days (see Annex 1).

Fig. 3. Mortality rates from road traffic injuries per 100 000 population, WHO European Region[a,b]

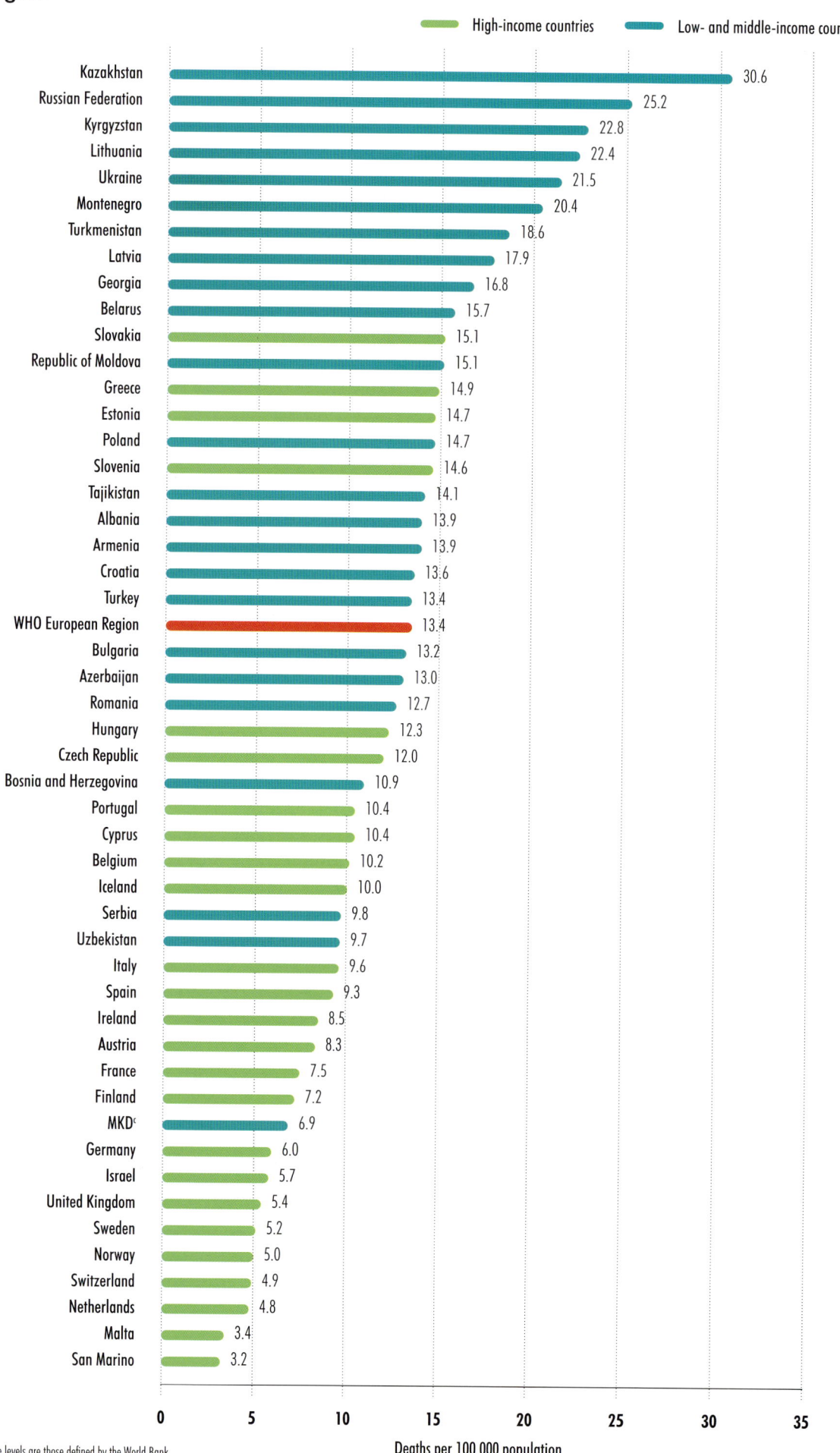

[a] Income levels are those defined by the World Bank.
[b] Modelled mortality rates. Annex 1 presents details on modelling.
[c] MKD is the International Organization for Standardization abbreviation for the former Yugoslav Republic of Macedonia; this is used in figures throughout this publication.

3.2 Very many non-fatal injuries

Every year 2.4 million people are injured in road crashes in the Region. Thus, for every fatality about 20 people are injured. Comparing this at the country level, the ratio of non-fatal injuries for every fatality ranges from 80 in the United Kingdom to 8 in the Russian Federation and 4 in Ukraine (see Annex 3 and country profiles). This may be due to gross underreporting of non-fatal road traffic injuries in some countries but also because of wide inconsistencies in how countries define injuries. Some countries define road traffic injuries as all those requiring treatment in emergency departments, whereas other countries classify injuries as those requiring hospitalization. Despite the large number of non-fatal injuries, little is known about the temporary and permanent consequences of these injuries. Due to the costs of health care, social welfare payments, production loss and the large number of injuries, the costs of non-fatal injuries tend to be higher than the costs of fatalities at the country level.

3.3 Vulnerable road users are at risk

Vulnerable road users, including pedestrians, cyclists and users of motorized two-wheelers, are at greater risk of serious injury in road crashes because they do not have a protective shell. Fig. 4 shows the distribution of deaths by road user categories for the European Region, the CIS and the EU. For the Region as a whole, vulnerable road users account for 39% of road traffic deaths. This is slightly less than the global figure of 46% *(5)*. The distribution of vulnerable road users within the Region differs notably. In the EU, the largest proportions of victims are motorized two-wheeler riders and cyclists. Greece, Malta, Cyprus, Italy and France have the highest proportions of deaths of motorized two-wheeler users among victims of road crashes, exceeding 1 in 4 deaths (Annex 3). This is partly because of the greater use of motorized two-wheelers in these countries, especially in urban areas, and because the licensing age for drivers is less than 18 years *(26,27)*.

The CIS has the highest proportion of pedestrian fatalities: 37% of all road deaths. Ukraine, Tajikistan and Kyrgyzstan have the highest shares of pedestrian victims in the Region (56%, 44% and 43%, respectively). One reason is the fact that urban design in many CIS cities dates back to when motorized traffic was very limited and professional drivers did most driving. Improvements in road infrastructure, driver training and enforcement have failed to adapt to the increase in motorization. The needs of

Fig. 4. Distribution of road traffic injury deaths by road user category, WHO European Region, CIS and EU

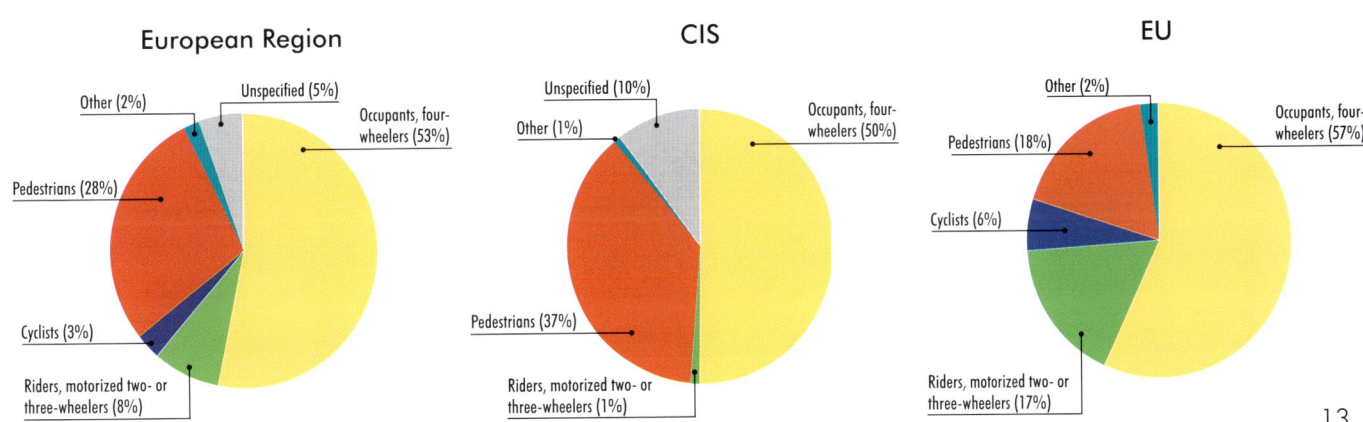

vulnerable road users have not yet been properly taken into account. For example, most CIS countries still have urban speed limits of 60 km/h (see section 3.7.1).

This finding is reflected somewhat in Fig. 5, showing that the proportion of pedestrians killed increases as the gross national income per person decreases. This is partly explained by greater exposure as pedestrians in low- and middle-income countries, which rely less on car transport, but also because of less investment in infrastructure and other measures promoting pedestrian safety than in high-income countries.

Fig. 5. Pedestrians as a proportion of total road traffic deaths, by gross national income per person, WHO European Region[a]

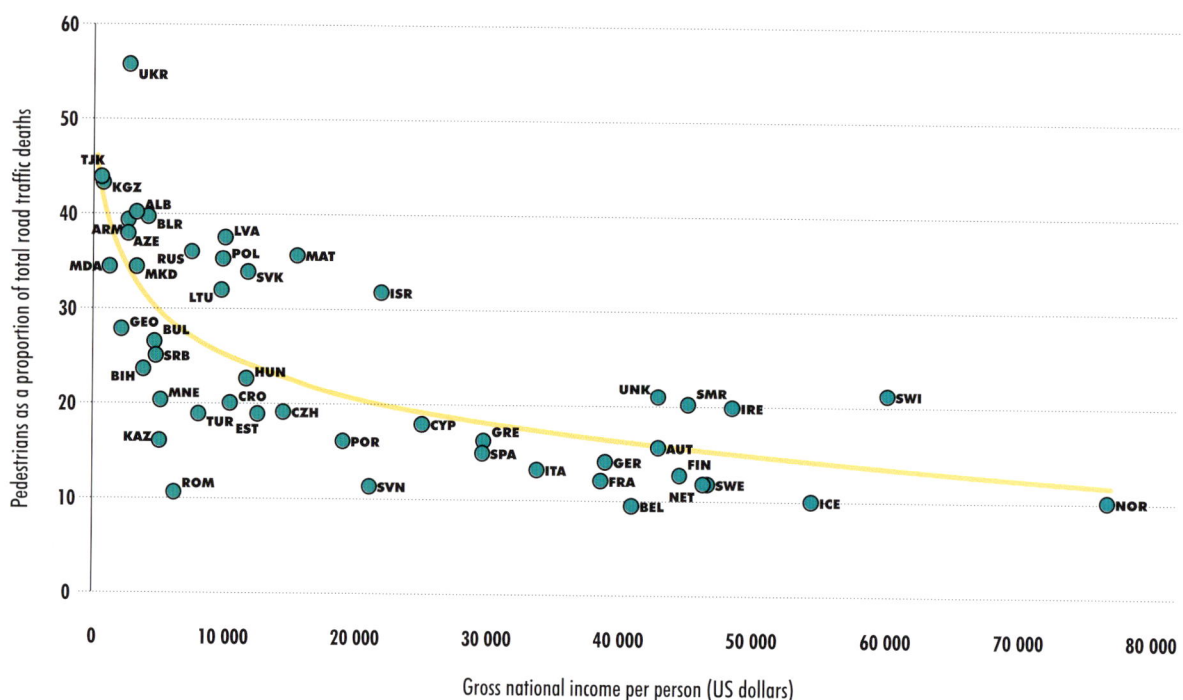

[a] The International Organization for Standardization acronyms are used in this figure: ALB: Albania; ARM: Armenia; AUT: Austria; AZE: Azerbaijan; BEL: Belgium; BIH: Bosnia and Herzegovina; BLR: Belarus; BUL: Bulgaria; CRO: Croatia; CYP: Cyprus; CZH: Czech Republic; DEU: Germany; EST: Estonia; FIN: Finland; FRA: France; GEO: Georgia; GRE: Greece; HUN: Hungary; ICE: Iceland; IRE: Ireland; ISR: Israel; ITA: Italy; KAZ: Kazakhstan; KGZ: Kyrgyzstan; LVA: Latvia; LTU: Lithuania; MDA: Republic of Moldova; MKD: The former Yugoslav Republic of Macedonia; MLT: Malta; MNE: Montenegro; NET: Netherlands; NOR: Norway; POL: Poland; POR: Portugal; ROM: Romania; RUS: Russian Federation; SMR: San Marino; SPA: Spain; SRB: Serbia; SVK: Slovakia; SVN: Slovenia; SWE: Sweden; SWI: Switzerland; TKM: Turkmenistan; TUR: Turkey; TJK: Tajikistan; UKR: Ukraine; UNK: United Kingdom.
Gross national income per person is from World Bank data for 2007.

Key actions
to protect vulnerable road users

- ✓ A maximum urban speed limit of 50 km/h should be set.
- ✓ Local authorities should be empowered to lower the speed limit in residential areas to 30 km/h.
- ✓ Police need to strictly enforce speed limits.
- ✓ Comprehensive laws requiring helmet use for all riders of all motorized two-wheelers need to be passed and enforced.
- ✓ Town planners and road engineers need to invest in infrastructure such as pedestrian-only zones, traffic-calming measures, upgrading marked pedestrian crossings, pedestrian bridges and underpasses and cycle lanes.

3.4 Health information systems need to be improved

Although all countries surveyed collect data on road traffic injuries, the quality of these data varies. Seven countries (14%) do not have readily available basic statistics on the sex and age of victims or trend data on fatalities and cannot provide any additional information besides death. Further, uniformity of terms is limited. For example, 10 of 49 countries apply definitions different from the international standard of road crash deaths as those occurring within 30 days, but instead use death at the scene or within 7 days of the crash (Annex 3). Similarly, 10% of deaths in CIS countries are not categorized by road user type. This makes international comparisons difficult. Even among countries with good data, there are discrepancies between health sector data from death certification and hospitalization compared with police reports.

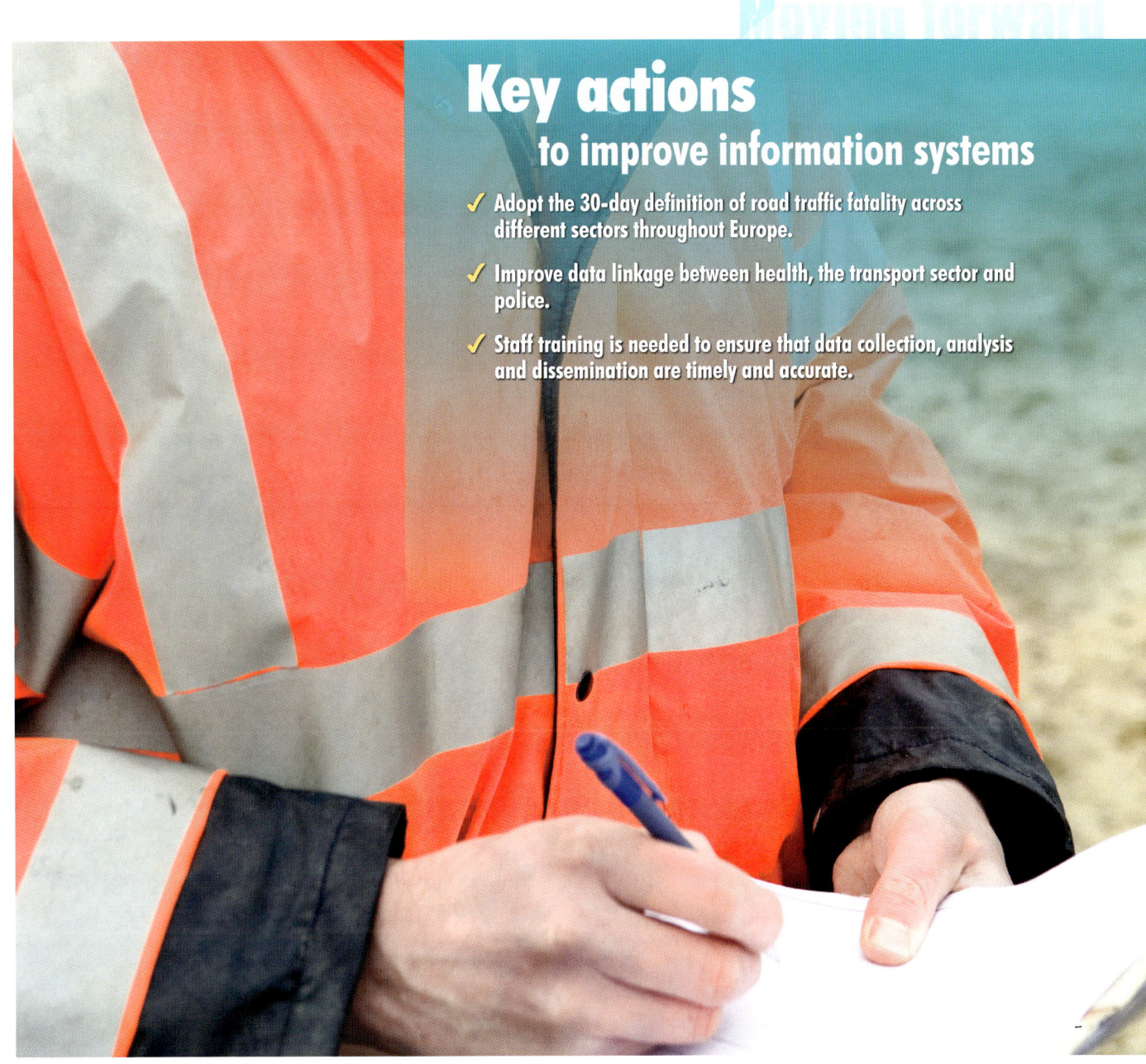

Key actions to improve information systems

- ✓ Adopt the 30-day definition of road traffic fatality across different sectors throughout Europe.
- ✓ Improve data linkage between health, the transport sector and police.
- ✓ Staff training is needed to ensure that data collection, analysis and dissemination are timely and accurate.

3.5 The economic costs of road traffic injuries

Road traffic deaths and injuries have vast costs. Data are collected using several methods, but 14 of the countries use a similar method.[3] This shows that the economic burden per person of road traffic injuries varies greatly across the Region and is usually higher in countries with higher income (Fig. 6). There could, however, still be differences in interpreting definitions. This limits the reliability of comparison between countries. Although these are rough estimates, their greatest value is in comparing within-country costs of road traffic injuries with expenditure on strategies for prevention (see section 3.6.2).

The estimated economic burden of road traffic injury ranges from 0.4% to 3.1% of GDP. Some countries also reported estimated costs per death in an attempt to express the cost of a human life in monetary terms (Annex 6).

[3] Gross output method: the cost components can be divided into the costs of resources consumed because of a crash (property damage costs, health care costs and administration costs) and costs resulting from a loss of future output (absence from work, long-term disability or death). Economic costs reported by countries were adjusted for inflation using 2007 as a base year and converted into euros at the exchange rate on 31 July 2008.

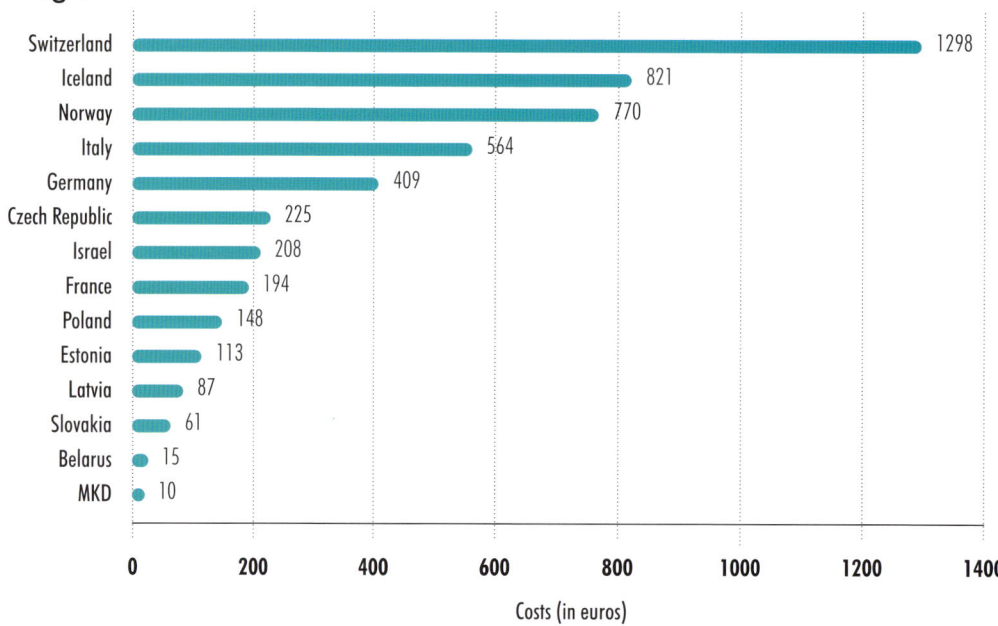

Fig. 6. Costs (in euros) of road traffic deaths and injuries per person, gross output method, selected countries in the WHO European Region[a]

- Switzerland: 1298
- Iceland: 821
- Norway: 770
- Italy: 564
- Germany: 409
- Czech Republic: 225
- Israel: 208
- France: 194
- Poland: 148
- Estonia: 113
- Latvia: 87
- Slovakia: 61
- Belarus: 15
- MKD: 10

[a] Data have been adjusted for inflation, applying, where necessary, a proper inflation or discount rate and using 2007 as the base year. Conversion to euros was performed using the exchange rate of 31 July 2008.

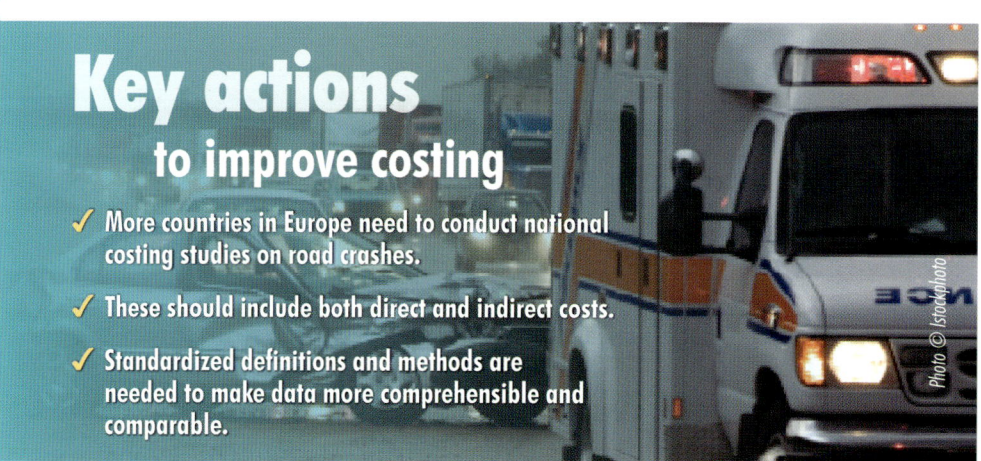

Key actions to improve costing

- ✓ More countries in Europe need to conduct national costing studies on road crashes.
- ✓ These should include both direct and indirect costs.
- ✓ Standardized definitions and methods are needed to make data more comprehensible and comparable.

3.6 Lead agency and national strategy on road safety

3.6.1 More countries need a national strategy for road safety

A lead agency on road safety has been proposed as being important for coordinating a multisectoral response *(4)*.

Ninety per cent of the countries surveyed have a lead agency (Table 2). Generally, these are either interministerial bodies or operate within a single ministry. In the latter case, almost all the lead agencies operate within the transport ministry, except for CIS countries, where the lead agencies operate within the interior ministry.

Only 76% of the countries surveyed have a multisectoral and multidisciplinary strategy on road safety, as recommended by the *World report on road traffic injury prevention (4)*. One quarter either have no strategy or have a strategy that does not engage other parties. Fewer low- and middle-income countries than high-income countries have a multisectoral strategy or a funded road safety agency (Table 2).

Box 6 presents an example from Norway's Ministry of Transport and Communications, which effectively coordinates road safety efforts through interagency activities and joint planning.

Setting short- and long-term targets using a measurable indicator helps road safety agencies and bodies in measuring and monitoring the implementation of a strategy. For example, all EU countries have agreed to implement the 50% reduction in road traffic injury deaths by 2010 compared with 2000 as highlighted in the European Road Safety Action Programme *(25)*. Having such a target has proven to be a useful stimulus for action, and a mid-term review *(29)* concluded that countries needed more concerted action to achieve the reduction in mortality. However, many other countries in the Region do not have easily measurable targets (Annex 5), creating difficulty in monitoring and evaluating implementation. Further, some national strategies do not have clear budgets indicating how certain activities will be funded. Israel's national strategy *(30)* presents a good example of a budget plan (Box 7).

Table 2. Lead agency and national strategy on road safety by country income level

	High income	Low and middle income	Total n	%
Lead agency				
Interministerial	7	11	18	37
Within government	13	7	20	41
Other	3	3	6	12
No agency	2	3	5	10
Total	25	24	49	100
Agency funded				
Yes	22	15	37	85
No	1	6	7	15
Countries with agency	23	21	44	100
National strategy				
Yes, formally approved	22	13	35	72
Yes, not endorsed	1	1	2	4
Multiple	2	6	8	16
No	0	4	4	8
Total	25	24	49	100

Box 6. Lead agency: the example of Norway

Norway's Ministry of Transport and Communications has assumed the role of an agency that effectively coordinates and oversees national road safety efforts through a multisectoral, integrated approach. By employing the help of national and local bodies (such as the police, Ministry of Education and Research, Ministry of Health and Care Services, Public Roads Administration, nongovernmental organizations and schools) it has made efficient use of all available resources. The Liaison Committee for Traffic Safety and the National Road Safety Forum provide all parties with an opportunity to draw on each other's qualifications and experiences through exchange and dissemination of information. To ensure cooperation between various levels of government, the Public Roads Administration has developed a road safety handbook and guidelines to be used by the municipalities. Similarly, the Ministry of Transport and Communications supports nongovernmental organizations, such as the Norwegian Council for Road Safety, in their educational work in schools and kindergartens. Finally, the Public Roads Administration has been developing guidelines requiring safe transport services to be used within the Administration, and private companies can adopt them.

Source: Vision, strategy and targets for road traffic safety in Norway 2006–2015 (28).

Box 7. Cost–benefit analysis as the basis for road safety measures: the case of Israel

Israel's National Road Safety Plan contains a good example of a straightforward financing strategy. Right from the start, the authors of the Plan acknowledge the significance of responsible resource allocation and a detailed budget breakdown to the success of road safety activities. They designate two separate agencies to carry out the proposed activities. The National Road Safety Authority is responsible for implementing and financing all the existing activities and upgrading urban road safety. The Israel National Roads Company is responsible for upgrading the interurban safety infrastructure. The two agencies have separate annual budgets, which are, in turn, broken down and earmarked for specific activities. The Authority's budget comes from two sources: the government and the compulsory insurance fee for all vehicles. The latter is said to be offset by the eventual reduction in insurance costs (due to the decrease in road crashes), which will result in reimbursement for drivers. The Israel National Roads Company receives funding from the national budget. A detailed cost–benefit analysis is provided for each agency's activity and serves to justify the proposed road safety measures.

Source: The national road safety plan. Major elements of the plan (30).

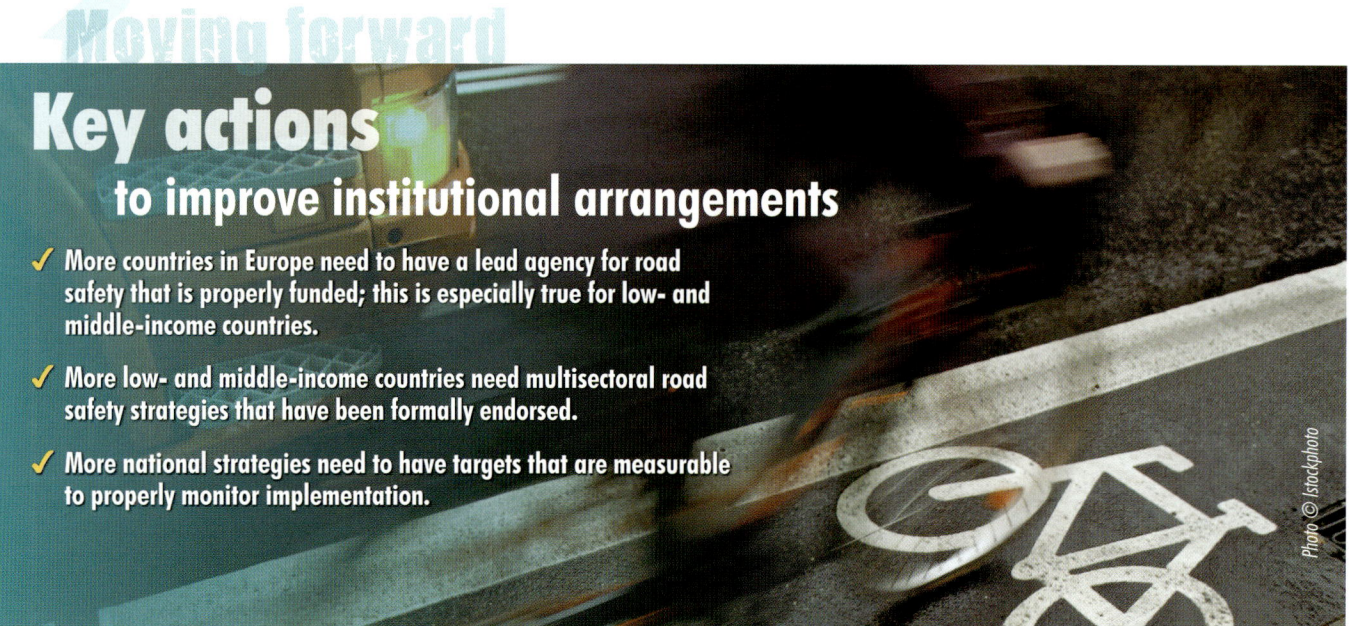

Moving forward

Key actions
to improve institutional arrangements

- ✓ More countries in Europe need to have a lead agency for road safety that is properly funded; this is especially true for low- and middle-income countries.
- ✓ More low- and middle-income countries need multisectoral road safety strategies that have been formally endorsed.
- ✓ More national strategies need to have targets that are measurable to properly monitor implementation.

3.6.2 Expenditure on road safety varies greatly, and this expenditure is far less than the costs of road traffic injuries

Reported government expenditure on national road safety strategies varies greatly across the Region. Countries in the Region on average spend €8.5 per person on implementing road safety strategies, but this varies widely.[4] Comparing countries' expenditure on road safety strategies is unreliable unless identical methods have been used. The countries surveyed differed considerably in the methods used. Nevertheless, the expenditure on road safety is much less than the costs incurred from road crashes (Table 3). Cost–benefit analysis can help to make a case for investing in road safety (Box 8).

---
[4] Government expenditure on national strategies was adjusted for inflation using 2007 as a base year and converted into euros at the exchange rate on 31 July 2008.

Box 8. Road safety: the use of cost–benefit analysis in Switzerland

An effective approach to advocating for and implementing a road safety strategy is to measure the potential economic benefits. The use of cost–benefit analysis helped policy-makers in assessing the feasibility of Via Sicura, Switzerland's road safety action programme *(31)*. The action programme outlines the costs associated with implementation, their allocation and the eventual savings that would accrue both to the private and public domains. A comprehensive table details the benefits of the programme (in the number of lives saved and injuries prevented) and the average road crash cost avoided. It shows that the estimated expenditure is far lower than the expected economic benefits. Knowing this allows policy-makers to charge private individuals for some of the costs; these are expected to be offset later by reductions in insurance premiums and thus contribute to the budget for implementing the plan.

Source: Via sicura. Federal action programme for greater road safety (31).

Table 3. Expenditure on implementing national strategies on road safety versus the costs of road crashes in selected countries in the WHO European Region[a]

	Expenditure on national strategy per person (euros)	Costs of road crashes per person (euros)
Iceland	12	821
Norway	23	770
Israel	15	208
France	38	194
Poland	17	148
Estonia	12	113
Latvia	3	87

[a] These calculations are based on the gross output method. The cost components can be divided into the costs of resources consumed because of a crash (property damage costs, health care costs and administration costs) and costs resulting from a loss of future output (absence from work, long-term disability or death). Economic costs reported by countries were adjusted for inflation using 2007 as a base year and converted into euros at the exchange rate on 31 July 2008.

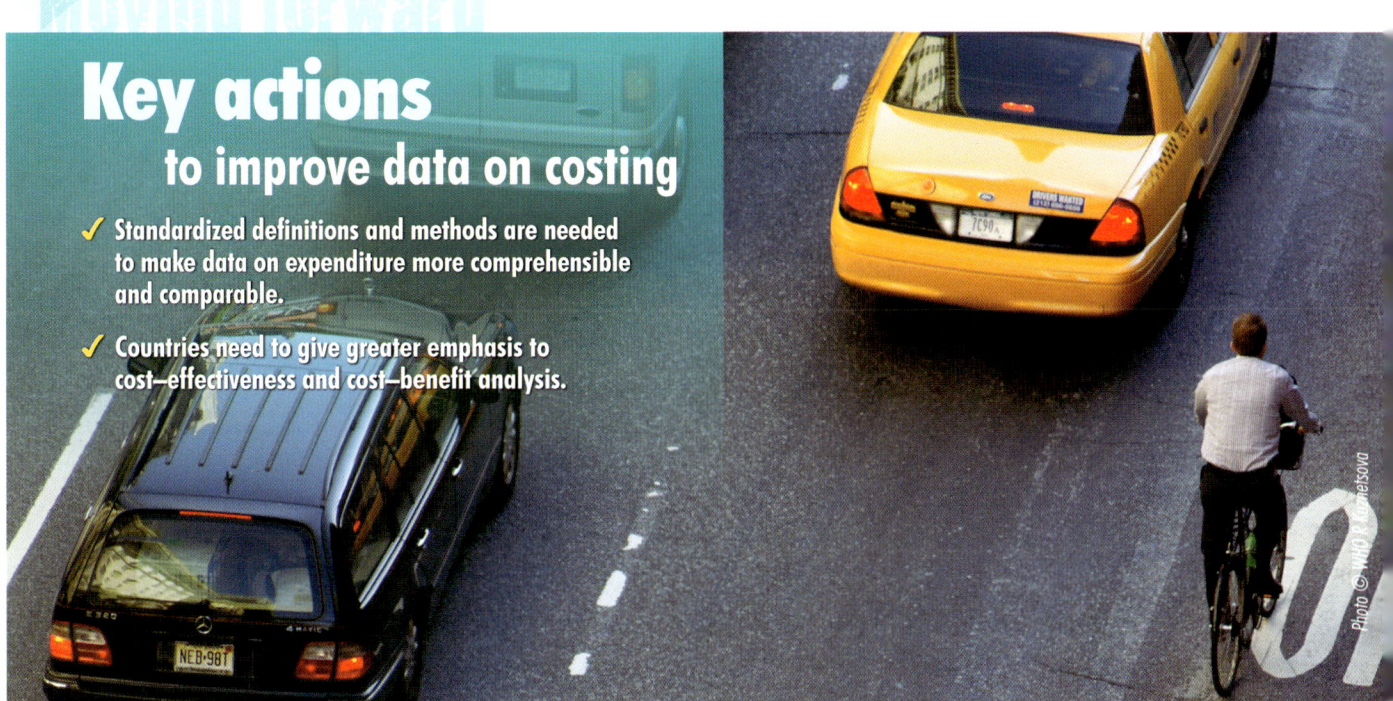

Moving forward

Key actions to improve data on costing

- ✓ Standardized definitions and methods are needed to make data on expenditure more comprehensible and comparable.
- ✓ Countries need to give greater emphasis to cost–effectiveness and cost–benefit analysis.

3.7 Legislation on and enforcement of risk factors

The *World report on road traffic injury prevention (4)* identifies high speed, drink–driving and disregard for the use of seat-belts, child car restraints and helmets (for riders of motorized two-wheelers) as major factors for road traffic injuries. Legislation is an effective way to discourage risky behaviour and increase road safety. Nevertheless, legislative measures alone are not enough to curb non-compliant behaviour. To be more effective, these measures should be well publicized and consistently enforced. Effective enforcement requires ensuring that the perceived risk of punishment for violations remains high by making the penalties sufficiently severe and imposing them quickly and efficiently. Table 4 summarizes legislative measures in countries that address these risk factors.

Table 4. Legislation on risk factors for road traffic injuries and its perceived level of enforcement by country income level as classified by the World Bank

	High income	Low and middle income	Total	
	n=25	n=24	n=49	%
Legislation on speed				
Countries with an urban speed limit ≤50 km/h	24	9	33	67
Countries reporting speed-limit enforcement ≥8 (scale of 1 to 10)	2	6	8	19[a]
Countries not allowing local authorities to modify national speed limits	3	7	10	20
Countries with a national urban speed limit ≤50 km/h and that allow local authorities to reduce it	21	9	30	61
Countries with a national urban speed limit ≤50 km/h and enforcement ≥8 (scale of 1 to 10)	2	2	4	8
Drink–driving				
Countries with national or subnational laws on drink–driving	25	24	49	100
Countries with a drink–driving law that imposes blood or breath alcohol concentration ≤0.05 g/dl	22	20	42	86
Countries with no alcohol limit stipulated	0	3	3	6
Countries with drink–driving enforcement ≥8 (scale of 1 to 10)	6	9	15	34[a]
Countries that have lower blood alcohol concentration limits for young or novice drivers	6	5	11	22
Data available on crashes attributable to alcohol	20	20	40	82
Helmet use for riders of motorized two-wheelers				
Countries with national or subnational laws	25	23	48	98
Countries with a helmet law that applies to all riders, all road types and all engine types with no exceptions	12	15	27	55
Countries with a helmet law applying to all riders and all engines without exceptions and requiring helmets to meet standards	8	3	11	22
Countries with the above plus enforcement ≥8 (scale of 1 to 10)	7	0	7	16[a]
Countries with no data on helmet-wearing rates	8	20	28	57
Seat-belt use				
Countries with national or subnational laws	25	24	49	100
Countries in which all car occupants are required to use seat-belts	25	19	44	90
Countries with comprehensive law and enforcement ≥8 (scale of 1 to 10)	9	5	14	31[a]
Countries with no data on rates of seat-belt use, front seats	2	18	20	41
Countries with no data on rates of seat-belt use, rear seats	2	20	22	45
Child car restraints				
Countries with legislation on child car restraints	25	17	42	86
Countries with enforcement of child car restraint law ≥8 (scale of 1 to 10)	7	3	10	26[a]

[a] These percentages are computed on countries where a consensus on the effectiveness of law enforcement was reached.

3.7.1 Speed control needs to be improved and more widespread

Controlling speed in densely populated urban environments is a critical factor in reducing mortality among vulnerable road users. In this survey, legislative measures for speed control are considered comprehensive if they limit speed in urban areas to 50 km/h or less and allow local authorities to reduce it.

The survey results show that only two thirds of countries in the Region have an urban speed limit ≤50 km/h (Table 4). All CIS countries have an urban speed limit of 60 km/h, except for Uzbekistan, in which the urban speed limit is 70 km/h. In one fifth of the countries, local authorities are not allowed to modify the speed limit, such as lowering it to calm traffic around schools or in residential areas. The effectiveness of speed control enforcement was reported as suboptimal in the Region, with only 8% of the countries being satisfied with it (≥8 on a scale of 1 to 10). This suggests that greater priority needs to be given to changing and enforcing speed control laws to protect all road users.

3.7.2 Controlling drink–driving is a priority

Driving under the influence of alcohol is an important risk factor for road traffic injuries and deaths. A blood alcohol concentration of or less than 0.05 g/dl is the recommended limit. The crash risk for young and novice drivers starts to increase substantially at lower blood alcohol concentrations than for more experienced drivers, and a limit of 0.02g/dl is recommended for young drivers.

The survey found that, whereas all countries in the Region have legislation that prohibits driving under the influence of alcohol, three countries have not set a blood alcohol concentration limit. In Kazakhstan, Kyrgyzstan and Uzbekistan, enforcing legislation is difficult without a legally mandated blood alcohol concentration limit. Four countries still have a legal blood alcohol concentration limit of 0.08 g/dl: Armenia, Ireland, Malta and the United Kingdom. Twenty-one countries (43%) have set the blood alcohol concentration limit for young and novice drivers at ≤0.02 g/dl. Many countries (66%) reported that enforcement was suboptimal (≤7 on a scale of 1 to 10).

Many countries (82%) have data on the proportion of injuries or deaths attributable to drink–driving. Although intercountry comparisons cannot be made as different methods are used, these data highlight that drink–driving is a severe hazard in the Region. For example, in Estonia 48% of all road traffic deaths are attributed to drink–driving (see country profile and Annex 7).

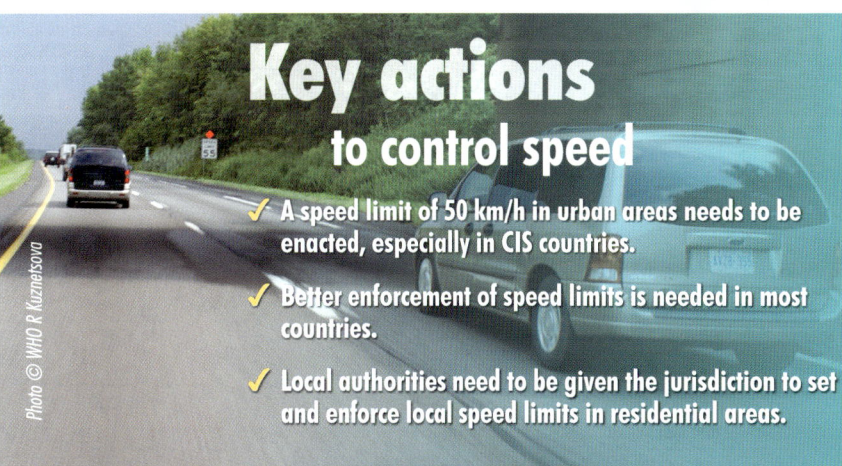

Key actions to control speed
- ✓ A speed limit of 50 km/h in urban areas needs to be enacted, especially in CIS countries.
- ✓ Better enforcement of speed limits is needed in most countries.
- ✓ Local authorities need to be given the jurisdiction to set and enforce local speed limits in residential areas.

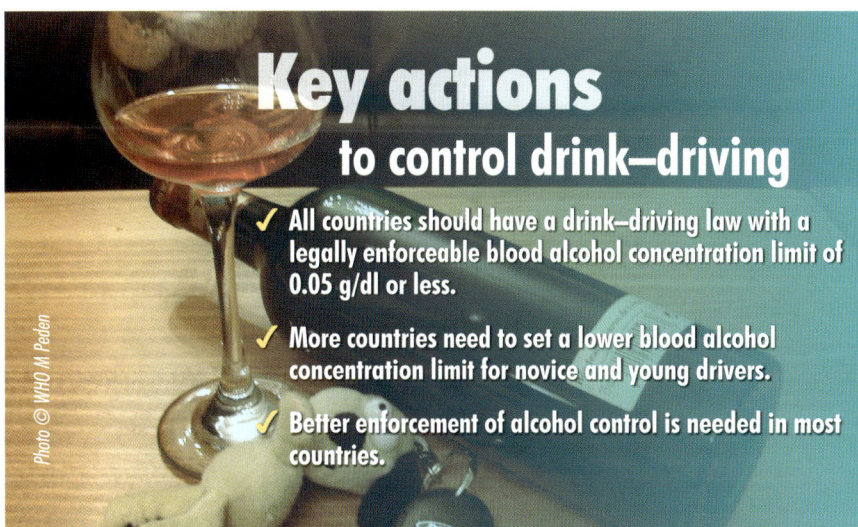

Key actions to control drink–driving
- ✓ All countries should have a drink–driving law with a legally enforceable blood alcohol concentration limit of 0.05 g/dl or less.
- ✓ More countries need to set a lower blood alcohol concentration limit for novice and young drivers.
- ✓ Better enforcement of alcohol control is needed in most countries.

3.7.3 Wearing helmets

Wearing helmets protects the brain and face from serious injury if motorized two-wheelers crash and can save life. A comprehensive law on helmet use applies to all riders of all motorized two-wheelers on all roads and irrespective of age, religion or engine size.

This survey found that only half the countries in the Region have such a law. Further, only 21 countries (43%) conduct surveys on the use of helmets to monitor implementation. Universal helmet use has been reported as achieved only in Norway and Switzerland; in other countries, such as the former Yugoslav Republic of Macedonia, almost no one is reported to wear a helmet (Annex 10).

3.7.4 There is much room for improvement in wearing seat-belts and using child car restraints

Seat-belt use is the most effective way to reduce the chance of injury or death for both front and rear car occupants.

The survey found that all countries in the Region have legislation mandating the use of seat-belts, but 10% have not yet made the use of seat-belts compulsory in rear seats (Table 4). These are low- and middle-income countries. Estimates of seat-belt usage are available for most countries (65%). These range from 98% in France to 30% in Albania for front-seat occupants. Less than one third of countries report seat-belt wearing rates higher than 90% (Annex 8). The rate of seat-belt use among rear-seat passengers is as low as one ninth that among front-seat occupants (Annex 8). Enforcement was reported as suboptimal (≤7 on a scale of 1 to 10) in 71% of countries. Of the CIS countries, only the Russian Federation has data on the use of seat-belts: 33% among front-seat occupants.

Using child car restraints is mandatory in all high-income countries, but legislation is lacking in 30% of low- and middle-income countries (Table 4). Even in the countries with legislation on child car restraints, the level of enforcement is considered ineffective in the great majority. Box 9 describes a newspaper published in the Russian Federation that is used as a communication tool specifically dedicated to improving the knowledge of children and their parents on road safety. Such tools are only successful if they are part of a communication campaign that accompanies enforcement.

Key actions on wearing helmets

- ✓ All countries should enact a comprehensive law requiring helmet usage for all riders of all ages on all types of motorized two-wheelers.
- ✓ Better enforcement of helmet wearing is needed in many countries.
- ✓ More countries should collect data on helmet wearing to better monitor enforcement.

Key actions to improve use of seat-belts and restraints

- ✓ Seat-belt laws should also be compulsory for rear-seat drivers.
- ✓ Better enforcement of seat-belt wearing is needed in most countries.
- ✓ More countries need to enact legislation requiring the use of child car restraints, and enforcement needs to be much improved in most countries.
- ✓ More countries need to conduct surveys on seat-belt usage to monitor enforcement.

Box 9. Tools to communicate with children and carers

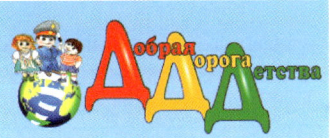

The happy road of childhood is a newspaper dedicated to preventing road traffic injuries among children. The biweekly newspaper is published in the Russian Federation and has a circulation of 30 000 copies. It serves as a creative and accessible tool for targeting a population group that is most vulnerable to road traffic injuries. The newspaper offers several approaches to educating readers about the problem and protecting children from road traffic injuries. Parents can receive advice on teaching their children about safety behaviour; teachers are offered tips on how to incorporate road safety education into their curriculum; and most importantly, the newspaper organizes engaging activities for the children themselves. The Ministry of Education and the State Automobile Inspection of the Russian Federation have recommended the newspaper to the regional authorities as an educational tool.

Source: [The happy road of childhood] [web site] *(32).*

3.7.5 Better legislation and enforcement are needed

In this survey, comprehensive legislation for all five main risk factors was considered as having an urban speed limit ≤50 km/h (and with local authorities authorized to modify this), a blood alcohol concentration while driving of ≤0.05 g/dl, compulsory helmet use for all riders of all motorized two-wheelers on any road and compulsory seat-belt or child car restraint use for all occupants. The great majority of countries (86%) have legislation on speed limits, drink–driving and use of seat-belts, child restraints and helmets. However, less than one third have comprehensive laws that control all five risk factors together. Further, only three countries reported that legislation on all five issues is being effectively enforced (≥8 on a scale of 1 to 10).

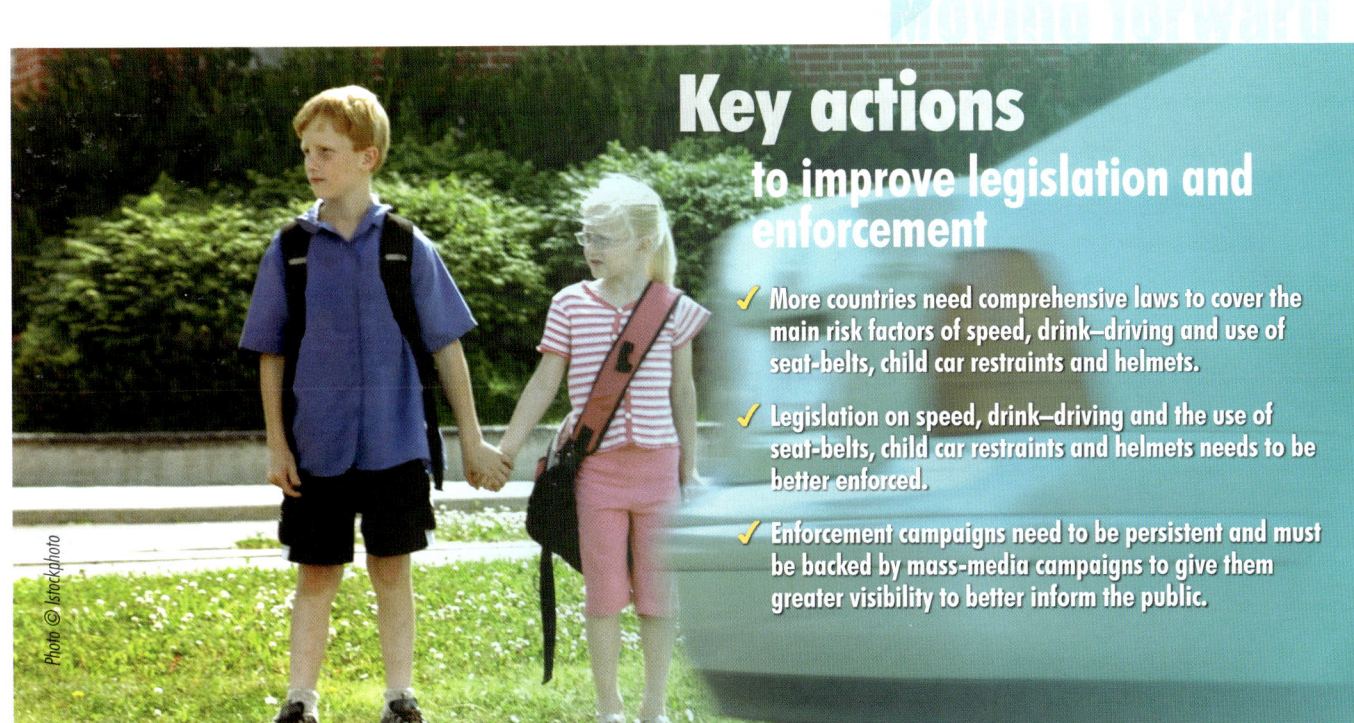

Moving forward

Key actions to improve legislation and enforcement

- ✓ More countries need comprehensive laws to cover the main risk factors of speed, drink–driving and use of seat-belts, child car restraints and helmets.
- ✓ Legislation on speed, drink–driving and the use of seat-belts, child car restraints and helmets needs to be better enforced.
- ✓ Enforcement campaigns need to be persistent and must be backed by mass-media campaigns to give them greater visibility to better inform the public.

3.8 Road safety management

3.8.1 Better transport and urban policy to improve mobility and road safety

Government policies on transport and fiscal matters determine the modes of transport people use and therefore influence exposure to different types of risk as well as environmental damage. For example, policies can encourage non-motorized modes of transport by investing in safe bicycling and pedestrian facilities (such as bicycle lanes, foot paths, pedestrianized areas and street crossings), discouraging the use of private cars (such as by introducing congestion charges and increased fuel prices as disincentives) and investing in public transport.

This survey found that car ownership in the Region is high, with an average of 3.4 private cars for every 10 people. It ranges from more than 6 cars per 10 people in countries such as Iceland, Italy and Malta to less than 1 per 10 people in countries such as Albania, Azerbaijan and Tajikistan, suggesting that dependence on private cars varies widely (Fig. 7). Car ownership is correlated with gross national income.

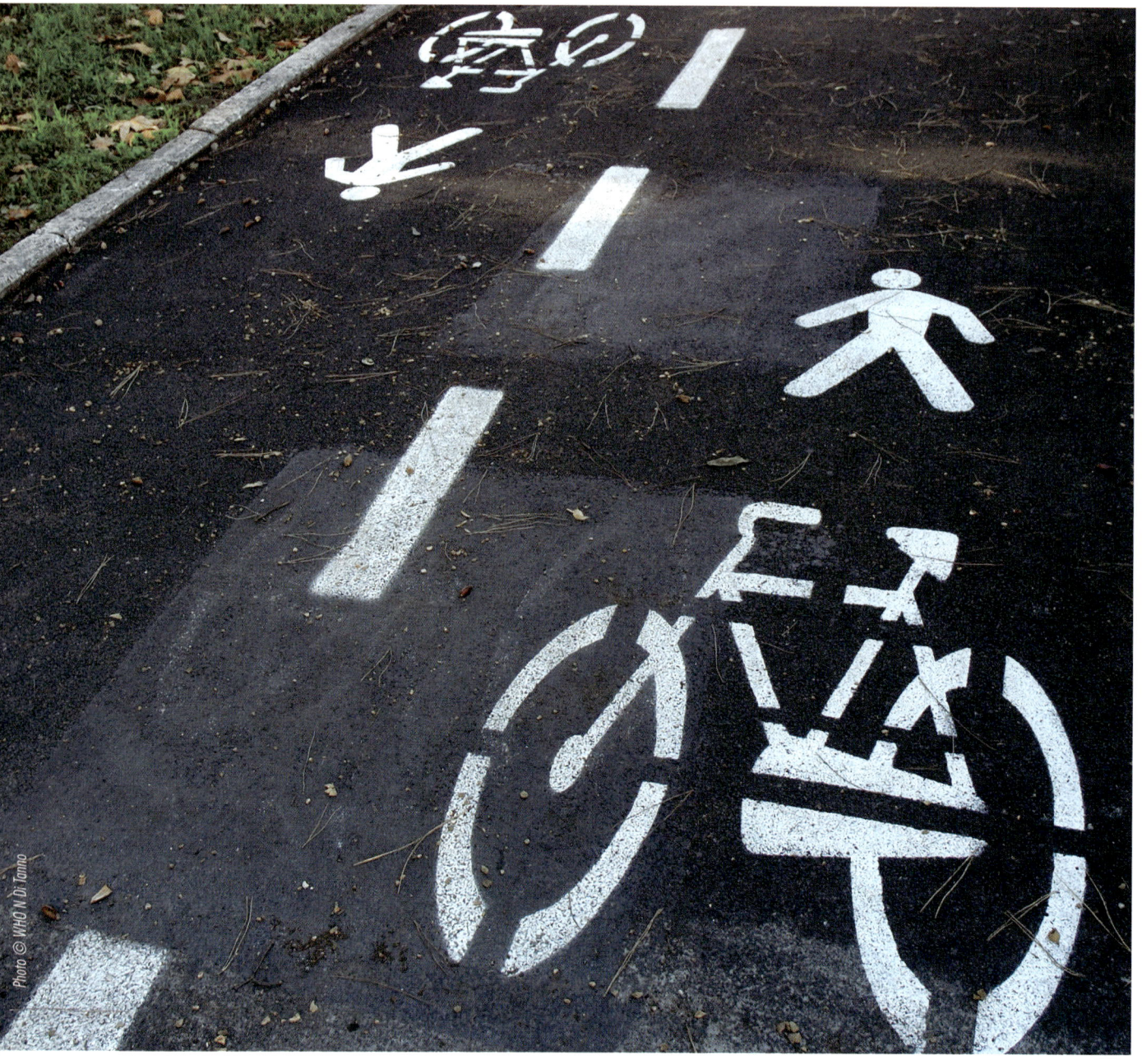

Fig. 7. Passenger car ownership per 1000 population, WHO European Region, 2008 or most recent year available[a]

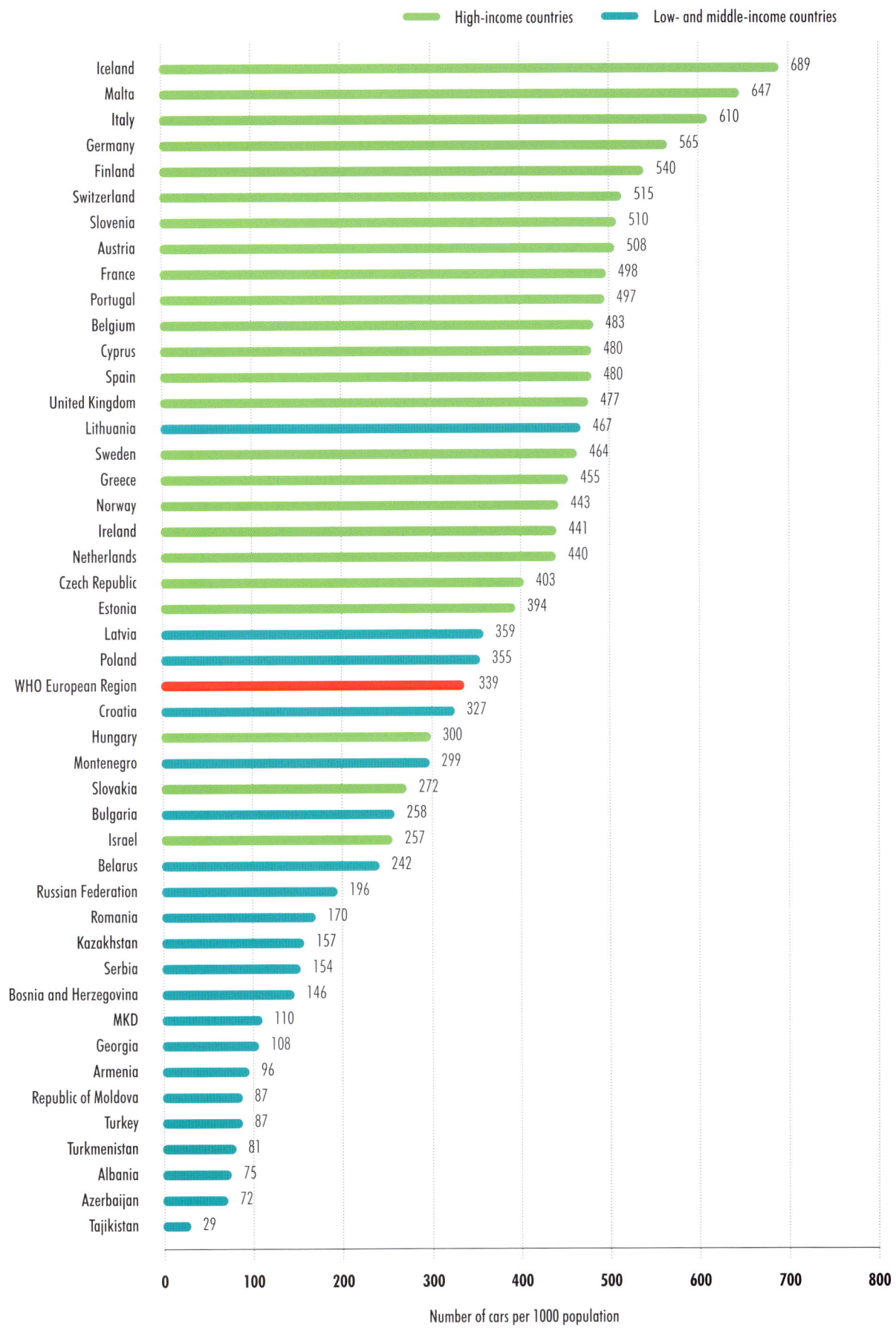

[a] Income levels are those defined by the World Bank. The Czech Republic, Ireland, Latvia, Lithuania, Poland, Portugal, Spain and the United Kingdom reported data for 2006. Estonia, France, Georgia, Italy, Kazakhstan, Romania, Turkey and Turkmenistan reported data for 2008. All other countries in the figure reported data for 2007. The figure for the European Region is an average.

Only 41% of countries have national policies on walking and/or cycling (Fig. 8) In some countries the municipalities are responsible for these. Among the countries that have national policies on walking and/or cycling, the most frequently implemented measures are bicycle lanes and traffic-calming interventions (Fig. 9). A good example of this is Finland, where active government intervention has successfully achieved safer conditions for pedestrians and cyclists (Box 10).

Nearly two thirds of countries have national policies promoting investment in public transport. A large proportion of countries have subsidized pricing of public transport services (94%) and investment in improving the frequency and coverage of public transport services (71%). However, only a quarter of respondents have policies with disincentives aimed at discouraging private car use. An example of such a policy is the London congestion charge (Box 11), which has reduced road traffic but has also encouraged cycling, public transport use and walking.

Fig. 8. Countries with policies on walking and/or cycling and on public transport[a]

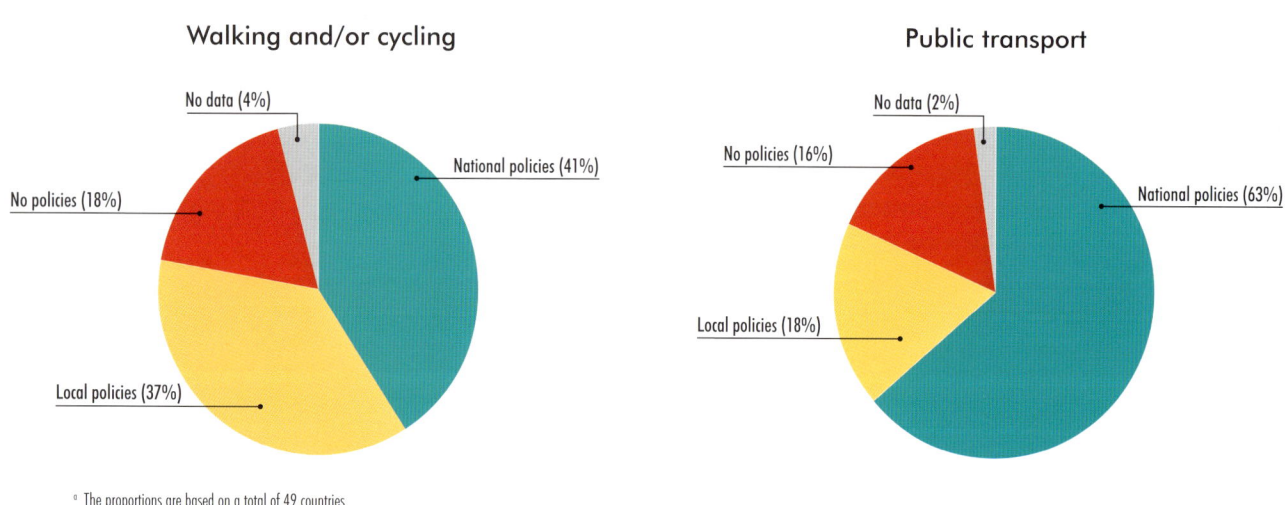

[a] The proportions are based on a total of 49 countries.

Fig. 9. Policies to promote walking and/or cycling and public transport

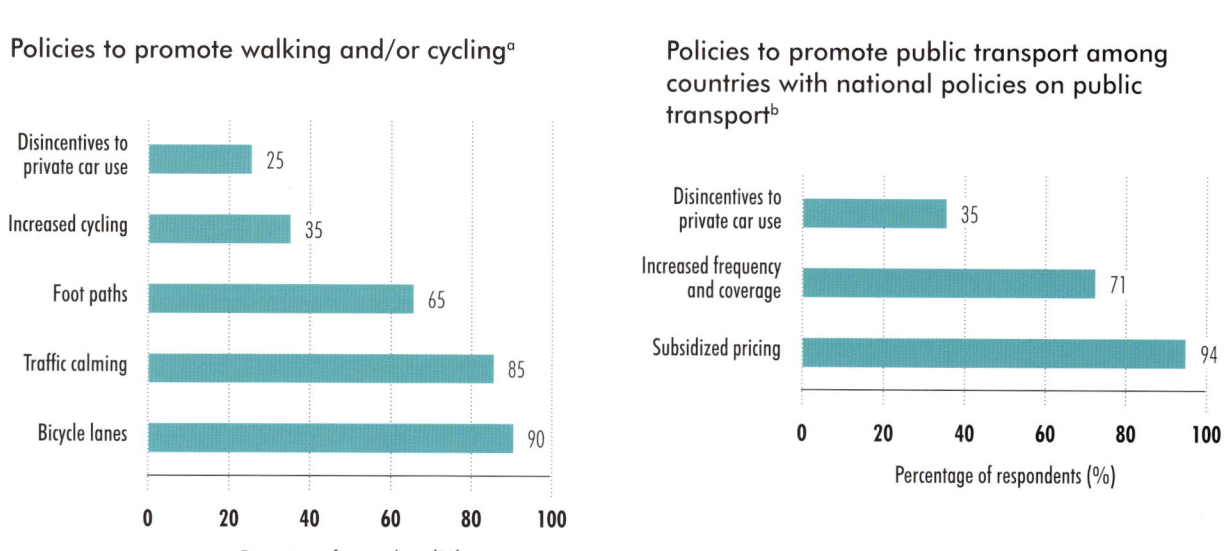

[a] The proportions are based on a total of 20 countries.
[b] The proportions are based on a total of 31 countries.

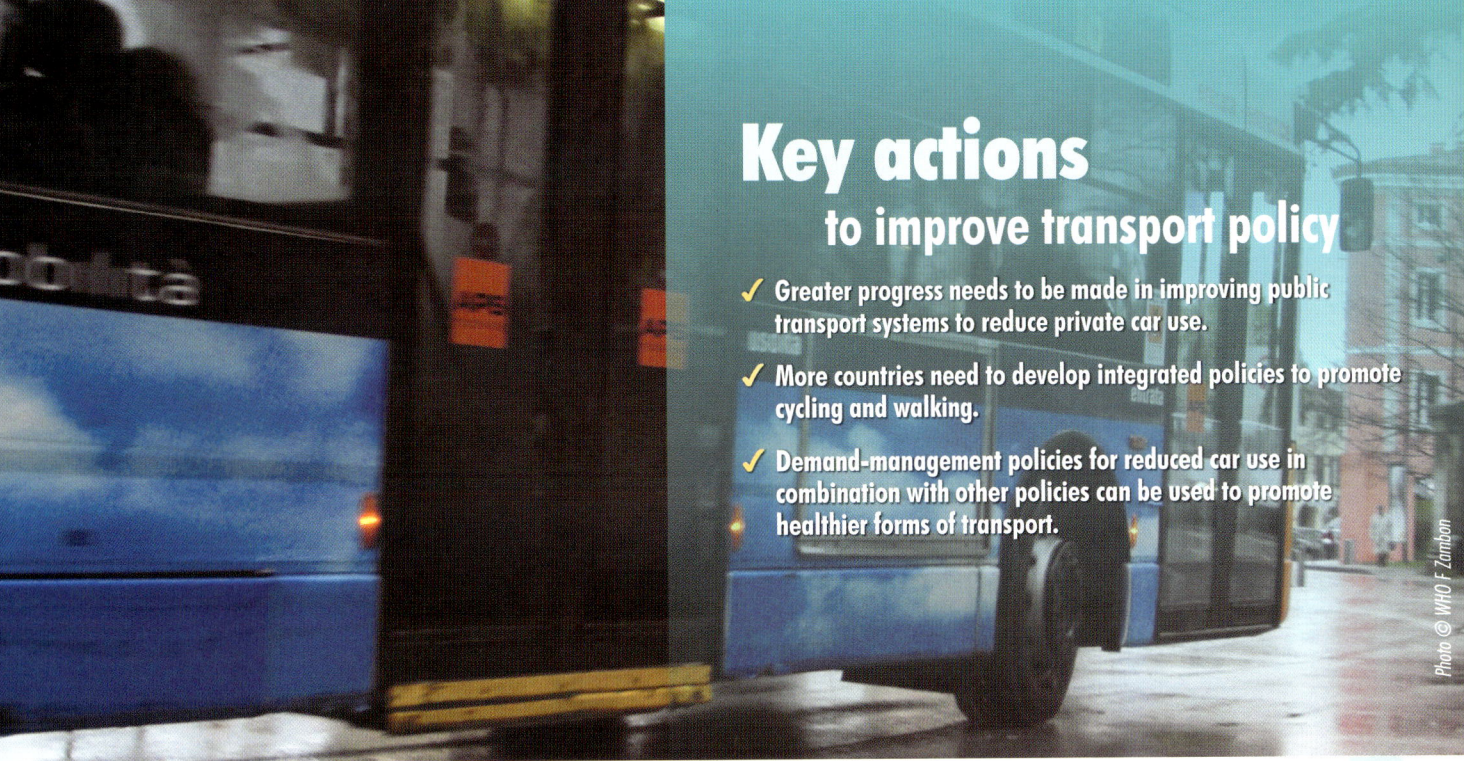

Key actions
to improve transport policy

✓ Greater progress needs to be made in improving public transport systems to reduce private car use.

✓ More countries need to develop integrated policies to promote cycling and walking.

✓ Demand-management policies for reduced car use in combination with other policies can be used to promote healthier forms of transport.

Box 10. Protecting pedestrians and cyclists in Finland

Providing safer conditions for pedestrians and cyclists is an integral part of ensuring the sustainability of Finland's road safety management plan *(33)*. The measures proposed are ambitious but realistic and have made dramatic improvement. These include: decreasing the speed limit in busy pedestrian areas to 30 km/h, developing road design features to curb traffic speed, making road signs and markings more understandable for motorists, creating more pedestrian-friendly environments, designating and improving pedestrian, cyclist and school routes, pursuing integrated land-use planning to efficiently reconcile busy urban areas and heavy-traffic networks, developing educational campaigns for children and fostering productive cooperation between local authorities and the Finnish Road Administration to ensure that these actions are taken. Provisional evaluation of the programme shows very promising results.

Box 11. Congestion charge: a disincentive for car use in London

The London congestion charge was introduced in 2003. Cars are charged to enter a zone in the city centre *(34)*. There has also been investment to improve public transport and road infrastructure generally, partly funded by revenue raised from the charge. The charge has resulted in reduced motorized traffic in and around the charging zone. It has also increased cycle journeys by 20%, reduced road crashes by 7% and improved air quality. There has also been an increase in walking as a result of the increased number of journeys in public transport and an increase in the number of journeys on foot. This simple intervention has had beneficial effects on public health, and the overall benefits have outweighed the costs. Other cities are introducing similar measures elsewhere in the Region, such as Manchester, Milan and Stockholm.

3.8.2 Other aspects of road safety management

As emphasized in the *World report on road traffic injury prevention (4)*, road safety audits are key in identifying and reducing the potential of the road network to lead to road crashes. Similarly, vehicle safety checks are also important. Most countries in the Region have periodic inspections to ensure that motor vehicles fulfil minimum safety standards and to check for the installation of seat-belts (Table 5). These checks are lacking on motorized two-wheelers in 9 of the 25 high-income countries. Less than two thirds of the countries perform regular road safety audits on either new or existing road projects.

Another aspect of road and vehicle management relates to vehicle insurance systems. Great progress has been made in this, and Armenia, Georgia and Kyrgyzstan are the only countries in the Region that do not have compulsory vehicle insurance.

Table 5. Road safety management and policies by country income

	High income	Low and middle income	Total n=49	%
Countries performing formal road safety audits on new and existing roads				
Yes	9	22	31	63
No	16	2	18	37
Total	25	24	49	100
Countries with a compulsory vehicle insurance system				
Yes	25	21	46	94
No	0	3	3	6
Total	25	24	49	100
Countries with car manufacturers in the country				
Yes	16	10	26	53
Standard on fuel consumption	7	6	13	50
Seat-belt installation required (all seats)	15	8	23	88
No	9	14	23	47
Total	25	24	49	100
Countries with periodic vehicle inspections for:				
Motorcars	25	23	48	98
Motorized two-wheelers	16	23	39	80
Minibuses, pick-up trucks, vans	25	23	48	98
Lorries	25	24	49	100
Buses	25	24	49	100

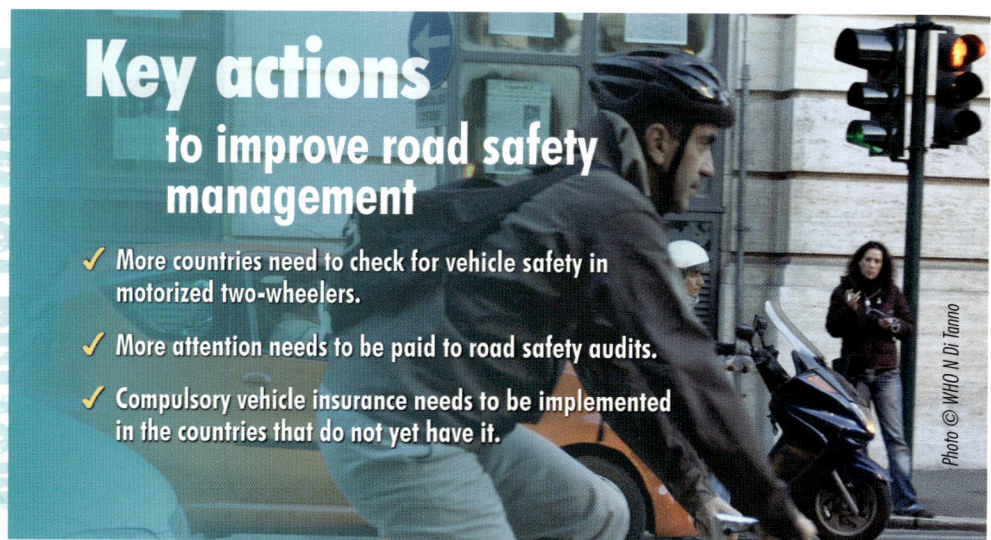

Key actions to improve road safety management

- ✓ More countries need to check for vehicle safety in motorized two-wheelers.
- ✓ More attention needs to be paid to road safety audits.
- ✓ Compulsory vehicle insurance needs to be implemented in the countries that do not yet have it.

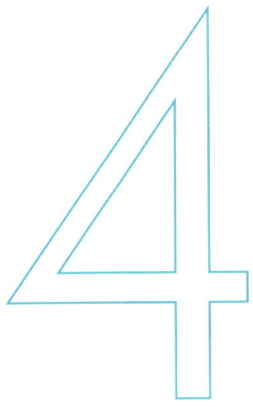

Conclusions

This survey is the first comprehensive assessment of policies and practices in road safety across the WHO European Region. Responses from national data coordinators in 49 of the 53 Member States have been collated. These show great disparities in the Region in the scale of the problem and that governments could do much more to improve road safety. The survey encouraged intersectoral work because respondents from different sectors came together and reached consensus for their country response. For some countries, this occurred for the first time. Regular assessments such as this will help governments and intergovernmental bodies in measuring progress towards fulfilling the goal of improving road safety in the Region. This survey thus represents an important baseline of data collated using standardized methods involving different sectors and can be used for future comparisons.

Some limitations of the survey methods need to be considered, such as differences in interpretation of the terms used in various countries, which may limit the reliability of comparisons between countries. Self-administered questionnaires may be susceptible to subjectivity and bias, although this was minimized by using a consensus panel in each country. Further, the requirement for national-level data may limit capturing some of the actions enacted locally, especially those related to regulatory and enforcement practices. In addition, this survey did not collect exposure data. Despite these minor limitations, the survey has led to some important findings relevant to policy-makers and practitioners concerned with reducing the burden of road traffic injuries. These are summarized below.

4.1 Key findings

This survey has shown that road traffic injuries cause 120 000 deaths and 2.4 million injuries annually in the Region, confirming data from other sources (1). Many of these deaths and injuries can be prevented. Despite the great achievements of some countries in the Region, others continue to have staggeringly high mortality rates from road traffic injuries, and some countries have an upward trend. A systems approach, strong coordination among stakeholders, clearly outlined responsibilities, accountability and effective law enforcement are all key factors present in countries that show the best performance in road safety management. The results that this survey has produced can be translated into some key findings and areas for action.

1. Road traffic injuries remain a major problem, and the vast disparities between countries need to be addressed

Road traffic injuries are a public health threat throughout the Region and the leading cause of death among people aged 5–29 years. Mortality rates for road traffic injuries differ widely between countries, with rates being twice as high in low- and middle-income countries as in high-income countries in the Region. Mortality rates in the CIS countries are up to 4 times higher than those in the Nordic countries. Trends have been falling in many high-income countries but not in low- and middle-income countries, many of which are in the CIS.

2. Vulnerable road users account for a large proportion of road traffic injuries

Pedestrians, cyclists and riders of motorized two-wheelers constitute 39% of all road traffic deaths in the WHO European Region. They are more likely to be more seriously injured. The proportion of pedestrians involved in road crashes is highest in the CIS countries. Rapid road traffic and urban design put these road users at increased risk.

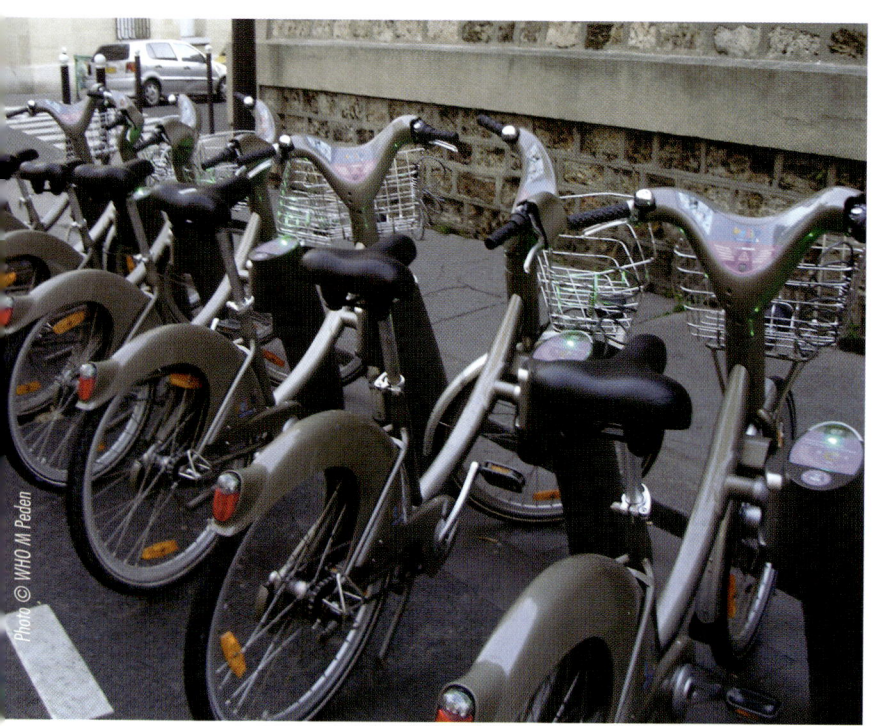

3. Some countries have inadequate information systems to measure the scale and costs of road traffic injuries

Fourteen per cent of the countries in the WHO European Region do not have readily available basic statistics on road traffic injuries. Many more do not collect information according to standard definitions. Reliable statistics are essential for assessing the scale of the problem, targeting those at risk and monitoring the implementation of national road safety strategies and achievement of targets. Methods for costing studies, when these have been done, vary considerably.

4. Institutional frameworks for road safety are weak in many countries

Many countries do not have a multisectoral body in charge of road safety (10%) or have one but this is not funded to conduct its duties (15%). About one third of the countries do not have a national, multisectoral strategy on road safety. Not all countries have measurable targets that can be properly monitored.

5. The legislative framework and enforcement are weak for important risk factors

Many countries have inadequate legislation to control speed in urban areas, drink–driving and use of helmets, seat-belts and child car restraints. Even well-designed legislation can have no effect if it is not properly enforced. In most countries in the Region, the current enforcement of laws on speed control, drink–driving and use of helmets, seat-belts and child car restraints is reported as not being effective enough.

6. Many countries can gain from investment in sustainable and healthy transport policies

Most countries subsidize public transport, but only 63% have a national policy encouraging investment and 41% have a national policy to promote cycling and/or walking. Moreover, only one quarter have measures to manage demand for private car use. Land-use and transport policies that encourage public transport, cycling and walking will provide multiple health gains by reducing injuries and emissions of greenhouse gases, air pollution and noise and by mitigating the negative effects of climate change, as highlighted by the Amsterdam Declaration *(35)*. Making roads safer for vulnerable road users through multisectoral stakeholder involvement and nongovernmental organizations will help ensure greater mobility by walking and cycling.

4.2 Key actions

1. Inequality in road traffic injury deaths should be reduced

More attention needs to be given to road safety throughout the Region. Some high-income countries have shown sustained political commitment and developed innovative strategies and technologies for reducing road traffic deaths and serious injuries. Countries with poorer road safety records need to take up this experience.

2. Vulnerable road users need better protection

Governments need to protect all road users and not neglect the needs of the most vulnerable ones. Road safety stakeholders need to work together to implement evidence-based action to guarantee better protection, especially in low- and middle-income countries.

3. More countries need a multisectoral road safety body that is well resourced to take forward a strategy for safety

Such a body should involve all stakeholders in developing a multisectoral strategy that should clearly designate responsibilities and authority as to who should do what, where and when.

4. Better enactment and enforcement of legislation on road safety could save lives

Governments need to ensure that comprehensive laws cover the main risk factors of speed, drink–driving and use of helmets, seat-belts and child car restraints. Enforcement of such legislation needs to be improved. This requires well-publicized enforcement campaigns, perceived certainty of being apprehended and making the penalties sufficiently severe and imposing them quickly and efficiently. Many countries need to put this winning combination in place.

5. Sustainable transport policies present a large untapped opportunity for health and environmental gains

This represents an important opportunity for contributing to the achievement of other public health and environmental goals. More countries could reap the multiple benefits of investing in policies that promote public transport, cycling and walking. Land-use and transport policies that encourage such modes of travel will provide multiple health gains by reducing injuries, decreasing respiratory illness, preventing noncommunicable disease through physical activity and mitigating the negative effects of climate change. Making roads safer for vulnerable road users will help to encourage greater mobility with walking and cycling. Transport policies that integrate road safety with environmental and health concerns are one way of achieving this.

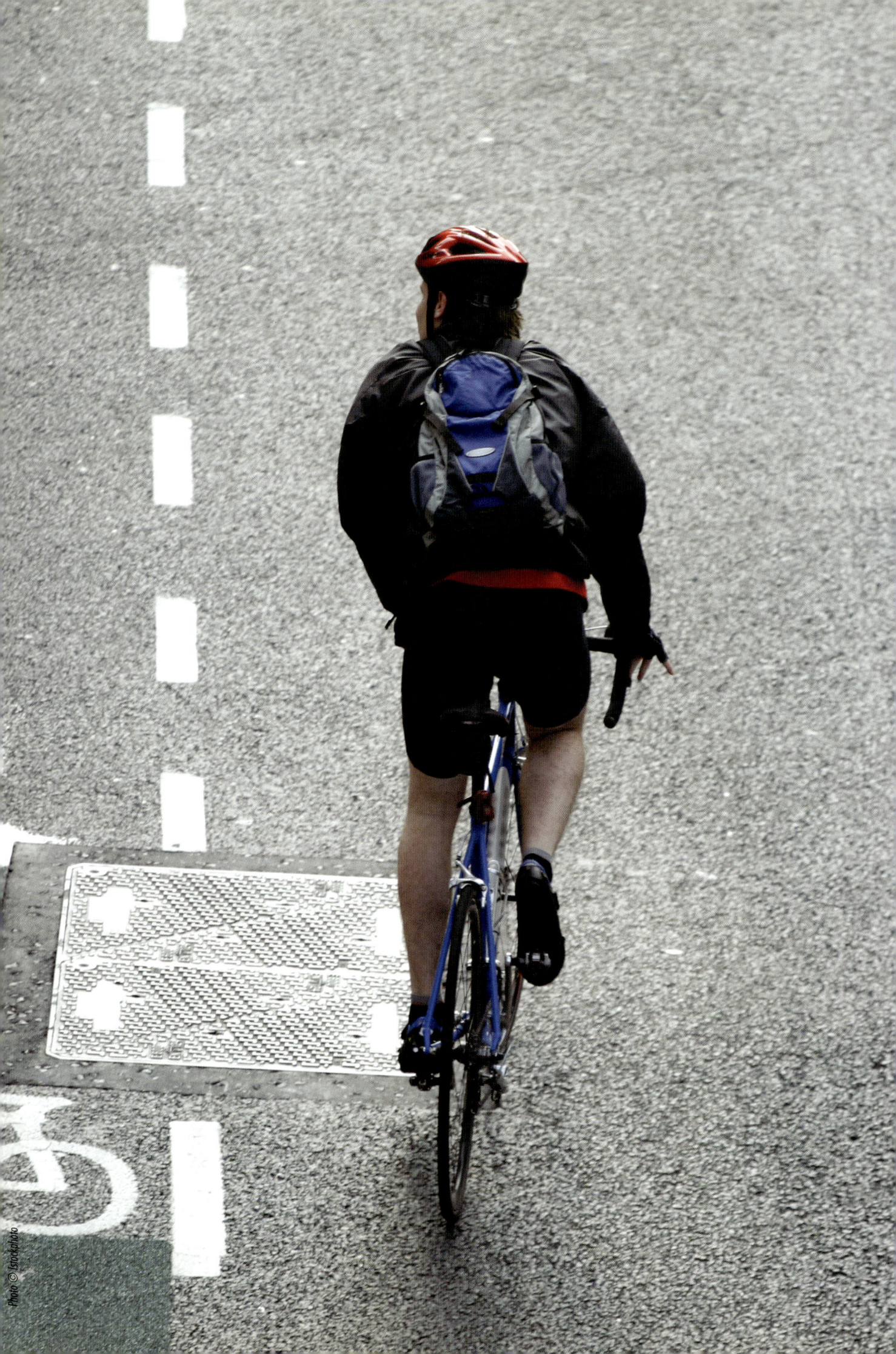

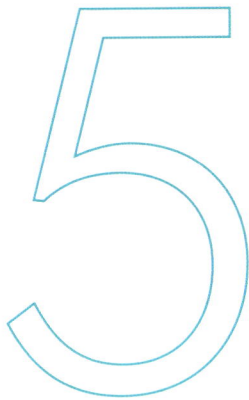

References

1. *The global burden of disease: 2004 update*. Geneva, World Health Organization, 2008 (http://www.who.int/healthinfo/global_burden_disease/GBD_report_2004update_AnnexA.pdf, accessed 23 July 2009).
2. Racioppi F et al. *Preventing road traffic injury: a public health perspective for Europe*. Copenhagen, WHO Regional Office for Europe, 2004 (http://www.euro.who.int/InformationSources/Publications/Catalogue/20041119_2, accessed 23 July 2009).
3. Peden M et al., eds. *World report on child injury prevention*. Geneva, World Health Organization and UNICEF, 2008 (http://www.who.int/violence_injury_prevention/child/injury/world_report/en, accessed 23 July 2009).
4. Peden M et al., eds. *World report on road traffic injury prevention*. Geneva, World Health Organization, 2004 (http://www.who.int/violence_injury_prevention/publications/road_traffic/world_report/en/index.html, accessed 23 July 2009).
5. *Global status report on road safety*. Geneva, World Health Organization, 2009 (http://www.who.int/violence_injury_prevention/road_safety–status/2009/en/index.html, accessed 23 July 2009).
6. *Faces behind the figures. Voices of road traffic crash victims and their families*. Geneva, World Health Organization, 2007 (http://www.who.int/violence_injury_prevention /road_traffic/activities/faces/en, accessed 23 July 2009).
7. Sethi D et al. *European report on child injury prevention*. Copenhagen, WHO Regional Office for Europe, 2008 (http://www.euro.who.int/violenceinjury/injuries/20081205_2, accessed 23 July 2009).
8. Jacobs G, Thomas AA, Astrop A. *Estimating global road fatalities*. Crowthorne, Transport Research Laboratory, 2000 (TRL report 445; http://www.trasnport-links.org/transport_links/filearea/publications/1_329_TRL445.pdf, accessed 23 July 2009).
9. Eksler V, Lassarre S, Thomas I. Regional analysis of road mortality in Europe. *Public Health*, 2008, 122:826–837.
10. European Health for All database [online database]. Copenhagen, WHO Regional Office for Europe, 2004 (http://www.euro.who.int/hfadb, accessed 23 July 2009).
11. Sethi D, Racioppi F, Mitis F. *Youth and road safety in Europe*. Copenhagen, WHO Regional Office for Europe, 2007 (http://www.euro.who.int/Document/E90142.pdf, accessed 23 July 2009).
12. Laflamme L et al. *Addressing the socioeconomic safety divide: a policy briefing*. Copenhagen, WHO Regional Office for Europe, 2009 (http://www.euro.who.int/Document/E92197.pdf, accessed 23 July 2009).
13. Edwards P et al. Deaths from injury in children and employment status in family: analysis of trends in class specific death rates. *British Medical Journal*, 2006, 333:119.
14. Sethi D et al. Reducing inequalities from injuries in Europe. *Lancet*, 2006, 368:2243–2250.
15. Towner E, Towner J. The hazards of daily life: an historical perspective on adult unintentional injuries. *Journal of Epidemiology and Community Health*, 2008, 62:952–956.

16. Kunzli N et al. Public-health impact of outdoor and traffic-related air pollution: a European assessment. *Lancet*, 2000, 356:795–801.
17. Roberts I, Hillman M. Climate change: the implications for policy on injury control and health promotion. *Injury Prevention*, 2005, 11:326–329.
18. WHO Regional Office for Europe and United Nations Economic Commission for Europe. *Ten years' work towards sustainable and healthy transport in Europe: key achievements and the way forward.* Copenhagen, WHO Regional Office for Europe and Geneva, United Nations Economic Commission for Europe, 2009 (http://www.euro.who.int/Document/mediacentre/FS_healthy_transport.pdf, accessed 23 July 2009).
19. *Climate for a transport change. TERM 2007: indicators tracking transport and environment in the European Union.* Copenhagen, European Environment Agency, 2008 (EEA Report, 1/2008).
20. *EMEP/CORINAIR emission inventory guidebook – 2006.* Copenhagen, European Environment Agency, 2006 (EEA Technical Report, No. 11/2006).
21. THE PEP – Transport, Health and Environment Pan-European Programme [web site]. Geneva, Transport, Health and Environment Pan-European Programme, 2009 (http://www.unece.org/thepep/en/welcome.htm, accessed 23 July 2009).
22. *Transport at a crossroads. TERM 2008: indicators tracking transport and environment in the European Union.* Copenhagen, European Environment Agency, 2009 (EEA Report No 3/2009; http://www.eea.europa.eu/publications/transport-at-a-crossroads, accessed 23 July 2009).
23. *Global road safety crisis.* New York, United Nations General Assembly, 2003 (http://www.who.int/violence_injury_prevention/media/en/un_general_assembly.pdf, accessed 23 July 2009).
24. *Global road safety crisis.* New York, United Nations General Assembly, 2003 (Resolution 57/309; http://www.unece.org/trans/roadsafe/docs/GA_R_57-309e.pdf, accessed 23 July 2009).
25. *European Road Safety Action Programme. Halving the number of road accident victims in the European Union by 2010: a shared responsibility.* Brussels, European Commission, 2003 (COM(2003)311 final).
26. Sethi D et al. *Progress in preventing injuries in the WHO European Region.* Copenhagen, WHO Regional Office for Europe, 2008 (http://www.euro.who.int/InformationSources/Publications/Catalogue/20080912_1, accessed 23 July 2009).
27. *Annual statistical report 2008.* Brussels, European Road Safety Observatory, 2008 (http://www.erso.eu/safetynet/fixed/WP1/2008/SafetyNet%20Annual%20Statistical%20Report%202008.pdf, accessed 23 July 2009).
28. *Vision, strategy and targets for road traffic safety in Norway 2006–2015.* Oslo, Norwegian Public Roads Administration, 2006.
29. *European Road Safety Action Programme – mid-term review.* Brussels, European Commission, 2006 (COM(2006)74 final).
30. *The national road safety plan. Major elements of the plan.* Tel Aviv, Committee for the Preparation of a National, Multi-year Road Safety Plan, 2005.
31. *Via sicura. Federal action programme for greater road safety.* Berne, Federal Roads Office, Switzerland, 2005.
32. [The happy road of childhood] [web site]. Moscow, Department of Road Safety, Ministry of Internal Affairs, 2009 (http://www.dddgazeta.ru, accessed 23 July 2009).
33. *Transport policy guidelines and transport network investment and financing programme until 2020. Government transport policy report to Parliament, 2008.* Helsinki, Ministry of Transport and Communication, Finland, 2008.
34. Evans R. *Central London Congestion Charging Scheme: ex-post evaluation of the quantified impacts of the original scheme. Prepared by Reg Evans, for Congestion Charging Modelling and Evaluation Team.* London, Transport for London, 2007.
35. *Amsterdam Declaration. Making THE link: transport choices for our health, environment and prosperity.* Geneva, United Nations Economic Commission for Europe and Copenhagen, WHO Regional Office for Europe, 2009 (http://www.euro.who.int/Document/E92356.pdf, accessed 23 July 2009).

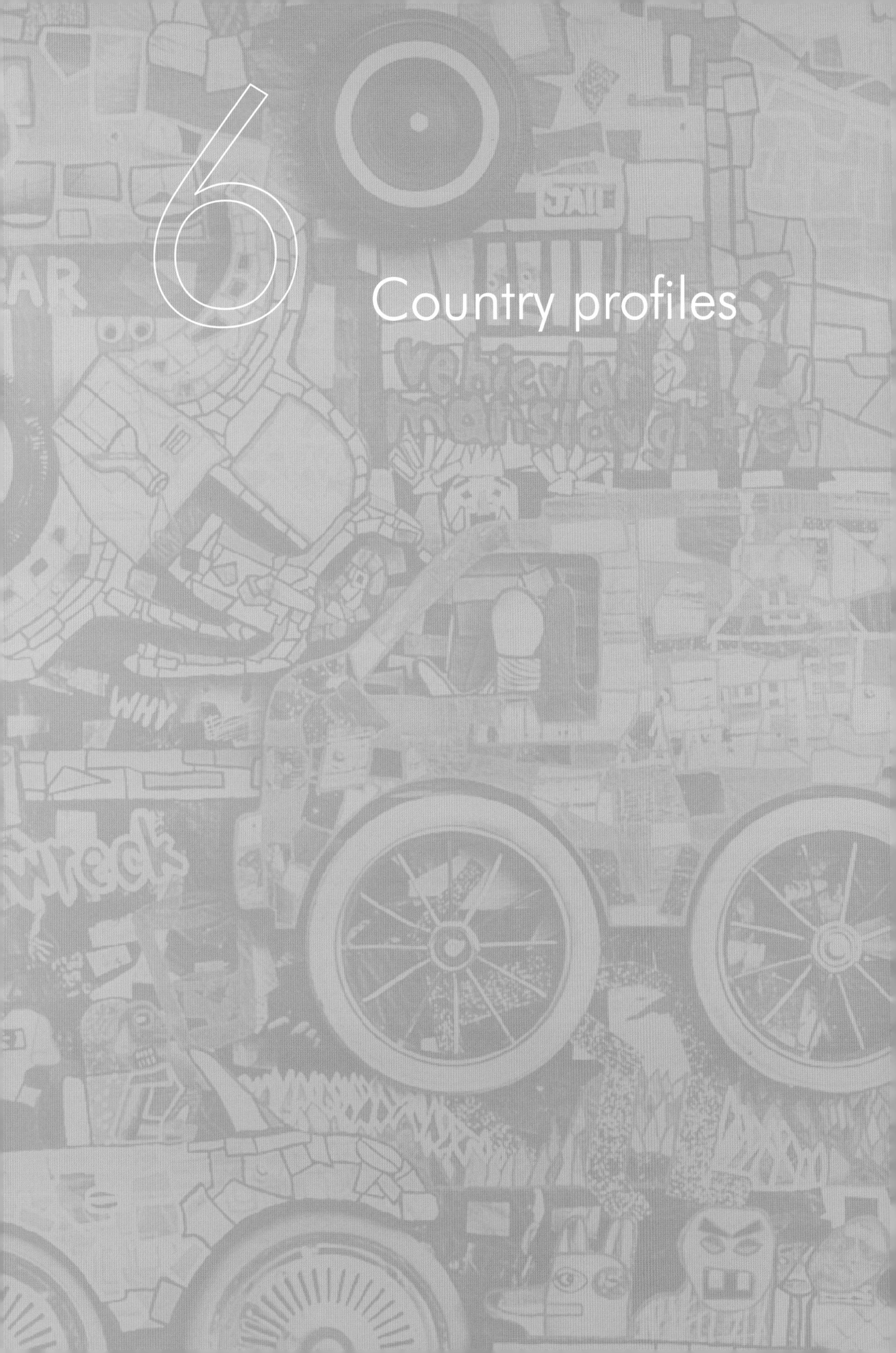

6 Country profiles

Explanatory notes

Background

The country profiles in this section of the report present selected information about road safety as reported by each of the 49 participating countries. Annexes 3–13 present additional national data. The country survey tools are available at: http://www.who.int/violence_injury_prevention/road_traffic/road_safety_status/2009.

Variation in methods

Forty-nine countries participated in the *European status report on road safety* (Annex 13). Most countries followed the standardized method (Annex 1), but the national data coordinators (Annex 13) in Kazakhstan, Ukraine and Uzbekistan completed the questionnaire without any consensus meeting. In Germany the questionnaire was completed by the Federal Highway Research Institute (BASt).

Population data are from the United Nations Population Division and refer to 2007. Income data, Human Development Index and CO_2 emissions per person per year are from the World Bank for the latest year available (2007 for income, 2006 for Human Development Index and 2004 for CO_2 emissions per person per year). Life expectancy and median age are from the WHO Statistical Information System (WHOSIS) for 2006.

Car ownership per 1000 population is calculated as: (the number of cars the country reported in the survey divided by the total population) times 1000.

Terms used

The following terms and issues should be considered when reviewing the individual country profiles.

- The questionnaire asked for information on several topics, with follow-up questions exploring each topic in further detail. For many topics, respondents were asked to skip follow-up questions depending on their answer to the top-level question. Consequently, the country profiles do not report information from follow-up questions if these should have been skipped.
- Road classifications (especially the definitions of an urban road, a rural road and a highway) vary greatly from country to country. Respondents were asked to report on the speed limits of different kinds of road according to the definitions used in the country concerned.
- Respondents were asked, as individuals, to rate the effectiveness of enforcement of various elements of national road safety legislation based on their professional opinion or perception. A scale of 0 to 10 was used, where 0 was "not effective" and 10 was "highly effective". The group of respondents then tried to reach consensus on an enforcement score. These scores are therefore subjective and should be seen only as indicating how enforcement is perceived in the country. Many respondents expressed difficulty in assessing enforcement at the national level since it often varies from region to region and the intensity of enforcement may vary.
- Blood alcohol concentration limits refer to the level above which a driver may be punished by law.
- If respondents provided explanatory information on rates of helmet wearing and/or seat-belt use – for instance, describing methods or geographical coverage – this information is reported in footnotes.
- A motorcycle helmet law is assessed as applying to all riders if the law requires drivers and passengers (both adults and children) to wear a helmet. Exceptions to these laws based on religion, health conditions or other reasons are indicated in a footnote.
- Respondents were asked to report on vehicle standards required for car manufacturers or assemblers in the country. Therefore, no information is included on vehicle standards for countries in which manufacture or assembly do not take place. Some countries apply stringent standards to imported vehicles, but this survey did not collect data on such standards.

Data presentation

Country profiles contain data on road traffic deaths and non-fatal injuries as reported by countries.
- Data from different countries are not necessarily comparable, as different definitions and time frames have been used.
- Due to space constraints in footnotes, the data source has been summarized as police, transport or health if the data are from the interior ministry, transport ministry or health ministry, respectively.

In the charts presenting data on deaths by road user category, proportions may not add up to 100% due to rounding. Some countries classify road traffic deaths according to the vehicle or road user "at fault" rather than according to who died or use categories different from those requested in the questionnaire. In these countries, deaths among vulnerable road users are even more likely to be underreported.

The standard colour coding of the pie charts used to represent the road user categories requested in the questionnaire is shown below. Non-standard colours represent additional categories.

- Drivers of four-wheeled vehicles
- Passengers of four-wheeled vehicles
- Occupants (drivers or passengers) of four-wheeled vehicles
- Riders (drivers or passengers) of motorized two- or three-wheelers
- Cyclists
- Pedestrians
- Other
- Unspecified

Age-specific mortality rates were computed according to the age categories provided by the country. Many country profiles therefore present age categories that are not directly comparable. Age-specific mortality rates for Tajikistan and Turkey are not reported due to underreporting (see the explanatory notes to the statistical annexes).

Trend graphs are shown either as road traffic death rates per 100 000 population (on a yellow background) or as an absolute number of road traffic deaths (on a blue background), depending on which figures the country supplied. Due to space constraints, an arbitrary starting-point of 1970 was applied for the few countries that provided many decades of trend data.

If the primary source of information for both the pie and trend graphs was not stipulated, the source has been reported as "country questionnaire".

Information about the number of vehicles in the country includes only registered vehicles and the proportions of various types of such vehicles. These proportions may not add up to 100% due to rounding. In some countries, respondents noted that much of the vehicle fleet may not be registered.

Albania

Population: 3.19 million (2007)

Median age: 29 years

Life expectancy at birth: 71 years

Income group:[a] middle

Gross national income per person: US$ 3290   Rank: 40 of 49[b]

Human Development Index:[c] 0.807   Rank: 35 of 49[b]

Private car ownership per 1000 population:[d] 74.5

CO_2 emissions (tonnes) per person per year:[a] 1.2

[a] World Bank data.
[b] Rank among the 49 countries in the WHO European Region participating in the survey.
[c] United Nations Development Programme data.
[d] WHO European Region average: 339.

Institutional framework for road safety

Lead agency: Interministerial Committee on Road Safety	
Status of the agency	Interministerial
Funded in national budget	No
National road safety strategy	**No**
Measurable targets	NA
Implementation funded	NA
Money allocated (in € (year))	NA

Key data

Reported number of road traffic deaths (2007)	384[a] (77% males, 23% females)
Reported number of non-fatal road traffic injuries (2007)	1344[b]
Road traffic deaths involving alcohol	5.2%[c]
Wearing motorcycle helmets	No information
Using seat-belts in cars	
Overall	No information
Front-seat occupants	30%[d]
Rear-seat occupants	No information
Costing study available	**No**
Annual estimated costs (in € (year))	NA
Study included deaths, injuries or both	NA
Methods used	NA

[a] Police data, defined as died at the crash scene.
[b] Police data.
[c] 2007, Traffic Police Directorate, Ministry of the Interior.
[d] 1996, Citizen Society of Road Safety, data from pilot cities.

NA: not applicable

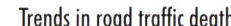

Trends in road traffic deaths

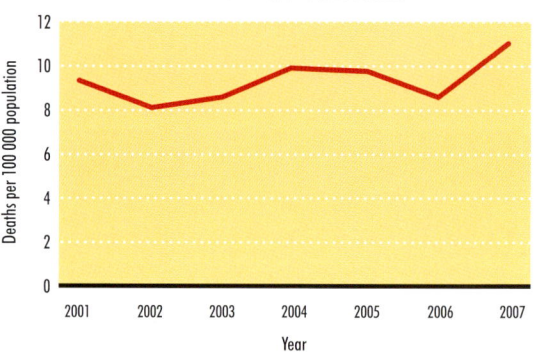

Source: Traffic Police Directorate, Ministry of the Interior

Age-specific mortality rates from road traffic injuries

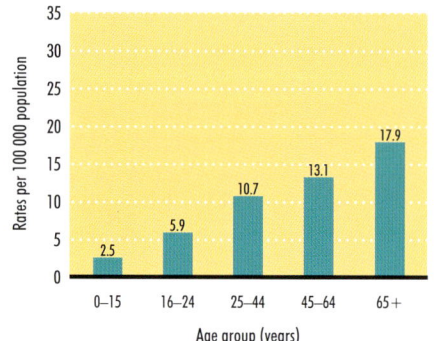

Source: 2006, Ministry of the Interior

Deaths by road user category

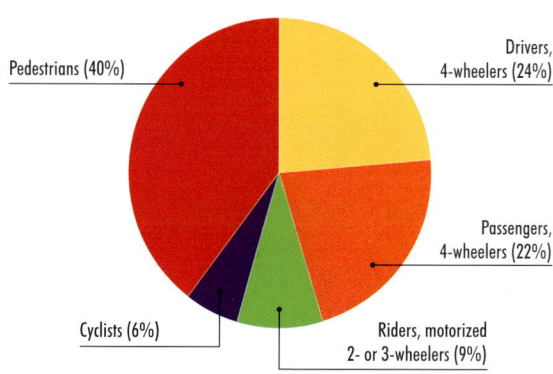

Source: 2006, Ministry of Public Works, Transport and Telecommunications

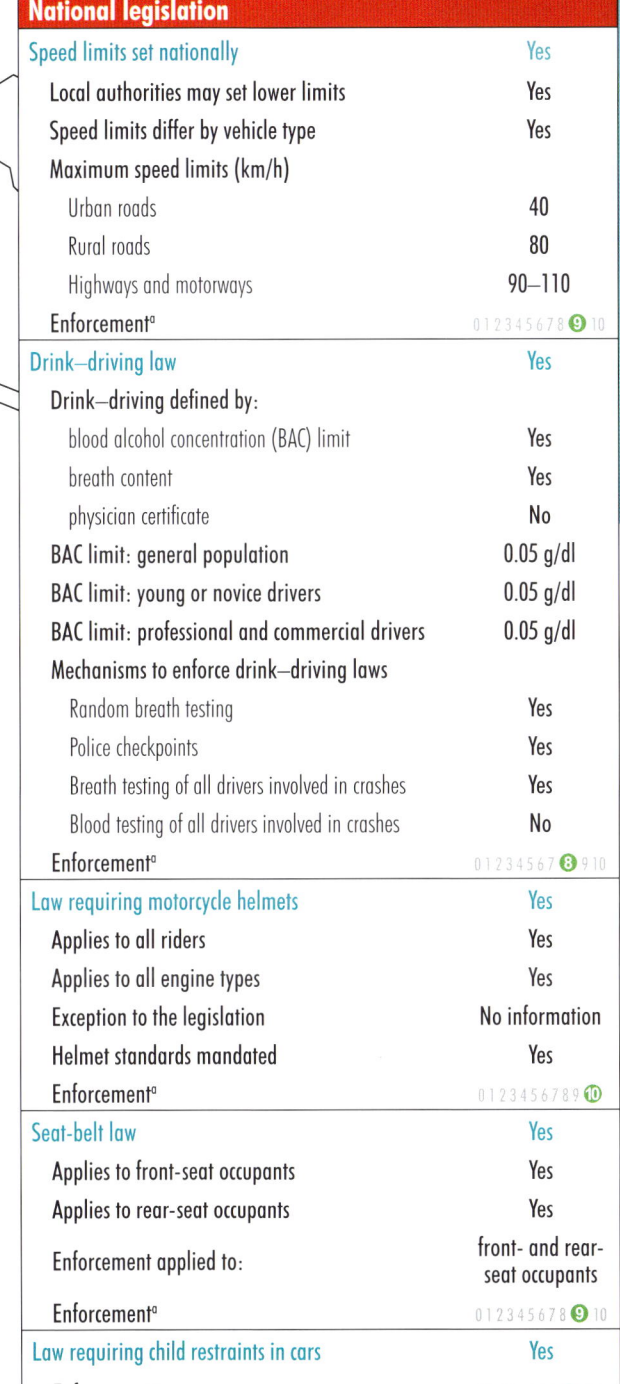

National legislation	
Speed limits set nationally	Yes
Local authorities may set lower limits	Yes
Speed limits differ by vehicle type	Yes
Maximum speed limits (km/h)	
Urban roads	40
Rural roads	80
Highways and motorways	90–110
Enforcement[a]	0 1 2 3 4 5 6 7 8 **9** 10
Drink–driving law	Yes
Drink–driving defined by:	
blood alcohol concentration (BAC) limit	Yes
breath content	Yes
physician certificate	No
BAC limit: general population	0.05 g/dl
BAC limit: young or novice drivers	0.05 g/dl
BAC limit: professional and commercial drivers	0.05 g/dl
Mechanisms to enforce drink–driving laws	
Random breath testing	Yes
Police checkpoints	Yes
Breath testing of all drivers involved in crashes	Yes
Blood testing of all drivers involved in crashes	No
Enforcement[a]	0 1 2 3 4 5 6 7 **8** 9 10
Law requiring motorcycle helmets	Yes
Applies to all riders	Yes
Applies to all engine types	Yes
Exception to the legislation	No information
Helmet standards mandated	Yes
Enforcement[a]	0 1 2 3 4 5 6 7 8 9 **10**
Seat-belt law	Yes
Applies to front-seat occupants	Yes
Applies to rear-seat occupants	Yes
Enforcement applied to:	front- and rear-seat occupants
Enforcement[a]	0 1 2 3 4 5 6 7 8 **9** 10
Law requiring child restraints in cars	Yes
Enforcement[a]	0 1 2 3 4 5 6 7 **8** 9 10

[a] The enforcement score represents a consensus based on the professional opinion of respondents on a scale of 0 to 10, where 0 is not effective and 10 is highly effective.

Road safety audits	
Formal audits required for major new road construction projects	Yes
Regular audits of existing road infrastructure	No

Vehicle standards	
No car manufacturers	

Promoting transport alternatives to cars	
National policies to promote walking or cycling	No
Investment in bicycle lanes	NA
Investment in foot paths	NA
Traffic-calming measures	NA
Investment for increasing cycling	NA
Disincentives for private car use	NA
National policies to promote public transport	Yes
Subsidized pricing of public transport	Yes
Improving the frequency and coverage of public transport	No
Disincentives for private car use	No

Vehicle regulations	
Compulsory insurance for vehicles	Yes
Periodic vehicle inspection for:	
cars	Yes
motorized 2- or 3-wheeled vehicles	Yes
minibuses and vans	Yes
lorries	Yes
buses	Yes

Registered motor vehicles	
Total (2007)	349 646
Cars	68%
Motorized 2- and 3-wheelers	7%
Minibuses, vans, etc. (seating <20 people)	8%
Lorries	12%
Buses	5%

Source: Ministry of Public Works, Transport and Telecommunications

Care after road crashes	
Formal, publicly available prehospital care system	Yes
National universal access telephone number	Subnational number (2253364)

Acknowledgements

Authority approving the data for publication: Ministry of Health
National data coordinator: Maksim Bozo, Ministry of Health
Respondents: Fatos Olldashi, University Military Hospital, Tirana; Maksim Tasho, Ministry of Public Works, Transport and Telecommunications; Demir Osmani, Citizen Society of Road Safety; Luri Balla, General State Police Directorate; Gentiana Qirjako, Faculty of Medicine, University of Tirana

Armenia

- Population: **3.00** million
- Median age: **32** years
- Life expectancy at birth: **69** years
- Income group:[a] **middle**
- Gross national income per person: **US$ 2640**   Rank: **41** of 49[b]
- Human Development Index:[c] **0.777**   Rank: **41** of 49[b]
- Private car ownership per 1000 population:[d] **95.9**
- CO_2 emissions (tonnes) per person per year:[a] **1.2**

[a] World Bank data.
[b] Rank among the 49 countries in the WHO European Region participating in the survey.
[c] United Nations Development Programme data.
[d] WHO European Region average: 339.

Institutional framework for road safety

Lead agency: Road Police of the Police of the Republic of Armenia	
Status of the agency	Directly under the Government
Funded in national budget	Yes
National road safety strategy	**No**
Measurable targets	NA
Implementation funded	NA
Money allocated (in € (year))	NA

Key data

Reported number of road traffic deaths (2007)	371[a] (75% males, 25% females)
Reported number of non-fatal road traffic injuries (2007)	2720[b]
Road traffic deaths involving alcohol	6.1%[c]
Wearing motorcycle helmets	No information
Using seat-belts in cars	
Overall	No information
Front-seat occupants	No information
Rear-seat occupants	No information
Costing study available	**No**
Annual estimated costs (in € (year))	NA
Study included deaths, injuries or both	NA
Methods used	NA

[a] Police data, no specified time period.
[b] Police data.
[c] 2007, Road Police of the Police of the Republic of Armenia.

NA: not applicable

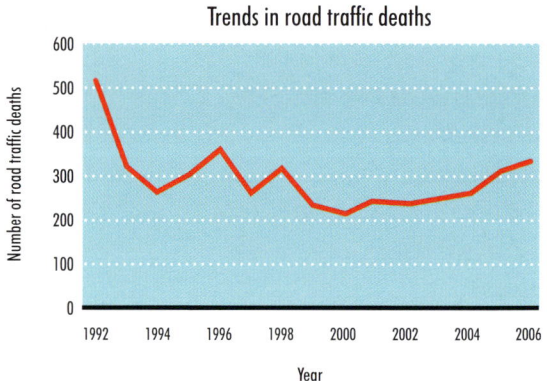

Trends in road traffic deaths

Source: Road Police of the Police of the Republic of Armenia

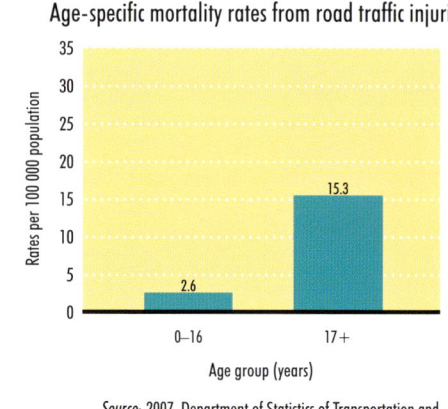

Age-specific mortality rates from road traffic injuries

Source: 2007, Department of Statistics of Transportation and Communication of National Statistical Service

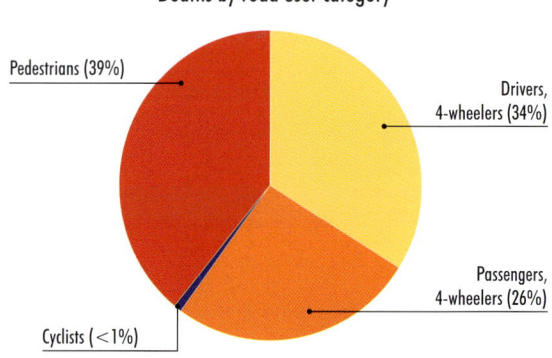

Deaths by road user category
- Pedestrians (39%)
- Drivers, 4-wheelers (34%)
- Passengers, 4-wheelers (26%)
- Cyclists (<1%)

Source: 2007, Road Police of the Police of the Republic of Armenia

National legislation	
Speed limits set nationally	Yes
Local authorities may set lower limits	Yes
Speed limits differ by vehicle type	Yes
Maximum speed limits (km/h)	
Urban roads	60
Rural roads	60
Highways and motorways	90–110
Enforcement[a]	5 (0–10)
Drink–driving law	Yes
Drink–driving defined by:	
blood alcohol concentration (BAC) limit	Yes
breath content	Yes
physician certificate	No
BAC limit: general population	0.08 g/dl
BAC limit: young or novice drivers	0.08 g/dl
BAC limit: professional and commercial drivers	0.08 g/dl
Mechanisms to enforce drink–driving laws	
Random breath testing	Yes
Police checkpoints	No
Breath testing of all drivers involved in crashes	Yes
Blood testing of all drivers involved in crashes	Yes
Enforcement[a]	5 (0–10)
Law requiring motorcycle helmets	Yes
Applies to all riders	Yes
Applies to all engine types	Yes
Exception to the legislation	No
Helmet standards mandated	No
Enforcement[a]	5 (0–10)
Seat-belt law	Yes
Applies to front-seat occupants	Yes
Applies to rear-seat occupants	Yes
Enforcement applied to:	front- and rear-seat occupants
Enforcement[a]	3 (0–10)
Law requiring child restraints in cars	Yes
Enforcement[a]	5 (0–10)

[a] The enforcement score represents a consensus based on the professional opinion of respondents on a scale of 0 to 10, where 0 is not effective and 10 is highly effective.

Road safety audits	
Formal audits required for major new road construction projects	Yes
Regular audits of existing road infrastructure	Yes

Vehicle standards	
No car manufacturers	

Promoting transport alternatives to cars	
National policies to promote walking or cycling	No
Investment in bicycle lanes	NA
Investment in foot paths	NA
Traffic-calming measures	NA
Investment for increasing cycling	NA
Disincentives for private car use	NA
National policies to promote public transport	No
Subsidized pricing of public transport	NA
Improving the frequency and coverage of public transport	NA
Disincentives for private car use	NA

Vehicle regulations	
Compulsory insurance for vehicles	No
Periodic vehicle inspection for:	
cars	Yes
motorized 2- or 3-wheeled vehicles	Yes
minibuses and vans	Yes
lorries	Yes
buses	Yes

Registered motor vehicles	
Total (2007)	366 836
Cars	79%
Buses	7%
Other	15%

Source: Road Police of the Police of the Republic of Armenia

Care after road crashes	
Formal, publicly available prehospital care system	Yes
National universal access telephone number	Yes (103)

Acknowledgements

Authority approving the data for publication: Ministry of Health
National data coordinator: Lilit Avetisyan, State Hygiene and Anitiepidemic Inspectorate of Ministry of Health
Respondents: Ella Safaryan, Health Care Department Ministry of Health; Grigory Torosyan, National Statistical Service; Rubik Navoyan, Ministry of Transport and Communications; Vardan Petrosyan, Ministry of Jurisdiction; Vahe Petrosyan, Police of the Republic of Armenia; Mariam Gukasyan, State Hygiene and Anitiepidemic Inspectorate of Ministry of Health

Austria

Population: **8.36 million (2007)**

Median age: **40** years

Life expectancy at birth: **80** years

Income group:[a] **high**

Gross national income per person: **US$ 42 700** Rank: **9 of 49**[b]

Human Development Index:[c] **0.951** Rank: **9 of 49**[b]

Private car ownership per 1000 population:[d] **507.5**

CO_2 emissions (tonnes) per person per year:[a] **8.5**

[a] World Bank data.
[b] Rank among the 49 countries in the WHO European Region participating in the survey.
[c] United Nations Development Programme data.
[d] WHO European Region average: 339.

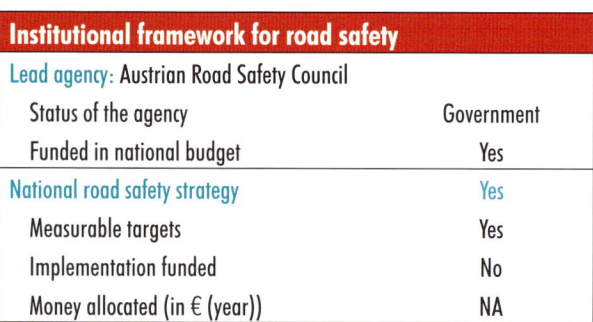

Institutional framework for road safety	
Lead agency: Austrian Road Safety Council	
Status of the agency	Government
Funded in national budget	Yes
National road safety strategy	Yes
Measurable targets	Yes
Implementation funded	No
Money allocated (in € (year))	NA

Key data	
Reported number of road traffic deaths (2007)	691[a] (77% males, 23% females)
Reported number of non-fatal road traffic injuries (2007)	53 211[b]
Road traffic deaths involving alcohol	8.1%[c]
Wearing motorcycle helmets	95%[d]
Using seat-belts in cars	
Overall	88%[d]
Front-seat occupants	89%[d]
Rear-seat occupants	49%[d]
Costing study available	Yes
Annual estimated costs (in € (2006))	9.92 billion
Study included deaths, injuries or both	Both deaths and injuries
Methods used	Willingness to pay

[a] Statistics Austria, defined as died within 30 days of the accident.
[b] Statistics Austria.
[c] 2007, Statistics Austria.
[d] 2007, Austrian Road Safety Board survey.

NA: not applicable

Trends in road traffic deaths

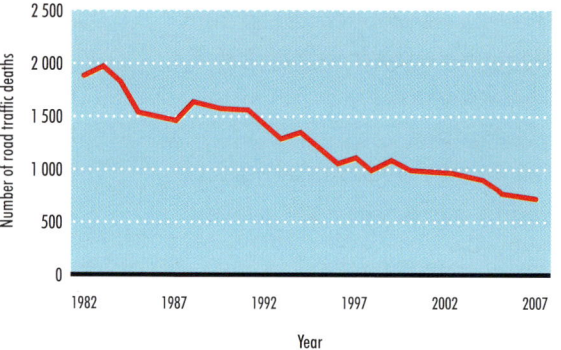

Source: Ministry of Internal Affairs, Statistics Austria

Age-specific mortality rates from road traffic injuries

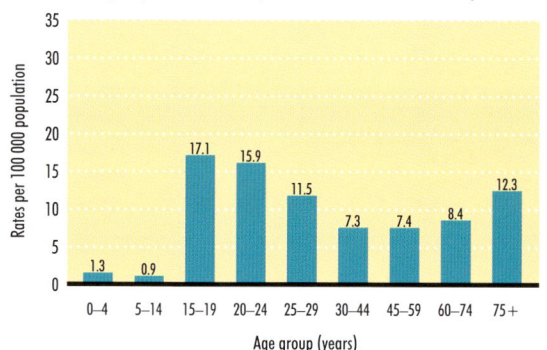

Source: 2007, *Road Accidents Statistics 2007*, Austrian Road Safety Board

Deaths by road user category

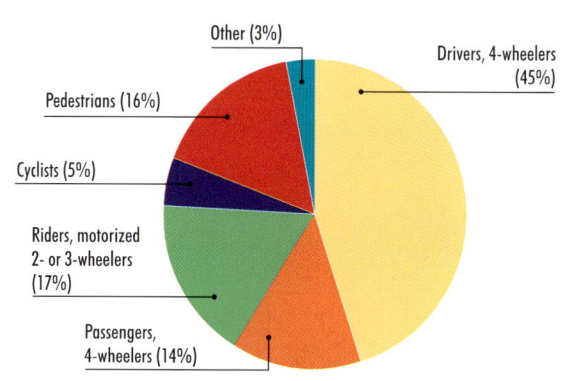

Source: 2007, Ministry of Internal Affairs, Statistics Austria

National legislation	
Speed limits set nationally	Yes
Local authorities may set lower limits	Yes
Speed limits differ by vehicle type	Yes
Maximum speed limits (km/h)	
Urban roads	50
Rural roads	100
Highways and motorways	100
Enforcement[a]	0 1 2 3 4 5 6 **7** 8 9 10
Drink–driving law	Yes
Drink–driving defined by:	
blood alcohol concentration (BAC) limit	Yes
breath content	Yes
physician certificate	No
BAC limit: general population	0.05 g/dl
BAC limit: young or novice drivers	0.01 g/dl
BAC limit: professional and commercial drivers	0.01 g/dl
Mechanisms to enforce drink–driving laws	
Random breath testing	Yes
Police checkpoints	Yes
Breath testing of all drivers involved in crashes	Yes
Blood testing of all drivers involved in crashes	Yes
Enforcement[a]	0 1 2 3 4 5 6 7 8 **9** 10
Law requiring motorcycle helmets	Yes
Applies to all riders	Yes
Applies to all engine types	Yes
Exception to the legislation	Yes[b]
Helmet standards mandated	Yes
Enforcement[a]	0 1 2 3 4 5 6 7 8 **9** 10
Seat-belt law	Yes
Applies to front-seat occupants	Yes
Applies to rear-seat occupants	Yes
Enforcement applied to:	front- and rear-seat occupants
Enforcement[a]	0 1 2 3 4 5 6 **7** 8 9 10
Law requiring child restraints in cars	Yes
Enforcement[a]	0 1 2 3 4 5 6 7 8 **9** 10

[a] The enforcement score represents a consensus based on the professional opinion of respondents on a scale of 0 to 10, where 0 is not effective and 10 is highly effective.
[b] Exceptions: constitutional impossibility and situations like parking.

Road safety audits	
Formal audits required for major new road construction projects	No
Regular audits of existing road infrastructure	Yes

Vehicle standards	
Car manufacturers required to adhere to standards on	
Fuel consumption	No
Seat-belt installation for all seats	Yes

Promoting transport alternatives to cars	
National policies to promote walking or cycling	Yes
Investment in bicycle lanes	Yes
Investment in foot paths	No
Traffic-calming measures	Yes
Investment for increasing cycling	No
Disincentives for private car use	No
National policies to promote public transport	Yes
Subsidized pricing of public transport	Yes
Improving the frequency and coverage of public transport	Yes
Disincentives for private car use	No

Vehicle regulations	
Compulsory insurance for vehicles	Yes
Periodic vehicle inspection for:	
cars	Yes
motorized 2- or 3-wheeled vehicles	Yes
minibuses and vans	Yes
lorries	Yes
buses	Yes

Registered motor vehicles	
Total (2007)	5 796 973
Cars	73%
Motorized 2- and 3-wheelers	11%
Lorries	14%
Buses	<1%
Other	2%

Source: Statistics Austria

Care after road crashes	
Formal, publicly available prehospital care system	Yes
National universal access telephone number	Yes (144)

Acknowledgements

Authority approving the data for publication: Federal Ministry of Health, Family and Youth
National data coordinator: Rupert Kisser, Austrian Road Safety Board
Respondents: Guenter Breyer, Federal Ministry of Traffic, Innovation and Technology; Martin Germ, Federal Ministry of Internal Affairs; Fritz Wagner, Federal Ministry of Health, Family and Youth; Martin Vergeiner, Austrian Road Safety Board; Thomas Fessl, Austrian Road Safety Board

Azerbaijan

Population: 8.47 million (2007)

Median age: 28 years

Life expectancy at birth: 64 years

Income group:[a] middle

Gross national income per person: US$ 2550 Rank: 42 of 49[b]

Human Development Index:[c] 0.758 Rank: 43 of 49[b]

Private car ownership per 1000 population:[d] 71.7

CO_2 emissions (tonnes) per person per year:[a] 3.8

[a] World Bank data.
[b] Rank among the 49 countries in the WHO European Region participating in the survey.
[c] United Nations Development Programme data.
[d] WHO European Region average: 339.

Institutional framework for road safety	
Lead agency: State Road Police	
Status of the agency	Government
Funded in national budget	Yes
National road safety strategy	Yes
Measurable targets	Yes
Implementation funded	Yes
Money allocated (in € (2007))	3.16 million

Key data	
Reported number of road traffic deaths (2007)	1107[a] (78% males, 22% females)
Reported number of non-fatal road traffic injuries (2007)	3432[b]
Road traffic deaths involving alcohol	2.7%[c]
Wearing motorcycle helmets	No information
Using seat-belts in cars	
Overall	No information
Front-seat occupants	No information
Rear-seat occupants	No information
Costing study available	No
Annual estimated costs (in € (year))	NA
Study included deaths, injuries or both	NA
Methods used	NA

[a] Police data, defined as died within 7 days of the crash.
[b] Police data.
[c] 2007, State Road Police.

NA: not applicable

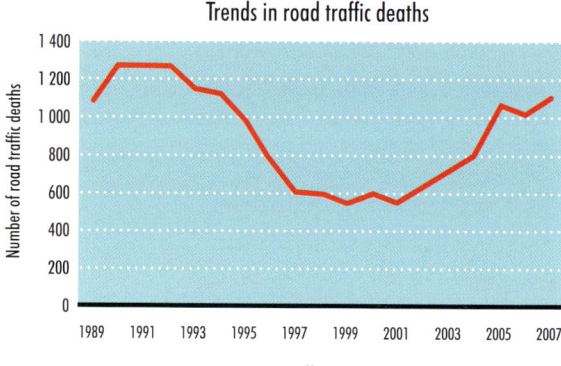

Trends in road traffic deaths

Source: Head Department of State Road Police

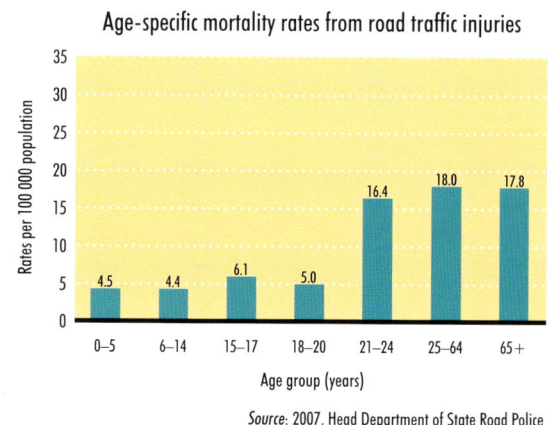

Age-specific mortality rates from road traffic injuries

Source: 2007, Head Department of State Road Police

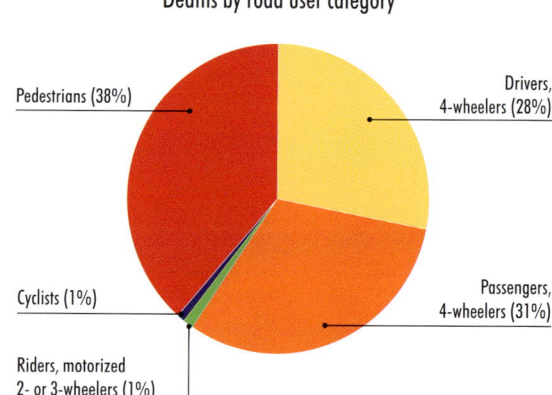

Deaths by road user category

Pedestrians (38%)
Drivers, 4-wheelers (28%)
Passengers, 4-wheelers (31%)
Riders, motorized 2- or 3-wheelers (1%)
Cyclists (1%)

Source: 2007, Head Department of State Road Police

National legislation

Speed limits set nationally	Yes
Local authorities may set lower limits	Yes
Speed limits differ by vehicle type	Yes
Maximum speed limits (km/h)	
Urban roads	60
Rural roads	90
Highways and motorways	110
Enforcement[a]	0 1 2 3 4 5 6 7 8 **9** 10
Drink–driving law	Yes
Drink–driving defined by:	
blood alcohol concentration (BAC) limit	Yes
breath content	Yes
physician certificate	Yes
BAC limit: general population	0.00 g/dl
BAC limit: young or novice drivers	0.00 g/dl
BAC limit: professional and commercial drivers	0.00 g/dl
Mechanisms to enforce drink–driving laws	
Random breath testing	Yes
Police checkpoints	Yes
Breath testing of all drivers involved in crashes	Yes
Blood testing of all drivers involved in crashes	Yes
Enforcement[a]	0 1 2 3 4 5 6 7 8 **9** 10
Law requiring motorcycle helmets	Yes
Applies to all riders	Yes
Applies to all engine types	Yes
Exception to the legislation	No
Helmet standards mandated	No
Enforcement[a]	0 1 2 3 4 5 6 7 8 **9** 10
Seat-belt law	Yes
Applies to front-seat occupants	Yes
Applies to rear-seat occupants	Yes
Enforcement applied to:	front- and rear-seat occupants
Enforcement[a]	0 1 2 3 4 5 6 7 8 **9** 10
Law requiring child restraints in cars	Yes
Enforcement[a]	0 1 2 3 4 5 6 7 8 **9** 10

[a] The enforcement score represents a consensus based on the professional opinion of respondents on a scale of 0 to 10, where 0 is not effective and 10 is highly effective.

Road safety audits

Formal audits required for major new road construction projects	Yes
Regular audits of existing road infrastructure	Yes

Vehicle standards

Car manufacturers required to adhere to standards on	
Fuel consumption	No
Seat-belt installation for all seats	No

Promoting transport alternatives to cars

National policies to promote walking or cycling	No
Investment in bicycle lanes	NA
Investment in foot paths	NA
Traffic-calming measures	NA
Investment for increasing cycling	NA
Disincentives for private car use	NA
National policies to promote public transport	Yes
Subsidized pricing of public transport	Yes
Improving the frequency and coverage of public transport	Yes
Disincentives for private car use	No

Vehicle regulations

Compulsory insurance for vehicles	Yes
Periodic vehicle inspection for:	
cars	Yes
motorized 2- or 3-wheeled vehicles	Yes
minibuses and vans	Yes
lorries	Yes
buses	Yes

Registered motor vehicles

Total (2007)	784 018
Cars	77%
Motorized 2- and 3-wheelers	<1%
Minibuses, vans, etc. (seating <20 people)	2%
Lorries	16%
Buses	4%
Non-motorized vehicles	<1%
Other	1%

Source: State Road Police

Care after road crashes

Formal, publicly available prehospital care system	Yes
National universal access telephone number	Yes[a] (103)

[a] Regional access number also available.

Acknowledgements

Authority approving the data for publication: Ministry of Health
National data coordinator: Rustam Talishinskiy, Traumatology and Orthopaedics Institute
Respondents: Hikmet Ibishov, Ministry of Justice; Ali Aliyarov, Ministry of Transport; Anar Orujov, State Statistical Committee; Rustam Humbetov, Ministry of Internal Affairs; Mamed Jafarov, Public Health; Arif Mirzoev, Public Health

Belarus

Population: **9.69** million (2007)
Median age: **38** years
Life expectancy at birth: **69** years
Income group:[a] **middle**
Gross national income per person: US$ **4220** Rank: **37** of 49[b]
Human Development Index:[c] **0.817** Rank: **33** of 49[b]
Private car ownership per 1000 population:[d] **241.7**
CO_2 emissions (tonnes) per person per year:[a] **6.6**

[a] World Bank data.
[b] Rank among the 49 countries in the WHO European Region participating in the survey.
[c] United Nations Development Programme data.
[d] WHO European Region average: 339.

Institutional framework for road safety

Lead agency: Standing Committee by Council of Ministers of Republic of Belarus, Ensuring Road Safety	
Status of the agency	Interministerial
Funded in national budget	No
National road safety strategy	Yes
Measurable targets	Yes
Implementation funded	Yes
Money allocated (in € (year))	No information

Key data

Reported number of road traffic deaths (2007)	1517[a] (74% males, 26% females)
Reported number of non-fatal road traffic injuries (2007)	7991[b]
Road traffic deaths involving alcohol	12.9%[c]
Wearing motorcycle helmets	No information
Using seat-belts in cars	
Overall	No information
Front-seat occupants	No information
Rear-seat occupants	No information
Costing study available	Yes
Annual estimated costs (in € (2003))	179.65 million
Study included deaths, injuries or both	Both deaths and injuries
Methods used	Gross output method

[a] Ministry of Home Affairs, defined as died within 30 days of the crash.
[b] Ministry of Home Affairs data.
[c] 2007, Ministry of Home Affairs.

NA: not applicable

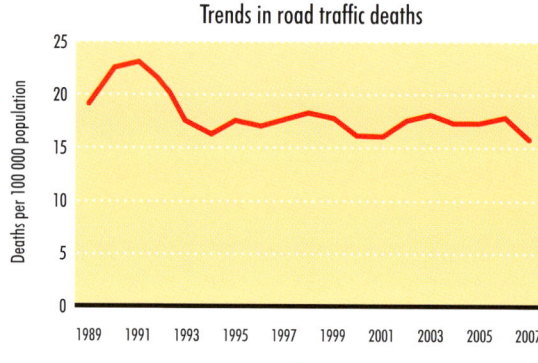

Trends in road traffic deaths
Source: Ministry of Home Affairs

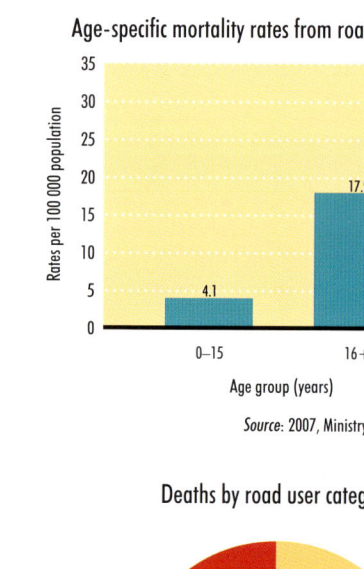

Age-specific mortality rates from road traffic injuries
Source: 2007, Ministry of Home Affairs

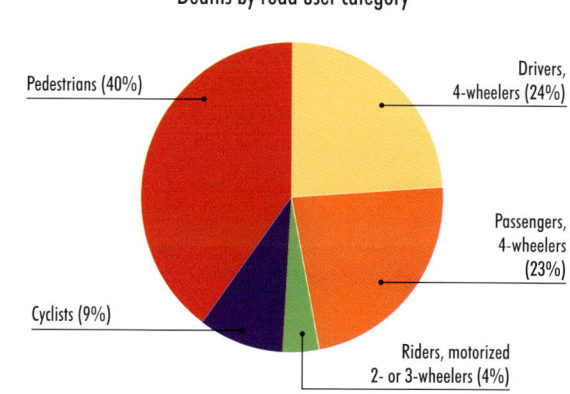

Deaths by road user category
Pedestrians (40%), Drivers, 4-wheelers (24%), Passengers, 4-wheelers (23%), Riders, motorized 2- or 3-wheelers (4%), Cyclists (9%)
Source: 2007, Ministry of Home Affairs

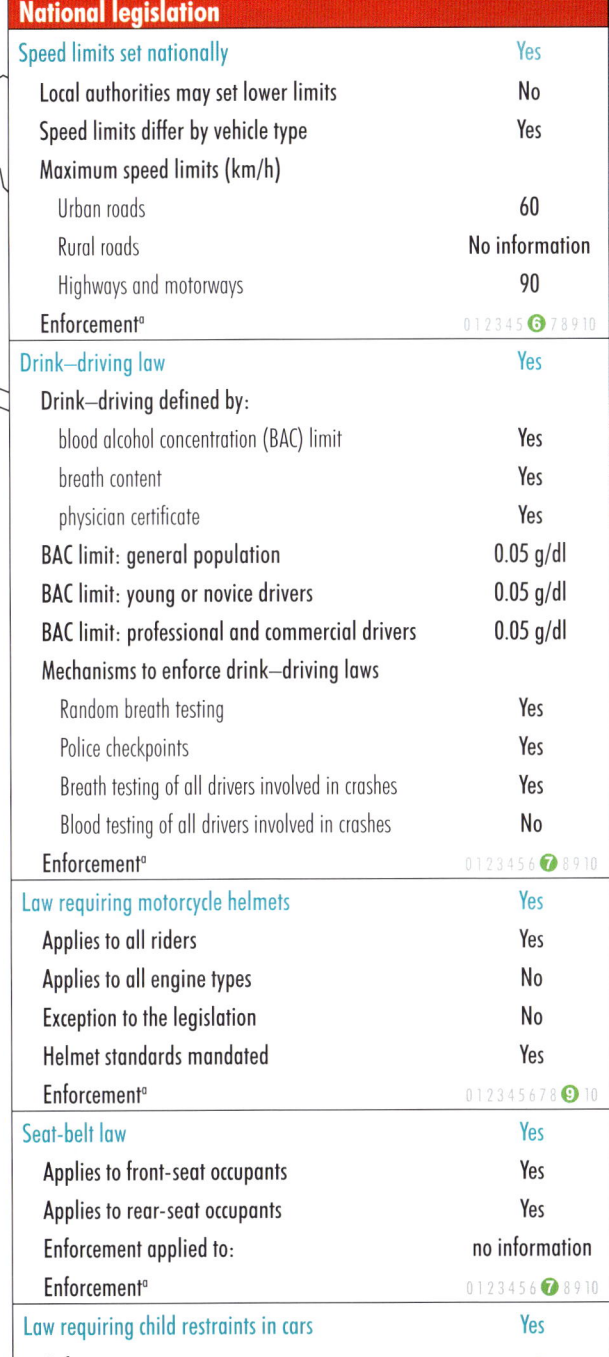

National legislation	
Speed limits set nationally	Yes
Local authorities may set lower limits	No
Speed limits differ by vehicle type	Yes
Maximum speed limits (km/h)	
Urban roads	60
Rural roads	No information
Highways and motorways	90
Enforcement[a]	0 1 2 3 4 5 **6** 7 8 9 10
Drink–driving law	Yes
Drink–driving defined by:	
blood alcohol concentration (BAC) limit	Yes
breath content	Yes
physician certificate	Yes
BAC limit: general population	0.05 g/dl
BAC limit: young or novice drivers	0.05 g/dl
BAC limit: professional and commercial drivers	0.05 g/dl
Mechanisms to enforce drink–driving laws	
Random breath testing	Yes
Police checkpoints	Yes
Breath testing of all drivers involved in crashes	Yes
Blood testing of all drivers involved in crashes	No
Enforcement[a]	0 1 2 3 4 5 6 **7** 8 9 10
Law requiring motorcycle helmets	Yes
Applies to all riders	Yes
Applies to all engine types	No
Exception to the legislation	No
Helmet standards mandated	Yes
Enforcement[a]	0 1 2 3 4 5 6 7 8 **9** 10
Seat-belt law	Yes
Applies to front-seat occupants	Yes
Applies to rear-seat occupants	Yes
Enforcement applied to:	no information
Enforcement[a]	0 1 2 3 4 5 6 **7** 8 9 10
Law requiring child restraints in cars	Yes
Enforcement[a]	0 1 2 3 4 5 **6** 7 8 9 10

[a] The enforcement score represents a consensus based on the professional opinion of respondents on a scale of 0 to 10, where 0 is not effective and 10 is highly effective.

Road safety audits	
Formal audits required for major new road construction projects	Yes
Regular audits of existing road infrastructure	Yes

Vehicle standards	
Car manufacturers required to adhere to standards on	
Fuel consumption	Yes
Seat-belt installation for all seats	Yes

Promoting transport alternatives to cars	
National policies to promote walking or cycling	Yes[a]
Investment in bicycle lanes	Yes
Investment in foot paths	Yes
Traffic-calming measures	Yes
Investment for increasing cycling	No
Disincentives for private car use	No
National policies to promote public transport	Yes[a]
Subsidized pricing of public transport	Yes
Improving the frequency and coverage of public transport	Yes
Disincentives for private car use	No

[a] Other policies are implemented in addition to those listed.

Vehicle regulations	
Compulsory insurance for vehicles	Yes
Periodic vehicle inspection for:	
cars	Yes
motorized 2- or 3-wheeled vehicles	Yes
minibuses and vans	Yes
lorries	Yes
buses	Yes

Registered motor vehicles	
Total (2007)	3 147 625
Cars	74%
Motorized 2- and 3-wheelers	12%
Lorries	12%
Buses	1%

Source: Ministry of Home Affairs

Care after road crashes	
Formal, publicly available prehospital care system	Yes
National universal access telephone number	Yes (103)

Acknowledgements

Authority approving the data for publication: Ministry of Health
National data coordinator: Ivan Pikirenia, Ministry of Health
Respondents: Pavel Bozhanov, Ministry of Transport and Services; Sergey Zarecky, Republican Theoretical and Practical Centre of Traumatology and Orthopaedics; Andrej Gusakov, Public Service of Medical Legal Expertises; Tatiana Goriainova, Ministry of Statistics and Analysis; Anatoly Sushko, Ministry of Home Affairs

Belgium

Population: **10.46 million (2007)**
Median age: **41** years
Life expectancy at birth: **79** years
Income group:[a] **high**
Gross national income per person: **US$ 40 710**   Rank: **11 of 49**[b]
Human Development Index:[c] **0.948**   Rank: **11 of 49**[b]
Private car ownership per 1000 population:[d] **482.8**
CO_2 emissions (tonnes) per person per year:[a] **9.7**

[a] World Bank data.
[b] Rank among the 49 countries in the WHO European Region participating in the survey.
[c] United Nations Development Programme data.
[d] WHO European Region average: 339.

Institutional framework for road safety

Lead agency: Interministerial Committee for Road Safety	
Status of the agency	Interministerial
Funded in national budget	Yes
National road safety strategy	Yes
Measurable targets	Yes
Implementation funded	Yes
Money allocated (in € (2008))	94.00 million[a]

[a] Figure indicates a supplementary allocation to enforcement.

Key data

Reported number of road traffic deaths (2007)	1067[a] (80% males, 20% females)
Reported number of non-fatal road traffic injuries (2007)	65 850[b]
Road traffic deaths involving alcohol	No information
Wearing motorcycle helmets	No information
Using seat-belts in cars	
Overall	No information
Front-seat occupants	79%[c]
Rear-seat occupants	46%[d]
Costing study available	No
Annual estimated costs (in € (year))	NA
Study included deaths, injuries or both	NA
Methods used	NA

[a] Statistics Belgium, defined as died within 30 days of the crash.
[b] Statistics Belgium estimate.
[c] 2007, Belgian Road Safety Institute observational study.
[d] 2006, Belgian Road Safety Institute self-report survey.

NA: not applicable

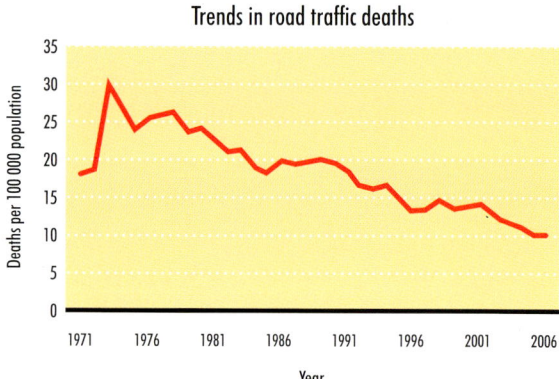

Trends in road traffic deaths

Source: Country questionnaire

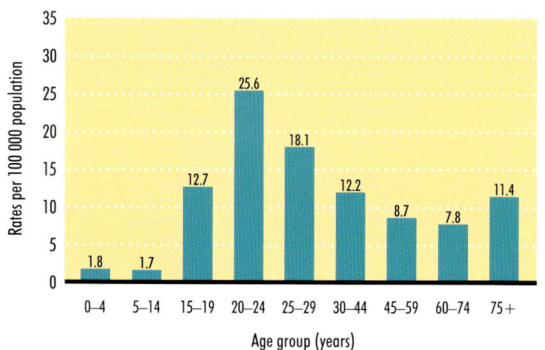

Age-specific mortality rates from road traffic injuries

Source: 2007, Statistics Belgium

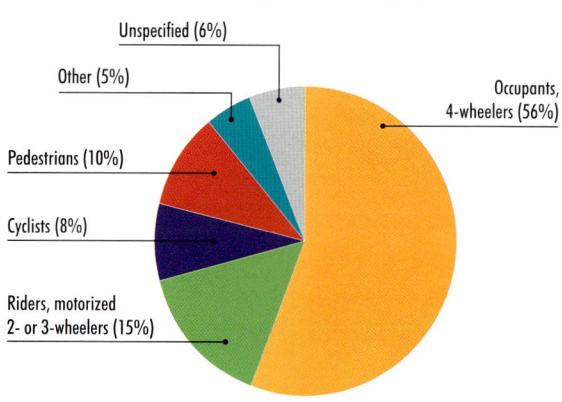

Deaths by road user category

- Occupants, 4-wheelers (56%)
- Riders, motorized 2- or 3-wheelers (15%)
- Cyclists (8%)
- Pedestrians (10%)
- Other (5%)
- Unspecified (6%)

Source: 2007, Statistics Belgium

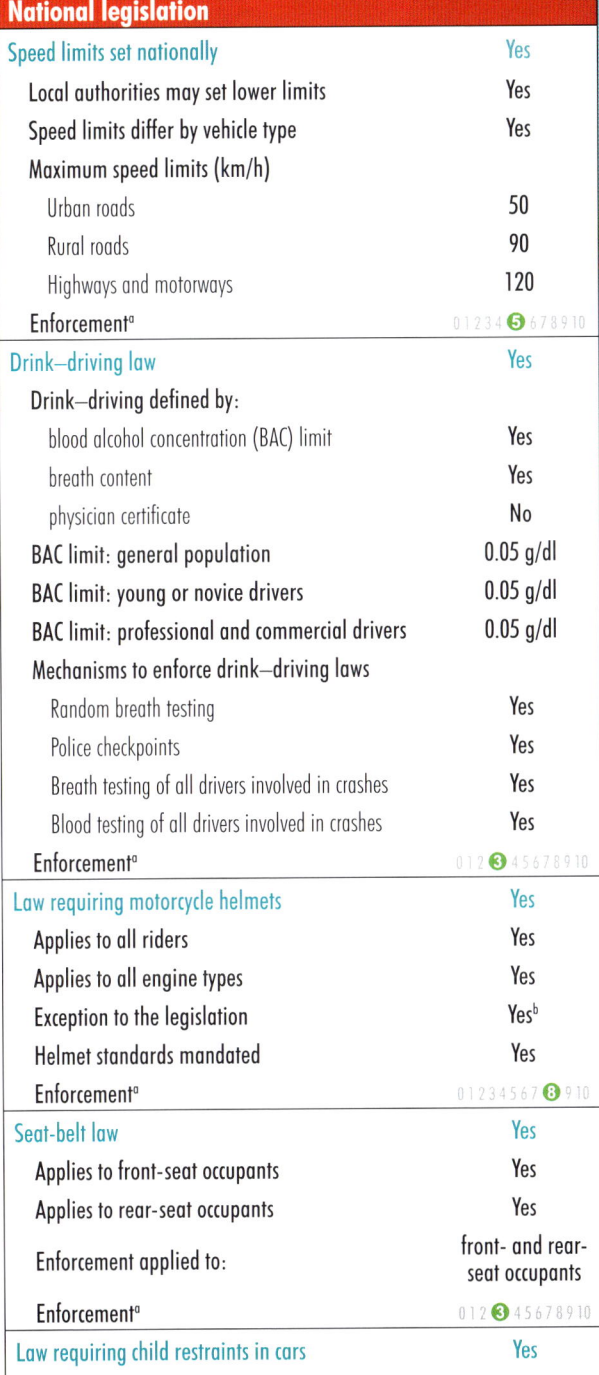

National legislation	
Speed limits set nationally	Yes
Local authorities may set lower limits	Yes
Speed limits differ by vehicle type	Yes
Maximum speed limits (km/h)	
Urban roads	50
Rural roads	90
Highways and motorways	120
Enforcement[a]	0 1 2 3 4 **5** 6 7 8 9 10
Drink–driving law	Yes
Drink–driving defined by:	
blood alcohol concentration (BAC) limit	Yes
breath content	Yes
physician certificate	No
BAC limit: general population	0.05 g/dl
BAC limit: young or novice drivers	0.05 g/dl
BAC limit: professional and commercial drivers	0.05 g/dl
Mechanisms to enforce drink–driving laws	
Random breath testing	Yes
Police checkpoints	Yes
Breath testing of all drivers involved in crashes	Yes
Blood testing of all drivers involved in crashes	Yes
Enforcement[a]	0 1 2 **3** 4 5 6 7 8 9 10
Law requiring motorcycle helmets	Yes
Applies to all riders	Yes
Applies to all engine types	Yes
Exception to the legislation	Yes[b]
Helmet standards mandated	Yes
Enforcement[a]	0 1 2 3 4 5 6 7 **8** 9 10
Seat-belt law	Yes
Applies to front-seat occupants	Yes
Applies to rear-seat occupants	Yes
Enforcement applied to:	front- and rear-seat occupants
Enforcement[a]	0 1 2 **3** 4 5 6 7 8 9 10
Law requiring child restraints in cars	Yes
Enforcement[a]	0 1 2 3 4 5 **6** 7 8 9 10

[a] The enforcement score represents a consensus based on the professional opinion of respondents on a scale of 0 to 10, where 0 is not effective and 10 is highly effective.
[b] Exceptions: post delivery at short distances.

Road safety audits	
Formal audits required for major new road construction projects	No
Regular audits of existing road infrastructure	No

Vehicle standards	
Car manufacturers required to adhere to standards on	
Fuel consumption	Yes
Seat-belt installation for all seats	Yes

Promoting transport alternatives to cars	
National policies to promote walking or cycling	Yes[a]
Investment in bicycle lanes	Yes
Investment in foot paths	Yes
Traffic-calming measures	Yes
Investment for increasing cycling	Yes
Disincentives for private car use	No
National policies to promote public transport	Yes[a]
Subsidized pricing of public transport	Yes
Improving the frequency and coverage of public transport	Yes
Disincentives for private car use	No

[a] Other policies are implemented in addition to those listed.

Vehicle regulations	
Compulsory insurance for vehicles	Yes
Periodic vehicle inspection for:	
cars	Yes
motorized 2- or 3-wheeled vehicles	No
minibuses and vans	Yes
lorries	Yes
buses	Yes

Registered motor vehicles	
Total (2007)	6 362 161
Cars	79%
Motorized 2- and 3-wheelers	6%
Buses	<1%
Lorries	10%
Other	4%

Source: Federal Public Service Mobility and Transport (Service of Vehicle Immatriculation)

Care after road crashes	
Formal, publicly available prehospital care system	Yes
National universal access telephone number	Yes (100)

Acknowledgements

Authority approving the data for publication: General Directorate for Mobility and Road Safety

National data coordinator: Anne Meerkens, Federal Public Service Mobility and Transport

Respondents: Leen Meulenbergs, Federal Public Service on Health, Food Chain Safety and Environment; Rudi Wagelmans, Permanent Commission of the Local Police Services; Miran Scheers, Belgian Road Safety Institute; Jan Robben, Federal Public Service Economy, Statistics Belgium; Denis Hendrichs, Federal Public Service Mobility and Transport; Anneliese Heeren, Federal Public Service Mobility and Transport; Paul Deblaere, Federal Police

Bosnia and Herzegovina

Population: **3.93 million (2007)**

Median age: **38** years

Life expectancy at birth: **75** years

Income group:[a] **middle**

Gross national income per person: **US$ 3790**   Rank: **38** of **49**[b]

Human Development Index:[c] **0.802**   Rank: **38** of **49**[b]

Private car ownership per 1000 population:[d] **145.8**

CO_2 emissions (tonnes) per person per year:[a] **4.0**

[a] World Bank data.
[b] Rank among the 49 countries in the WHO European Region participating in the survey.
[c] United Nations Development Programme data.
[d] WHO European Region average: 339.

Institutional framework for road safety

Lead agency: Ministry of Communication and Transport of Bosnia and Herzegovina	
Status of the agency	Government
Funded in national budget	Yes
National road safety strategy	Yes[a]
Measurable targets	Yes
Implementation funded	Yes
Money allocated (in € (2008))	0.026 million[b]

[a] Formally approved in the Federation of Bosnia and Herzegovina only (not in the Republic of Srpska).
[b] Financial incentives only for the development of Strategy in the Federation of Bosnia and Herzegovina and not for its implementation.

Key data

Reported number of road traffic deaths (2007)	428[a]
Reported number of non-fatal road traffic injuries (2007)	11 647[b]
Road traffic deaths involving alcohol	6.7%[c]
Wearing motorcycle helmets	No information
Using seat-belts in cars	
Overall	No information
Front-seat occupants	No information
Rear-seat occupants	No information
Costing study available	**No**
Annual estimated costs (in € (year))	NA
Study included deaths, injuries or both	NA
Methods used	NA

[a] Institute for Statistics of the Federation of Bosnia and Herzegovina, defined as died at crash scene; Ministry of Internal Affairs of the Republic of Srpska, defined as died within 30 days of the crash.
[b] Data from multiple sources.
[c] 2007, Ministry of Internal Affairs of the Republic of Srpska, data apply to Republic of Srpska only.

NA: not applicable

Trends in road traffic deaths

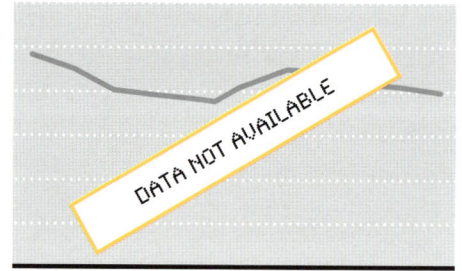

Age-specific mortality rates from road traffic injuries

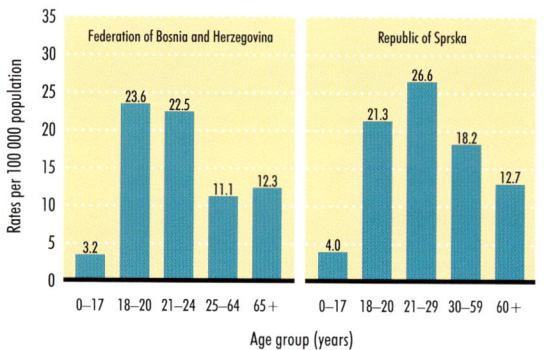

Source: 2007, Country questionnaire

Deaths by road user category

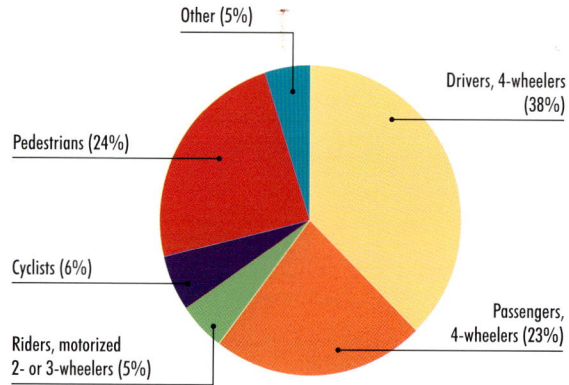

Source: 2007, Ministry of Internal Affairs of the Republic of Srpska, data apply to Republic of Srpska only

National legislation	
Speed limits set nationally	Yes
Local authorities may set lower limits	Yes
Speed limits differ by vehicle type	Yes
Maximum speed limits (km/h)	
Urban roads	60
Rural roads	No information
Highways and motorways	130
Enforcement[a]	0 1 2 3 4 5 **6** 7 8 9 10
Drink–driving law	Yes
Drink–driving defined by:	
blood alcohol concentration (BAC) limit	Yes
breath content	Yes
physician certificate	Yes
BAC limit: general population	0.03 g/dl
BAC limit: young or novice drivers	0.00 g/dl
BAC limit: professional and commercial drivers	0.00 g/dl
Mechanisms to enforce drink–driving laws	
Random breath testing	Yes
Police checkpoints	Yes
Breath testing of all drivers involved in crashes	Yes
Blood testing of all drivers involved in crashes	Yes
Enforcement[a]	0 1 2 3 4 5 **6** 7 8 9 10
Law requiring motorcycle helmets	Yes
Applies to all riders	Yes
Applies to all engine types	Yes
Exception to the legislation	No
Helmet standards mandated	No
Enforcement[a]	0 1 2 3 4 5 **6** 7 8 9 10
Seat-belt law	Yes
Applies to front-seat occupants	Yes
Applies to rear-seat occupants	Yes
Enforcement applied to:	front- and rear-seat occupants
Enforcement[a]	0 1 2 3 4 5 6 **7** 8 9 10
Law requiring child restraints in cars	Yes
Enforcement[a]	0 1 2 3 4 **5** 6 7 8 9 10

[a] The enforcement score represents a consensus based on the professional opinion of respondents on a scale of 0 to 10, where 0 is not effective and 10 is highly effective.

Road safety audits	
Formal audits required for major new road construction projects	Yes
Regular audits of existing road infrastructure	Yes

Vehicle standards	
Car manufacturers required to adhere to standards on[a]	
Fuel consumption	Yes
Seat-belt installation for all seats	Yes

[a] Data apply to the Federation of Bosnia and Herzegovina only.

Promoting transport alternatives to cars	
National policies to promote walking or cycling	No
Investment in bicycle lanes	NA
Investment in foot paths	NA
Traffic-calming measures	NA
Investment for increasing cycling	NA
Disincentives for private car use	NA
National policies to promote public transport	No
Subsidized pricing of public transport	NA
Improving the frequency and coverage of public transport	NA
Disincentives for private car use	NA

Vehicle regulations	
Compulsory insurance for vehicles	Yes
Periodic vehicle inspection for:	
cars	Yes
motorized 2- or 3-wheeled vehicles	Yes
minibuses and vans	Yes
lorries	Yes
buses	Yes

Registered motor vehicles	
Total (2007)	675 063
Cars	85%
Motorized 2- and 3-wheelers	1%
Lorries	9%
Buses	1%
Other	5%

Source: Ministry of Internal Affairs of the Republic of Srpska, Institute for Statistic of the Federation of Bosnia and Herzegovina

Care after road crashes	
Formal, publicly available prehospital care system	Yes
National universal access telephone number	Yes[a] (124)

[a] Regional access number also available.

Acknowledgements

Authority approving the data for publication: Ministry of Civil Affairs
National data coordinator: Jasminka Kovacevic, Emergency Medical Service Sarajevo; Alen Seranic, Ministry of Health and Social Welfare of Republika Srpska
Respondents: Munira Zahiragic, Institute for Statistics of the Federation of Bosnia and Herzegovina; Muhamed Ahmic, Ministry of Internal Affairs of the Federation of Bosnia and Herzegovina; Pavo Boban, Ministry for Traffic and Communication of the Federation of Bosnia and Herzegovina; Irena Jokic, Public Health Institute of the Federation of Bosnia and Herzegovina; Natasa Kostic, Ministry of Transport and Communications of the Republic of Srpska; Mira Bera, Ministry of Education and Culture of the Republic of Srpska; Zelimir Skrbic, Ministry of Internal Affairs of the Republic of Srpska; Jelena Glamocika, Institute of Statistics of the Republic of Srpska

Bulgaria

Population: **7.64 million (2007)**
Median age: **41** years
Life expectancy at birth: **73** years
Income group:[a] **middle**
Gross national income per person: **US$ 4590**   Rank: **36** of 49[b]
Human Development Index:[c] **0.834**   Rank: **29** of 49[b]
Private car ownership per 1000 population:[d] **258.2**
CO_2 emissions (tonnes) per person per year:[a] **5.5**

[a] World Bank data.
[b] Rank among the 49 countries in the WHO European Region participating in the survey.
[c] United Nations Development Programme data.
[d] WHO European Region average: 339.

Institutional framework for road safety

Lead agency: State-Public Consultative Commission on the Problems of Road Safety	
Status of the agency	Interministerial
Funded in national budget	Yes
National road safety strategy	Yes
Measurable targets	Yes
Implementation funded	Yes
Money allocated (in € (year))	No information

Key data

Reported number of road traffic deaths (2007)	1006[a] (73% males, 27% females)
Reported number of non-fatal road traffic injuries (2007)	9827[b]
Road traffic deaths involving alcohol	4.7%[c]
Wearing motorcycle helmets	No information
Using seat-belts in cars	
Overall	No information
Front-seat occupants	No information
Rear-seat occupants	No information
Costing study available	No
Annual estimated costs (in € (year))	NA
Study included deaths, injuries or both	NA
Methods used	NA

[a] Police data, defined as died within 30 days of the crash.
[b] Police data.
[c] 2007, Traffic Police Department, Ministry of Interior.

NA: not applicable

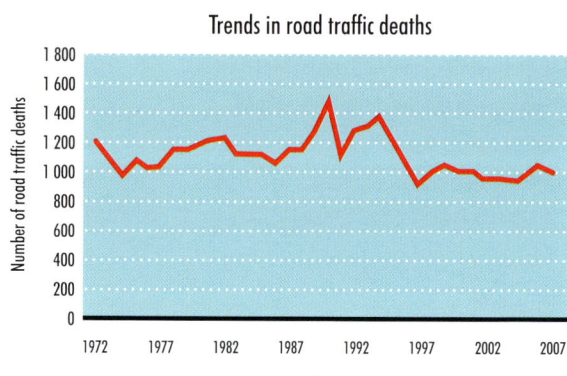

Trends in road traffic deaths

Source: Country questionnaire

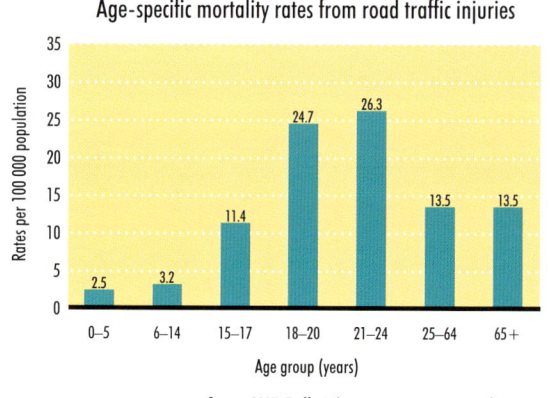

Age-specific mortality rates from road traffic injuries

Source: 2007, Traffic Police Department, Ministry of Interior

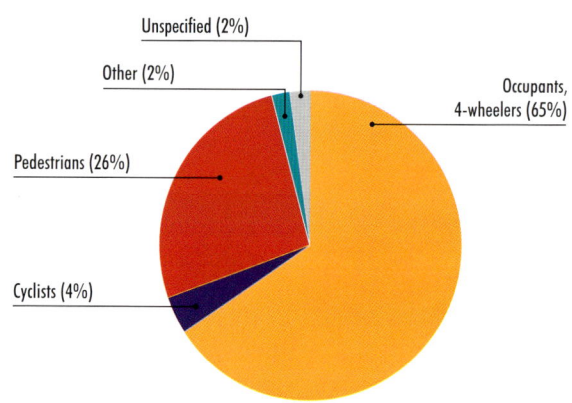

Deaths by road user category

Unspecified (2%)
Other (2%)
Occupants, 4-wheelers (65%)
Pedestrians (26%)
Cyclists (4%)

Source: 2007, Traffic Police Department, Ministry of Interior

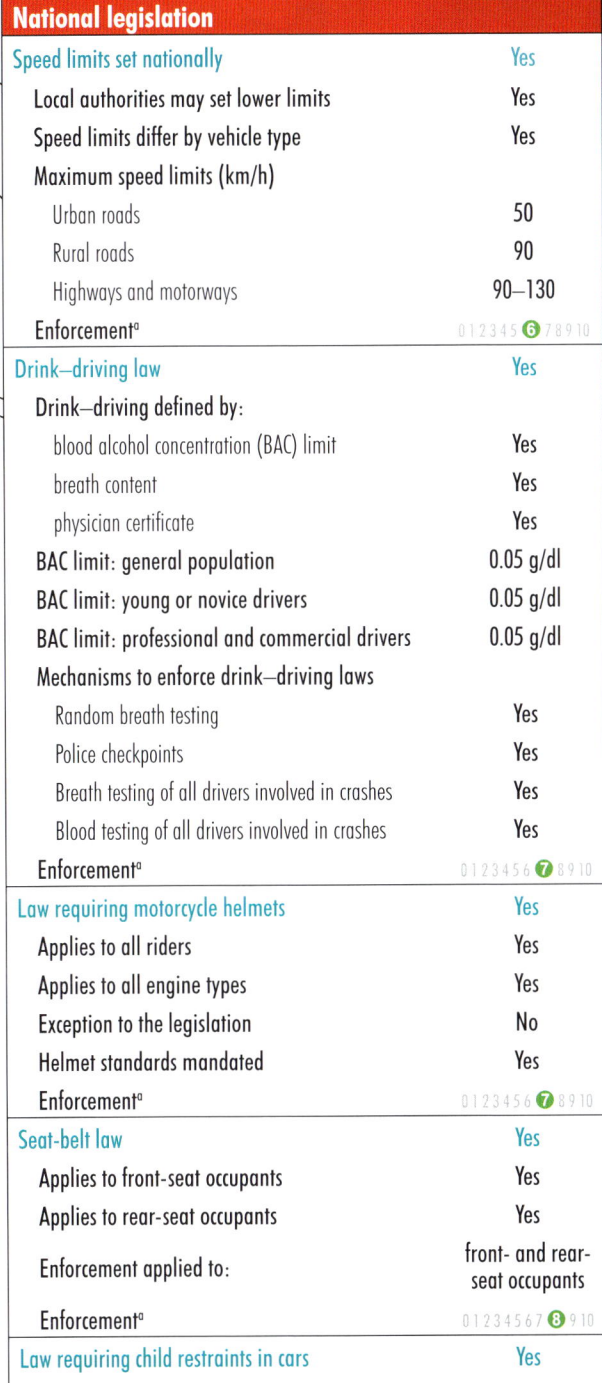

National legislation	
Speed limits set nationally	Yes
Local authorities may set lower limits	Yes
Speed limits differ by vehicle type	Yes
Maximum speed limits (km/h)	
Urban roads	50
Rural roads	90
Highways and motorways	90–130
Enforcement[a]	0 1 2 3 4 5 **6** 7 8 9 10
Drink–driving law	Yes
Drink–driving defined by:	
blood alcohol concentration (BAC) limit	Yes
breath content	Yes
physician certificate	Yes
BAC limit: general population	0.05 g/dl
BAC limit: young or novice drivers	0.05 g/dl
BAC limit: professional and commercial drivers	0.05 g/dl
Mechanisms to enforce drink–driving laws	
Random breath testing	Yes
Police checkpoints	Yes
Breath testing of all drivers involved in crashes	Yes
Blood testing of all drivers involved in crashes	Yes
Enforcement[a]	0 1 2 3 4 5 6 **7** 8 9 10
Law requiring motorcycle helmets	Yes
Applies to all riders	Yes
Applies to all engine types	Yes
Exception to the legislation	No
Helmet standards mandated	Yes
Enforcement[a]	0 1 2 3 4 5 6 **7** 8 9 10
Seat-belt law	Yes
Applies to front-seat occupants	Yes
Applies to rear-seat occupants	Yes
Enforcement applied to:	front- and rear-seat occupants
Enforcement[a]	0 1 2 3 4 5 6 7 **8** 9 10
Law requiring child restraints in cars	Yes
Enforcement[a]	0 1 2 3 **4** 5 6 7 8 9 10

[a] The enforcement score represents a consensus based on the professional opinion of respondents on a scale of 0 to 10, where 0 is not effective and 10 is highly effective.

Road safety audits	
Formal audits required for major new road construction projects	Yes
Regular audits of existing road infrastructure	Yes

Vehicle standards	
No car manufacturers	

Promoting transport alternatives to cars	
National policies to promote walking or cycling	No (subnational)
Investment in bicycle lanes	NA
Investment in foot paths	NA
Traffic-calming measures	NA
Investment for increasing cycling	NA
Disincentives for private car use	NA
National policies to promote public transport	Yes[a]
Subsidized pricing of public transport	No
Improving the frequency and coverage of public transport	No
Disincentives for private car use	No

[a] Other policies are implemented in addition to those listed.

Vehicle regulations	
Compulsory insurance for vehicles	Yes
Periodic vehicle inspection for:	
cars	Yes
motorized 2- or 3-wheeled vehicles	Yes
minibuses and vans	Yes
lorries	Yes
buses	Yes

Registered motor vehicles	
Total (2007)	2 628 680
Cars	75%
Motorized 2- and 3-wheelers	3%
Lorries	10%
Buses	1%
Other	10%

Source: Traffic Police Department, Ministry of Interior

Care after road crashes	
Formal, publicly available prehospital care system	Yes
National universal access telephone number	Yes (150)

Acknowledgements

Authority approving the data for publication: Ministry of Health
National data coordinator: Irina Kovacheva, Ministry of Health
Respondents: Valentin Panchev, Ministry of Transport; Evelin Jordanova, National Statistic Institute; Anton Antonov, Traffic Police, Ministry of Interior; George Petrishki, Traffic Police, Ministry of Interior; Diana Dimitrova, Ministry of Health

Croatia

Population: **4.56 million (2007)**

Median age: **41** years

Life expectancy at birth: **76** years

Income group:[a] **middle**

Gross national income per person: **US$ 10 460** Rank: **26** of **49**[b]

Human Development Index:[c] **0.862** Rank: **28** of **49**[b]

Private car ownership per 1000 population:[d] **327.5**

CO_2 emissions (tonnes) per person per year:[a] **5.3**

[a] World Bank data.
[b] Rank among the 49 countries in the WHO European Region participating in the survey.
[c] United Nations Development Programme data.
[d] WHO European Region average: 339.

Institutional framework for road safety	
Lead agency	Yes
Status of the agency	Interministerial
Funded in national budget	Yes
National road safety strategy	Yes
Measurable targets	Yes
Implementation funded	Yes
Money allocated (in € (2008))	2.08 million

Key data	
Reported number of road traffic deaths (2007)	619[a]
Reported number of non-fatal road traffic injuries (2007)	25 092[b]
Road traffic deaths involving alcohol	30.0%[c]
Wearing motorcycle helmets	No information
Using seat-belts in cars	
Overall	45%[d]
Front-seat occupants	No information
Rear-seat occupants	No information
Costing study available	No information
Annual estimated costs (in € (year))	NA
Study included deaths, injuries or both	NA
Methods used	NA

[a] Police data, defined as died within 30 days of the crash.
[b] Police data.
[c] 2007, Ministry of Interior.
[d] 2004, Ministry of Interior.

NA: not applicable

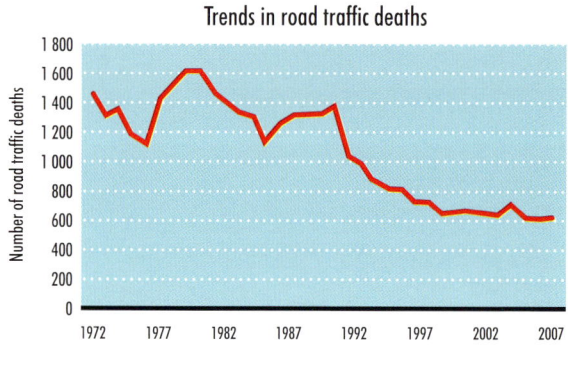

Trends in road traffic deaths

Source: Ministry of Interior

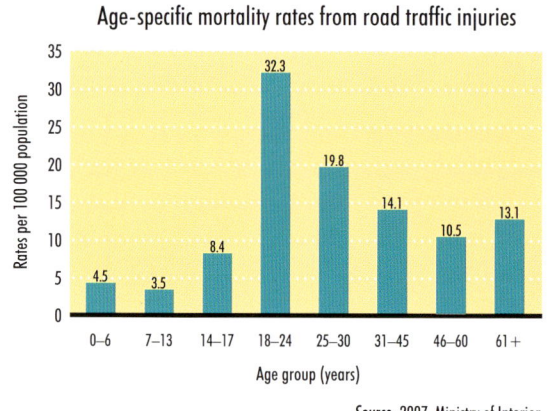

Age-specific mortality rates from road traffic injuries

Source: 2007, Ministry of Interior

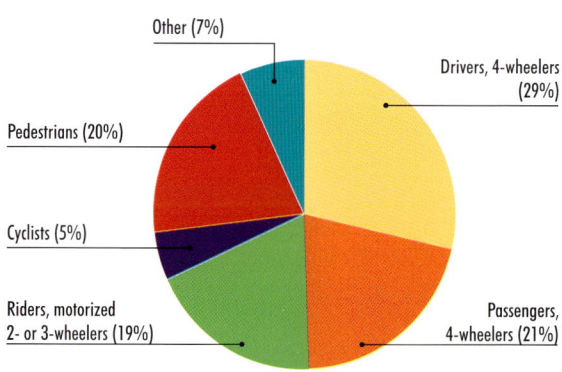

Deaths by road user category

Source: 2007, Ministry of Interior

National legislation

Speed limits set nationally	Yes
Local authorities may set lower limits	Yes
Speed limits differ by vehicle type	Yes
Maximum speed limits (km/h)	
Urban roads	50
Rural roads	90
Highways and motorways	130
Enforcement[a]	0 1 2 3 4 5 **6** 7 8 9 10
Drink–driving law	Yes
Drink–driving defined by:	
blood alcohol concentration (BAC) limit	Yes
breath content	Yes
physician certificate	Yes
BAC limit: general population	0.05 g/dl
BAC limit: young or novice drivers	0.00 g/dl
BAC limit: professional and commercial drivers	0.00 g/dl
Mechanisms to enforce drink–driving laws	
Random breath testing	Yes
Police checkpoints	Yes
Breath testing of all drivers involved in crashes	Yes
Blood testing of all drivers involved in crashes	No
Enforcement[a]	0 1 2 3 4 5 6 **7** 8 9 10
Law requiring motorcycle helmets	Yes
Applies to all riders	Yes
Applies to all engine types	Yes
Exception to the legislation	No
Helmet standards mandated	No
Enforcement[a]	0 1 2 3 4 5 **6** 7 8 9 10
Seat-belt law	Yes
Applies to front-seat occupants	Yes
Applies to rear-seat occupants	Yes
Enforcement applied to:	front- and rear-seat occupants
Enforcement[a]	0 1 2 3 4 5 6 **7** 8 9 10
Law requiring child restraints in cars	Yes
Enforcement[a]	0 1 2 3 4 **5** 6 7 8 9 10

[a] The enforcement score represents a consensus based on the professional opinion of respondents on a scale of 0 to 10, where 0 is not effective and 10 is highly effective.

Road safety audits

Formal audits required for major new road construction projects	Yes
Regular audits of existing road infrastructure	Yes

Vehicle standards

No car manufacturers	

Promoting transport alternatives to cars

National policies to promote walking or cycling	No
Investment in bicycle lanes	NA
Investment in foot paths	NA
Traffic-calming measures	NA
Investment for increasing cycling	NA
Disincentives for private car use	NA
National policies to promote public transport	No
Subsidized pricing of public transport	NA
Improving the frequency and coverage of public transport	NA
Disincentives for private car use	NA

Vehicle regulations

Compulsory insurance for vehicles	Yes
Periodic vehicle inspection for:	
cars	Yes
motorized 2- or 3-wheeled vehicles	Yes
minibuses and vans	Yes
lorries	Yes
buses	Yes

Registered motor vehicles

Total (2007)	1 949 936
Cars	77%
Motorized 2- and 3-wheelers	8%
Lorries	9%
Buses	<1%
Other	6%

Source: Ministry of Interior

Care after road crashes

Formal, publicly available prehospital care system	Yes
National universal access telephone number	Yes (112)

Acknowledgements

Authority approving the data for publication: National Institute of Public Health
National data coordinator: Ivana Brkić Biloš, Croatian National Institute of Public Health
Respondents: Tihomira Ivanda, Ministry of Health and Social Welfare; Ivica Franić, Ministry of Interior; Boris Orlović, Ministry of Interior; Dinka Rajčić, Ministry of Sea, Transport and Infrastructure; Željko Remenar, Ministry of Sea, Transport and Infrastructure

Cyprus

Population: **0.86 million (2007)**

Median age: **35** years

Life expectancy at birth: **80** years

Income group:[a] **high**

Gross national income per person: **US$ 24 940**   Rank: **17** of **49**[b]

Human Development Index:[c] **0.912**   Rank: **18** of **49**[b]

Private car ownership per 1000 population:[d] **480.4**

CO_2 emissions (tonnes) per person per year:[a] **No information**

[a] World Bank data.
[b] Rank among the 49 countries in the WHO European Region participating in the survey.
[c] United Nations Development Programme data.
[d] WHO European Region average: 339.

Institutional framework for road safety

Lead agency: Road Safety Council	
Status of the agency	Interministerial
Funded in national budget	Yes
National road safety strategy	**Yes**
Measurable targets	Yes
Implementation funded	Yes
Money allocated (in € (2008))	7.00 million

Key data

Reported number of road traffic deaths (2007)	89[a] (84% males, 16% females)
Reported number of non-fatal road traffic injuries (2007)	2119[b]
Road traffic deaths involving alcohol	18.0%[c]
Wearing motorcycle helmets	68% Drivers; 56% Passengers[d]
Using seat-belts in cars	
Overall	No information
Front-seat occupants	81%[e]
Rear-seat occupants	9%[e]
Costing study available	**Yes**
Annual estimated costs (in € (2001))	38.15 million
Study included deaths, injuries or both	Deaths only
Methods used	Gross output method

[a] Police data, defined as died within 30 days of the crash.
[b] Police data.
[c] 2007, Police records.
[d] 2007, Police in cooperation with the Government Statistical Service.
[e] 2007, Police records, national observational study.

NA: not applicable

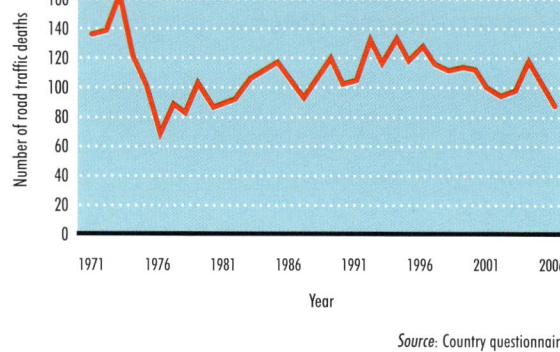

Trends in road traffic deaths

Source: Country questionnaire

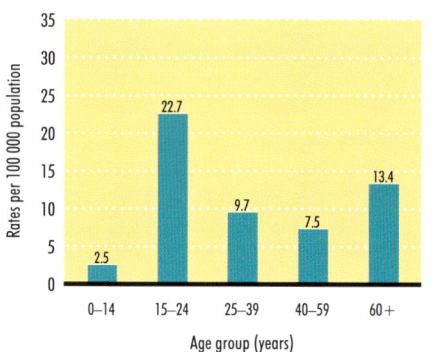

Age-specific mortality rates from road traffic injuries

Source: 2007, Police records

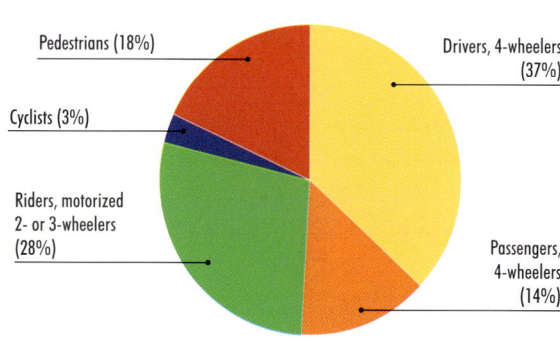

Deaths by road user category

- Pedestrians (18%)
- Cyclists (3%)
- Riders, motorized 2- or 3-wheelers (28%)
- Passengers, 4-wheelers (14%)
- Drivers, 4-wheelers (37%)

Source: 2007, Police records

National legislation

Speed limits set nationally	Yes
Local authorities may set lower limits	Yes
Speed limits differ by vehicle type	No
Maximum speed limits (km/h)	
Urban roads	50
Rural roads	80
Highways and motorways	100
Enforcement[a]	0 1 2 3 4 5 **6** 7 8 9 10
Drink–driving law	**Yes**
Drink–driving defined by:	
blood alcohol concentration (BAC) limit	Yes
breath content	Yes
physician certificate	No
BAC limit: general population	0.05 g/dl
BAC limit: young or novice drivers	0.05 g/dl
BAC limit: professional and commercial drivers	0.05 g/dl
Mechanisms to enforce drink–driving laws	
Random breath testing	Yes
Police checkpoints	No
Breath testing of all drivers involved in crashes	Yes
Blood testing of all drivers involved in crashes	Yes
Enforcement[a]	0 1 2 3 4 5 **6** 7 8 9 10
Law requiring motorcycle helmets	**Yes**
Applies to all riders	Yes
Applies to all engine types	Yes
Exception to the legislation	Yes[b]
Helmet standards mandated	Yes
Enforcement[a]	0 1 2 3 4 **5** 6 7 8 9 10
Seat-belt law	**Yes**
Applies to front-seat occupants	Yes
Applies to rear-seat occupants	Yes
Enforcement applied to:	front- and rear-seat occupants
Enforcement[a]	0 1 2 3 4 5 6 **7** 8 9 10
Law requiring child restraints in cars	**Yes**
Enforcement[a]	0 1 2 **3** 4 5 6 7 8 9 10

[a] The enforcement score represents a consensus based on the professional opinion of respondents on a scale of 0 to 10, where 0 is not effective and 10 is highly effective.
[b] Exceptions: children under 12 years old are not allowed on two-wheelers as passengers.

Road safety audits

Formal audits required for major new road construction projects	No
Regular audits of existing road infrastructure	Yes

Vehicle standards

No car manufacturers

Promoting transport alternatives to cars

National policies to promote walking or cycling	Yes
Investment in bicycle lanes	Yes
Investment in foot paths	Yes
Traffic-calming measures	Yes
Investment for increasing cycling	No
Disincentives for private car use	No
National policies to promote public transport	**Yes**
Subsidized pricing of public transport	Yes
Improving the frequency and coverage of public transport	No
Disincentives for private car use	No

Vehicle regulations

Compulsory insurance for vehicles	Yes
Periodic vehicle inspection for:	
cars	Yes
motorized 2- or 3-wheeled vehicles	No
minibuses and vans	Yes
lorries	Yes
buses	Yes

Registered motor vehicles

Total (2007)	592 480
Cars	69%
Motorized 2- and 3-wheelers	7%
Minibuses, vans, etc. (seating <20 people)	18%
Lorries	2%
Buses	1%
Other	4%

Source: Department of Road Transport

Care after road crashes

Formal, publicly available prehospital care system	Yes
National universal access telephone number	Yes[a] (199, 112)

[a] Regional access number also available.

Acknowledgements

Authority approving the data for publication: Ministry of Health
National data coordinator: Costas Antoniades, Accident and Emergency Deptartment of the Nicosia General Hospital, Ministry of Health; Olga Kalakouta, Medical and Public Health Services, Ministry of Health
Respondents: Soteris Koletias, Department of Road Transport; Stavros Cleanthous, Public Works Department, Ministry of Communication and Works; Andreas Kouppis, Ambulance Service of Nicosia General Hospital; George Morfakis, Road Safety Unit to the Ministry of Communication and Works; Charilaos Evripidou, Cyprus Police

Czech Republic

Population: **10.19 million (2007)**

Median age: **39** years

Life expectancy at birth: **77** years

Income group:[a] **high**

Gross national income per person: **US$ 14 450** Rank: **22** of 49[b]

Human Development Index:[c] **0.897** Rank: **20** of 49[b]

Private car ownership per 1000 population:[d] **403.2**

CO_2 emissions (tonnes) per person per year:[a] **11.5**

[a] World Bank data.
[b] Rank among the 49 countries in the WHO European Region participating in the survey.
[c] United Nations Development Programme data.
[d] WHO European Region average: 339.

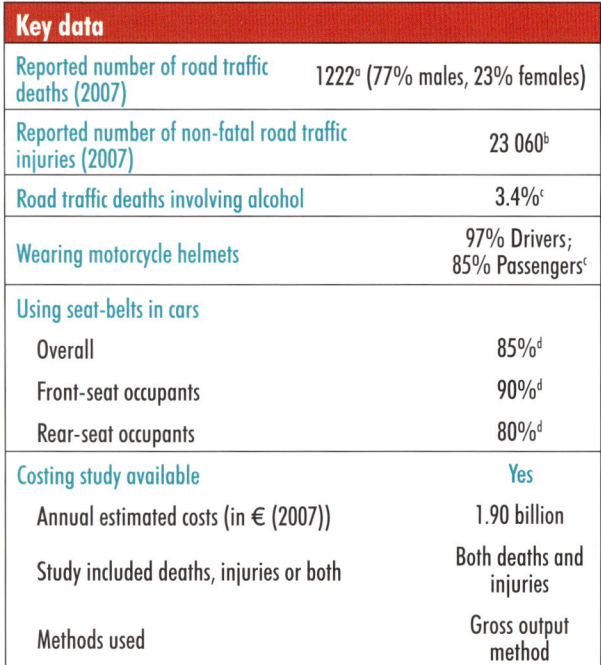

Institutional framework for road safety

Lead agency: Ministry of Transport	
Status of the agency	Government
Funded in national budget	Yes
National road safety strategy	**Yes**
Measurable targets	Yes
Implementation funded	No
Money allocated (in € (year))	NA

Key data

Reported number of road traffic deaths (2007)	1222[a] (77% males, 23% females)
Reported number of non-fatal road traffic injuries (2007)	23 060[b]
Road traffic deaths involving alcohol	3.4%[c]
Wearing motorcycle helmets	97% Drivers; 85% Passengers[c]
Using seat-belts in cars	
Overall	85%[d]
Front-seat occupants	90%[d]
Rear-seat occupants	80%[d]
Costing study available	**Yes**
Annual estimated costs (in € (2007))	1.90 billion
Study included deaths, injuries or both	Both deaths and injuries
Methods used	Gross output method

[a] Police data, defined as died within 30 days of the crash.
[b] Police data.
[c] 2007, Czech Police.
[d] 2006, Transport Research Centre.

NA: not applicable

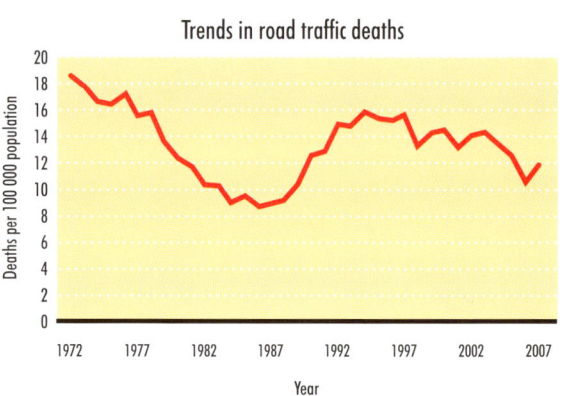

Trends in road traffic deaths

Source: Country questionnaire

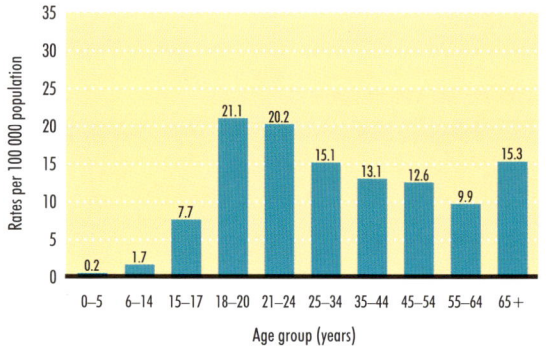

Age-specific mortality rates from road traffic injuries

Source: 2007, Czech Police

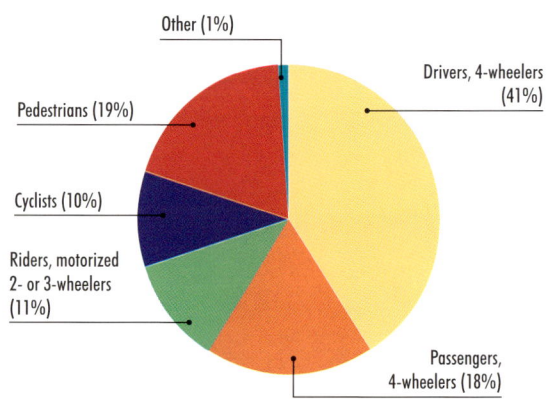

Deaths by road user category

Other (1%)
Drivers, 4-wheelers (41%)
Pedestrians (19%)
Cyclists (10%)
Riders, motorized 2- or 3-wheelers (11%)
Passengers, 4-wheelers (18%)

Source: 2007, Police Presidium of the Czech Republic, Directorate of Traffic Branch

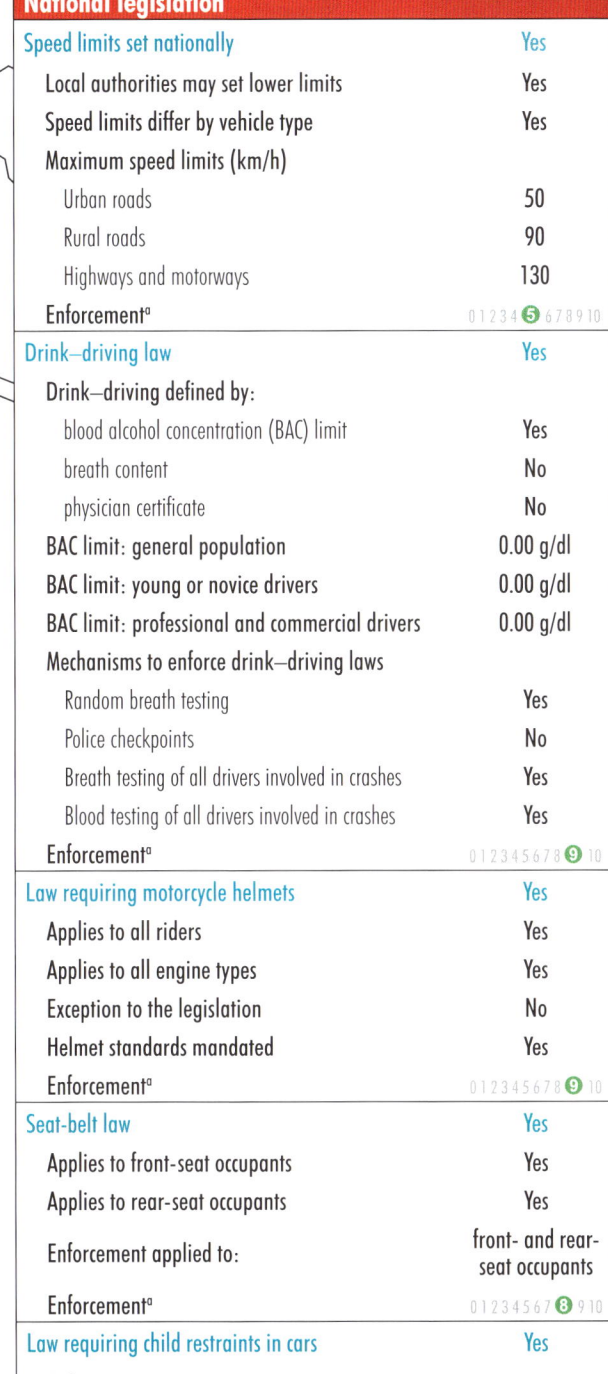

National legislation	
Speed limits set nationally	Yes
Local authorities may set lower limits	Yes
Speed limits differ by vehicle type	Yes
Maximum speed limits (km/h)	
Urban roads	50
Rural roads	90
Highways and motorways	130
Enforcement[a]	0 1 2 3 4 ⑤ 6 7 8 9 10
Drink–driving law	Yes
Drink–driving defined by:	
blood alcohol concentration (BAC) limit	Yes
breath content	No
physician certificate	No
BAC limit: general population	0.00 g/dl
BAC limit: young or novice drivers	0.00 g/dl
BAC limit: professional and commercial drivers	0.00 g/dl
Mechanisms to enforce drink–driving laws	
Random breath testing	Yes
Police checkpoints	No
Breath testing of all drivers involved in crashes	Yes
Blood testing of all drivers involved in crashes	Yes
Enforcement[a]	0 1 2 3 4 5 6 7 8 ⑨ 10
Law requiring motorcycle helmets	Yes
Applies to all riders	Yes
Applies to all engine types	Yes
Exception to the legislation	No
Helmet standards mandated	Yes
Enforcement[a]	0 1 2 3 4 5 6 7 8 ⑨ 10
Seat-belt law	Yes
Applies to front-seat occupants	Yes
Applies to rear-seat occupants	Yes
Enforcement applied to:	front- and rear-seat occupants
Enforcement[a]	0 1 2 3 4 5 6 7 ⑧ 9 10
Law requiring child restraints in cars	Yes
Enforcement[a]	0 1 2 3 4 5 6 ⑦ 8 9 10

[a] The enforcement score represents a consensus based on the professional opinion of respondents on a scale of 0 to 10, where 0 is not effective and 10 is highly effective.

Road safety audits	
Formal audits required for major new road construction projects	No
Regular audits of existing road infrastructure	No

Vehicle standards	
Car manufacturers required to adhere to standards on	
Fuel consumption	No
Seat-belt installation for all seats	Yes

Promoting transport alternatives to cars	
National policies to promote walking or cycling	Yes[a]
Investment in bicycle lanes	Yes
Investment in foot paths	Yes
Traffic-calming measures	Yes
Investment for increasing cycling	Yes
Disincentives for private car use	No
National policies to promote public transport	No (subnational)
Subsidized pricing of public transport	NA
Improving the frequency and coverage of public transport	NA
Disincentives for private car use	NA

[a] Other policies are implemented in addition to those listed.

Vehicle regulations	
Compulsory insurance for vehicles	Yes
Periodic vehicle inspection for:	
cars	Yes
motorized 2- or 3-wheeled vehicles	Yes
minibuses and vans	Yes
lorries	Yes
buses	Yes

Registered motor vehicles	
Total (2006)	5 455 110
Cars	75%
Motorized 2- and 3-wheelers	15%
Lorries	9%
Buses	<1%
Other	1%

Source: Transport Yearbook, Transport Research Centre

Care after road crashes	
Formal, publicly available prehospital care system	Yes
National universal access telephone number	Yes (112; 155)

Acknowledgements

Authority approving the data for publication: Ministry of Health
National data coordinator: Veronika Benesova, Charles University in Prague, 2nd Faculty of Medicine
Respondents: Sarka Kasalova Dankova, Institute of Health Information and Statistics, Ministry of Health; Josef Tesarik, Ministry of Interior; Zuzana Ambrozova, Ministry of Transport; Jaroslav Horin, Ministry of Interior

Estonia

Population: 1.34 million (2007)

Median age: 39 years

Life expectancy at birth: 73 years

Income group:[a] high

Gross national income per person: US$ 13 200   Rank: 23 of 49[b]

Human Development Index:[c] 0.871   Rank: 25 of 49[b]

Private car ownership per 1000 population:[d] 394.2

CO_2 emissions (tonnes) per person per year:[a] 14.0

[a] World Bank data.
[b] Rank among the 49 countries in the WHO European Region participating in the survey.
[c] United Nations Development Programme data.
[d] WHO European Region average: 339.

Institutional framework for road safety

Lead agency: The Road Safety Committee of the Government of the Republic of Estonia	
Status of the agency	Interministerial
Funded in national budget	Yes
National road safety strategy	**Yes**
Measurable targets	Yes
Implementation funded	Yes
Money allocated (in € (2008))	15.40 million

Key data

Reported number of road traffic deaths (2007)	196[a] (75% males, 25% females)
Reported number of non-fatal road traffic injuries (2007)	3270[b]
Road traffic deaths involving alcohol	48.0%[c]
Wearing motorcycle helmets	No information
Using seat-belts in cars	
Overall	88%[d]
Front-seat occupants	90%[d]
Rear-seat occupants	68%[d]
Costing study available	**Yes**
Annual estimated costs (in € (2007))	150.32 million
Study included deaths, injuries or both	Both deaths and injuries
Methods used	Gross output method

[a] Estonian National Road Administration data, defined as died within 30 days of the crash.
[b] Estonian National Road Administration data.
[c] 2007, Estonian National Road Adminstration.
[d] 2007, Traffic Behavioural Monitoring.

NA: not applicable

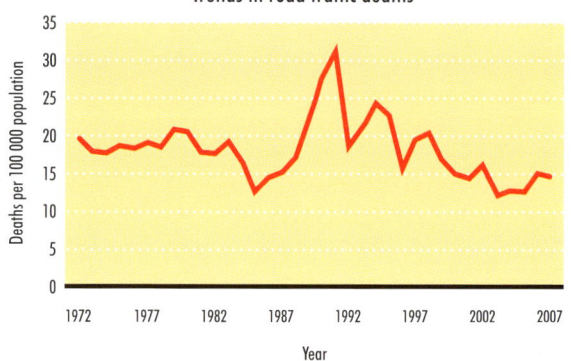

Trends in road traffic deaths

Source: Estonian National Road Administration

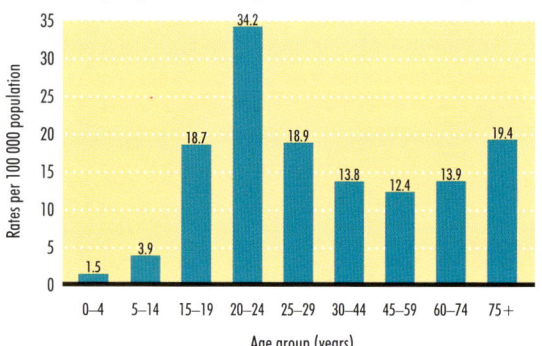

Age-specific mortality rates from road traffic injuries

Source: 2007, Statistics of Estonian Road Administration

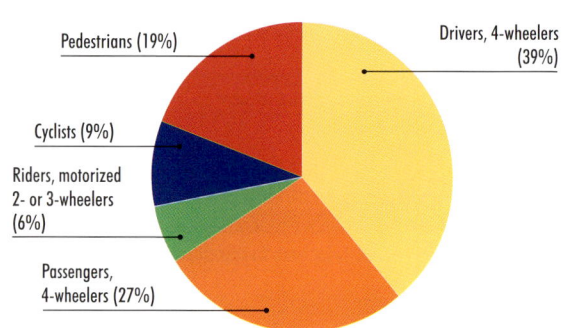

Deaths by road user category

- Pedestrians (19%)
- Drivers, 4-wheelers (39%)
- Cyclists (9%)
- Riders, motorized 2- or 3-wheelers (6%)
- Passengers, 4-wheelers (27%)

Source: 2007, Estonian National Road Administration

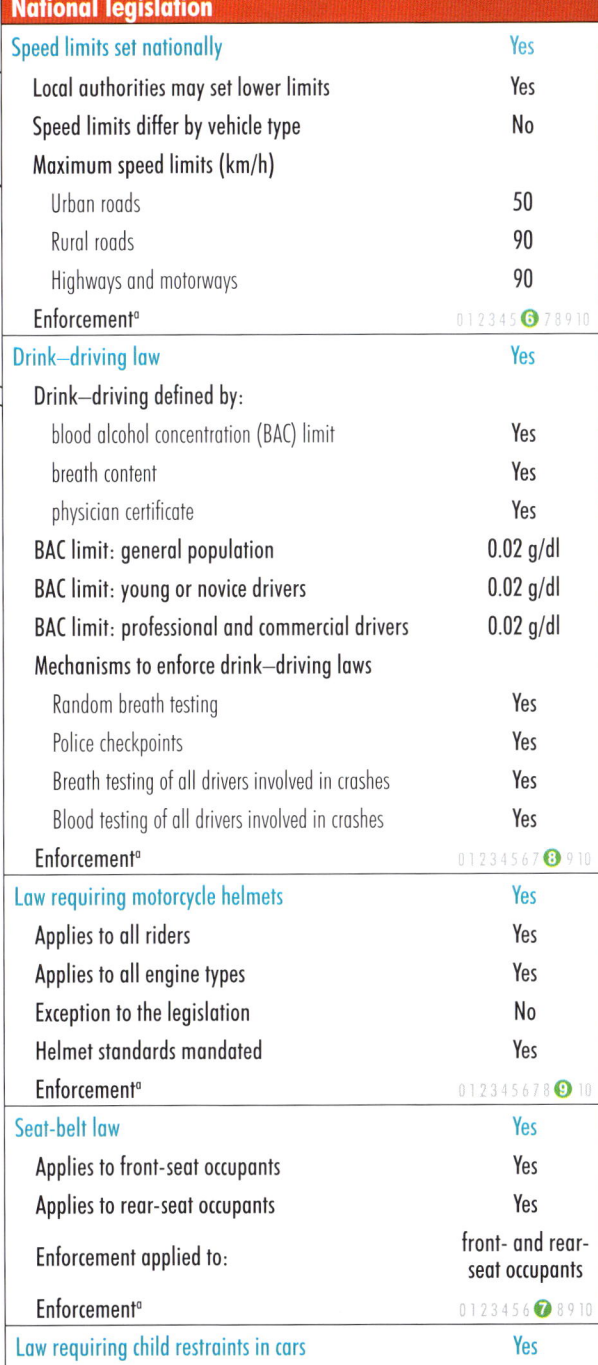

National legislation

Speed limits set nationally	Yes
Local authorities may set lower limits	Yes
Speed limits differ by vehicle type	No
Maximum speed limits (km/h)	
Urban roads	50
Rural roads	90
Highways and motorways	90
Enforcement[a]	0 1 2 3 4 5 **6** 7 8 9 10
Drink–driving law	Yes
Drink–driving defined by:	
blood alcohol concentration (BAC) limit	Yes
breath content	Yes
physician certificate	Yes
BAC limit: general population	0.02 g/dl
BAC limit: young or novice drivers	0.02 g/dl
BAC limit: professional and commercial drivers	0.02 g/dl
Mechanisms to enforce drink–driving laws	
Random breath testing	Yes
Police checkpoints	Yes
Breath testing of all drivers involved in crashes	Yes
Blood testing of all drivers involved in crashes	Yes
Enforcement[a]	0 1 2 3 4 5 6 7 **8** 9 10
Law requiring motorcycle helmets	Yes
Applies to all riders	Yes
Applies to all engine types	Yes
Exception to the legislation	No
Helmet standards mandated	Yes
Enforcement[a]	0 1 2 3 4 5 6 7 8 **9** 10
Seat-belt law	Yes
Applies to front-seat occupants	Yes
Applies to rear-seat occupants	Yes
Enforcement applied to:	front- and rear-seat occupants
Enforcement[a]	0 1 2 3 4 5 6 **7** 8 9 10
Law requiring child restraints in cars	Yes
Enforcement[a]	0 1 2 3 4 5 6 7 **8** 9 10

[a] The enforcement score represents a consensus based on the professional opinion of respondents on a scale of 0 to 10, where 0 is not effective and 10 is highly effective.

Road safety audits

Formal audits required for major new road construction projects	No
Regular audits of existing road infrastructure	Yes

Vehicle standards

No car manufacturers

Promoting transport alternatives to cars

National policies to promote walking or cycling	Yes[a]
Investment in bicycle lanes	Yes
Investment in foot paths	Yes
Traffic-calming measures	Yes
Investment for increasing cycling	Yes
Disincentives for private car use	Yes
National policies to promote public transport	Yes[a]
Subsidized pricing of public transport	Yes
Improving the frequency and coverage of public transport	Yes
Disincentives for private car use	Yes

[a] Other policies are implemented in addition to those listed.

Vehicle regulations

Compulsory insurance for vehicles	Yes
Periodic vehicle inspection for:	
cars	Yes
motorized 2- or 3-wheeled vehicles	Yes
minibuses and vans	Yes
lorries	Yes
buses	Yes

Registered motor vehicles

Total (2008)	708 794
Cars	74%
Motorized 2- and 3-wheelers	2%
Lorries	11%
Buses	1%
Other	12%

Source: Estonian Motor Vehicle Registration Centre (ARK)

Care after road crashes

Formal, publicly available prehospital care system	Yes
National universal access telephone number	Yes (112)

Acknowledgements

Authority approving the data for publication: Ministry of Social Affairs
National data coordinator: Ursel Kedars, Ministry of Social Affairs
Respondents: Dago Antov, Technical University of Tallinn; Erik Ernits, Estonian Traffic Insurance Fund; Jaak Kalda, Police Board under the Ministry of Interior; Alo Kirsimäe, Central Law Enforcement Police under the Ministry of Interior; Toomas Ernits, Estonian Road Administration under the Ministry of Economic Affairs and Communications

Finland

Population: **5.28 million (2007)**

Median age: **41** years

Life expectancy at birth: **79** years

Income group:[a] **high**

Gross national income per person: **US$ 44 400**   Rank: **7** of 49[b]

Human Development Index:[c] **0.954**   Rank: **8** of 49[b]

Private car ownership per 1000 population:[d] **540.0**

CO_2 emissions (tonnes) per person per year:[a] **12.6**

[a] World Bank data.
[b] Rank among the 49 countries in the WHO European Region participating in the survey.
[c] United Nations Development Programme data.
[d] WHO European Region average: 339.

Institutional framework for road safety

Lead agency: Ministry of Transport and Communications of Finland	
Status of the agency	Government
Funded in national budget	Yes
National road safety strategy	Yes
Measurable targets	Yes
Implementation funded	Yes
Money allocated (in € (year))	No information

Key data

Reported number of road traffic deaths (2007)	380[a] (73% males, 27% females)
Reported number of non-fatal road traffic injuries (2007)	8446[b]
Road traffic deaths involving alcohol	23.9%[b]
Wearing motorcycle helmets	95% Drivers[c]
Using seat-belts in cars	
Overall	No information
Front-seat occupants	89%[d]
Rear-seat occupants	80%[e]
Costing study available	Yes
Annual estimated costs (in € (2007))	2.53 billion
Study included deaths, injuries or both	Both deaths and injuries
Methods used	Gross output method; Willingness to pay

[a] *Road Traffic Accidents 2007*, Statistics Finland, Central Organization for Traffic Safety in Finland data, defined as died within 30 days of the crash.
[b] *Road Traffic Accidents 2007*, Statistics Finland, Central Organization for Traffic Safety in Finland data.
[c] Estimation by consensus group.
[d] 2007, Central Organization for Traffic Safety in Finland.
[e] 2007, Central Organization for Traffic Safety in Finland, data apply to urban areas only.

NA: not applicable

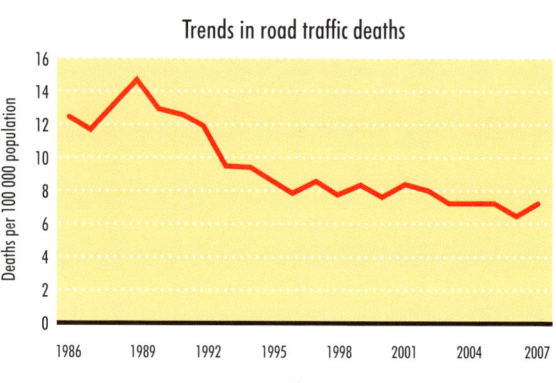

Trends in road traffic deaths

Source: *Road Traffic Accidents 2007*, Statistics Finland, Central Organization for Traffic Safety in Finland

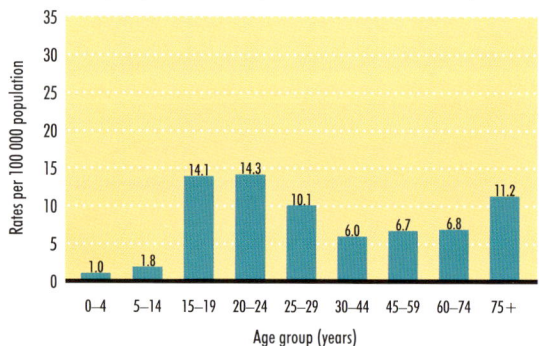

Age-specific mortality rates from road traffic injuries

Source: 2007, *Road Traffic Accidents 2007*, Statistics Finland, Central Organization for Traffic Safety in Finland

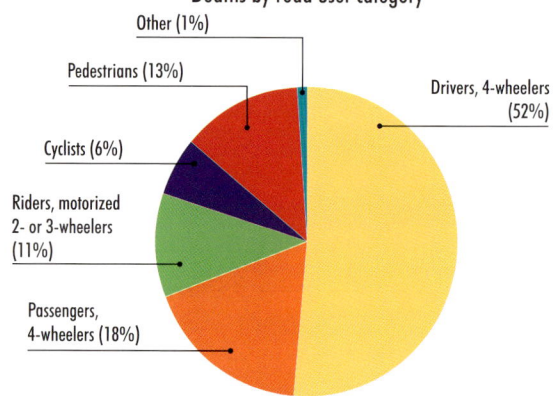

Deaths by road user category

- Other (1%)
- Pedestrians (13%)
- Cyclists (6%)
- Riders, motorized 2- or 3-wheelers (11%)
- Passengers, 4-wheelers (18%)
- Drivers, 4-wheelers (52%)

Source: 2007, *Road Traffic Accidents 2007*, Statistics Finland, Central Organization for Traffic Safety in Finland

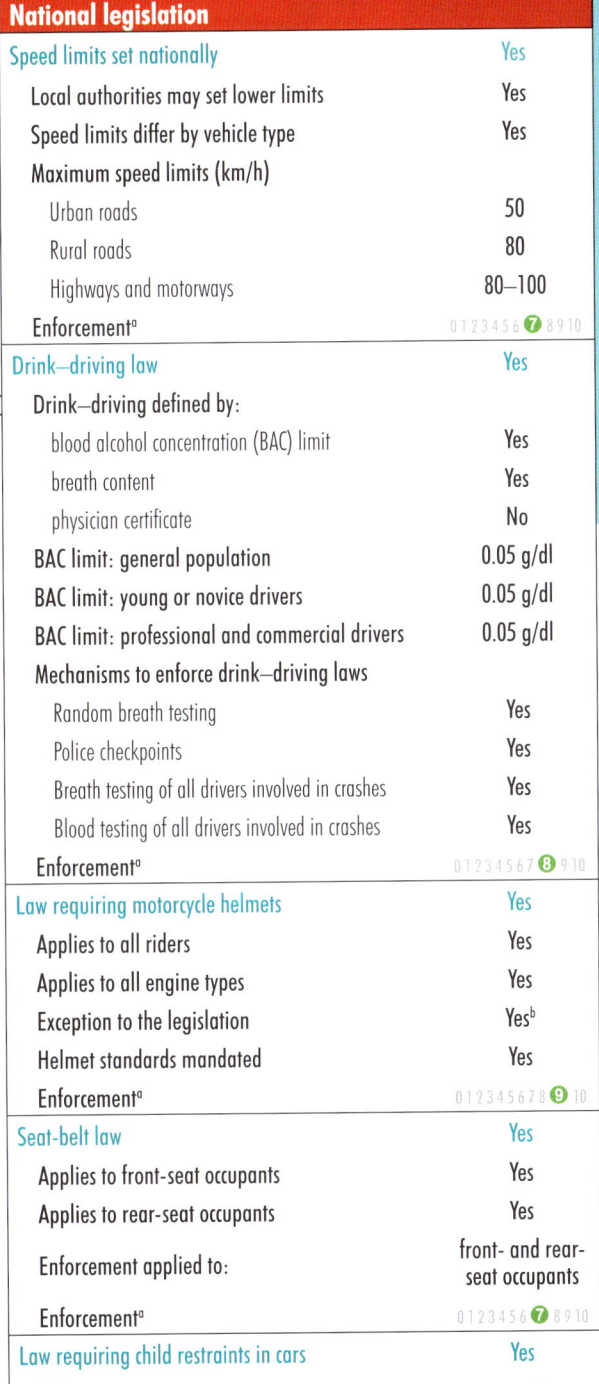

National legislation	
Speed limits set nationally	Yes
Local authorities may set lower limits	Yes
Speed limits differ by vehicle type	Yes
Maximum speed limits (km/h)	
Urban roads	50
Rural roads	80
Highways and motorways	80–100
Enforcement[a]	0 1 2 3 4 5 6 **7** 8 9 10
Drink–driving law	Yes
Drink–driving defined by:	
blood alcohol concentration (BAC) limit	Yes
breath content	Yes
physician certificate	No
BAC limit: general population	0.05 g/dl
BAC limit: young or novice drivers	0.05 g/dl
BAC limit: professional and commercial drivers	0.05 g/dl
Mechanisms to enforce drink–driving laws	
Random breath testing	Yes
Police checkpoints	Yes
Breath testing of all drivers involved in crashes	Yes
Blood testing of all drivers involved in crashes	Yes
Enforcement[a]	0 1 2 3 4 5 6 7 **8** 9 10
Law requiring motorcycle helmets	Yes
Applies to all riders	Yes
Applies to all engine types	Yes
Exception to the legislation	Yes[b]
Helmet standards mandated	Yes
Enforcement[a]	0 1 2 3 4 5 6 7 8 **9** 10
Seat-belt law	Yes
Applies to front-seat occupants	Yes
Applies to rear-seat occupants	Yes
Enforcement applied to:	front- and rear-seat occupants
Enforcement[a]	0 1 2 3 4 5 6 **7** 8 9 10
Law requiring child restraints in cars	Yes
Enforcement[a]	0 1 2 3 4 5 6 **7** 8 9 10

[a] The enforcement score represents a consensus based on the professional opinion of respondents on a scale of 0 to 10, where 0 is not effective and 10 is highly effective.
[b] Exceptions: specially equipped 2-, 3-, 4-wheeled vehicles, invalids and officers performing special duties.

Road safety audits	
Formal audits required for major new road construction projects	Yes
Regular audits of existing road infrastructure	Yes

Vehicle standards	
Car manufacturers required to adhere to standards on	
Fuel consumption	Yes
Seat-belt installation for all seats	Yes

Promoting transport alternatives to cars	
National policies to promote walking or cycling	Yes[a]
Investment in bicycle lanes	No
Investment in foot paths	No
Traffic-calming measures	No
Investment for increasing cycling	No
Disincentives for private car use	No
National policies to promote public transport	Yes
Subsidized pricing of public transport	Yes
Improving the frequency and coverage of public transport	Yes
Disincentives for private car use	No

[a] Other policies are implemented in addition to those listed.

Vehicle regulations	
Compulsory insurance for vehicles	Yes
Periodic vehicle inspection for:	
cars	Yes
motorized 2- or 3-wheeled vehicles	No
minibuses and vans	Yes
lorries	Yes
buses	Yes

Registered motor vehicles	
Total (2007)	4 656 370
Cars	61%
Motorized 2- and 3-wheelers	8%
Lorries	2%
Buses	<1%
Other	29%

Source: The Finnish Vehicle Administration

Care after road crashes	
Formal, publicly available prehospital care system	Yes
National universal access telephone number	Yes (112)

Acknowledgements

Authority approving the data for publication: Ministry of Social Affairs and Health
National data coordinator: Petri Jääskeläinen, Central Organization for Traffic Safety in Finland
Respondents: Merja Söderholm, Ministry of Social Affairs and Health; Leif Beilinson, Ministry of Transport and Communications; Pasi Kemppainen, The National Traffic Police; Marita Koivukoski, The Finnish Vehicle Administration

France

- Population: **61.65 million (2007)**
- Median age: **39** years
- Life expectancy at birth: **81** years
- Income group:[a] **high**
- Gross national income per person: **US$ 38 500**   Rank: **13** of 49[b]
- Human Development Index:[c] **0.955**   Rank: **6** of 49[b]
- Private car ownership per 1000 population:[d] **498.0**
- CO_2 emissions (tonnes) per person per year:[a] **6.2**

[a] World Bank data.
[b] Rank among the 49 countries in the WHO European Region participating in the survey.
[c] United Nations Development Programme data.
[d] WHO European Region average: 339.

Institutional framework for road safety

Lead agency: Interministerial Road Safety Task Force	
Status of the agency	Interministerial
Funded in national budget	Yes
National road safety strategy	Yes
Measurable targets	Yes
Implementation funded	Yes
Money allocated (in € (2007))	2.30 billion

Key data

Reported number of road traffic deaths (2007)	4620[a] (76% males, 24% females)
Reported number of non-fatal road traffic injuries (2007)	77 007[b]
Road traffic deaths involving alcohol	27.0%[c]
Wearing motorcycle helmets	95%[d]
Using seat-belts in cars	
Overall	No information
Front-seat occupants	98%[e]
Rear-seat occupants	83%[e]
Costing study available	Yes
Annual estimated costs (in € (2006))	11.60 billion
Study included deaths, injuries or both	Both deaths and injuries
Methods used	Gross output method

[a] Observatoire national interministériel de sécurité routière (ONISR) data, defined as died within 30 days of the crash.
[b] Observatoire national interministériel de sécurité routière (ONISR) data.
[c] 2006, Observatoire national interministériel de sécurité routière (ONISR).
[d] 2006, ONISR, Observational study, data apply to motorcyclists (99% for moped riders).
[e] 2006, ONISR, Observational study.

NA: not applicable

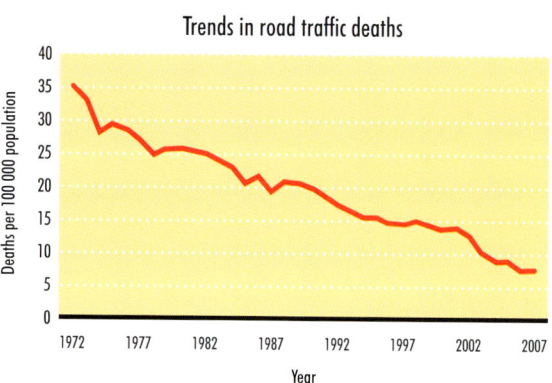

Trends in road traffic deaths

Source: Observatoire national interministériel de sécurité routière (ONISR)

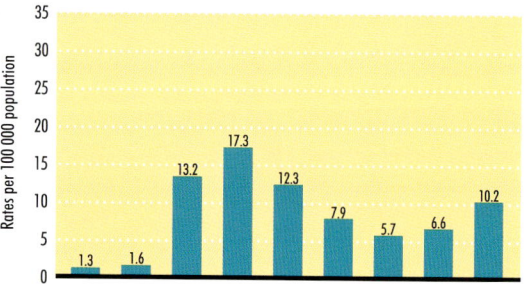

Age-specific mortality rates from road traffic injuries

Source: 2007, Observatoire national interministériel de sécurité routière (ONISR)

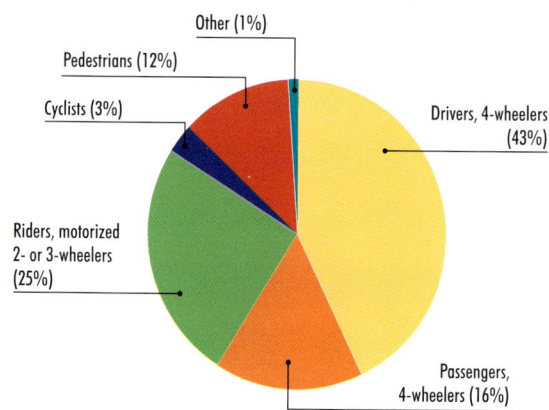

Deaths by road user category

Source: 2007, Observatoire national interministériel de sécurité routière (ONISR)

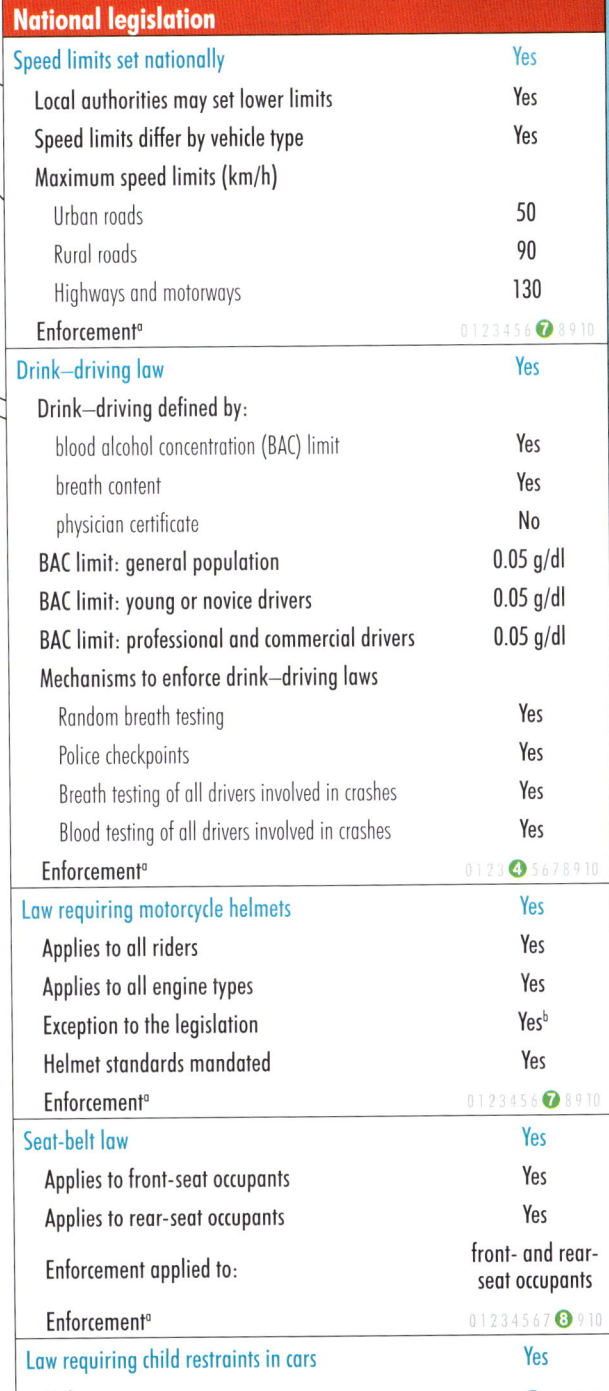

National legislation	
Speed limits set nationally	Yes
Local authorities may set lower limits	Yes
Speed limits differ by vehicle type	Yes
Maximum speed limits (km/h)	
Urban roads	50
Rural roads	90
Highways and motorways	130
Enforcement[a]	7 / 10
Drink–driving law	Yes
Drink–driving defined by:	
blood alcohol concentration (BAC) limit	Yes
breath content	Yes
physician certificate	No
BAC limit: general population	0.05 g/dl
BAC limit: young or novice drivers	0.05 g/dl
BAC limit: professional and commercial drivers	0.05 g/dl
Mechanisms to enforce drink–driving laws	
Random breath testing	Yes
Police checkpoints	Yes
Breath testing of all drivers involved in crashes	Yes
Blood testing of all drivers involved in crashes	Yes
Enforcement[a]	4 / 10
Law requiring motorcycle helmets	Yes
Applies to all riders	Yes
Applies to all engine types	Yes
Exception to the legislation	Yes[b]
Helmet standards mandated	Yes
Enforcement[a]	7 / 10
Seat-belt law	Yes
Applies to front-seat occupants	Yes
Applies to rear-seat occupants	Yes
Enforcement applied to:	front- and rear-seat occupants
Enforcement[a]	8 / 10
Law requiring child restraints in cars	Yes
Enforcement[a]	5 / 10

[a] The enforcement score represents a consensus based on the professional opinion of respondents on a scale of 0 to 10, where 0 is not effective and 10 is highly effective.
[b] Exceptions: motorized 2-wheeled vehicles equipped with seat-belts.

Road safety audits	
Formal audits required for major new road construction projects	Yes
Regular audits of existing road infrastructure	No

Vehicle standards	
Car manufacturers required to adhere to standards on	
Fuel consumption	No
Seat-belt installation for all seats	Yes

Promoting transport alternatives to cars	
National policies to promote walking or cycling	No (subnational)
Investment in bicycle lanes	NA
Investment in foot paths	NA
Traffic-calming measures	NA
Investment for increasing cycling	NA
Disincentives for private car use	NA
National policies to promote public transport	Yes
Subsidized pricing of public transport	Yes
Improving the frequency and coverage of public transport	No
Disincentives for private car use	No

Vehicle regulations	
Compulsory insurance for vehicles	Yes
Periodic vehicle inspection for:	
cars	Yes
motorized 2- or 3-wheeled vehicles	No
minibuses and vans	Yes
lorries	Yes
buses	Yes

Registered motor vehicles	
Total (2007)	39 926 000
Cars	77%
Motorized 2- and 3-wheelers	6%
Minibuses, vans, etc. (seating <20 people)	14%
Lorries	1%
Buses	<1%
Other	1%

Source: 2006, Chambre syndicale nationale du motocycle; 2007, Fichier central des automobiles; 2008, Comité des constructeurs français d'automobiles

Care after road crashes	
Formal, publicly available prehospital care system	Yes
National universal access telephone number	Yes (112)

Acknowledgements

Authority approving the data for publication: Interministerial Road Safety Task Force
National data coordinator: Bernard Laumon, Institut National de REcherche sur les Transports et leur Sécurité (INRETS)
Respondents: Jean Chapelon, Obervatoire national interministériel de sécurité routière (ONISR); Mireille Chiron, Institut National de REcherche sur les Transports et leur Sécurité (INRETS); Mouloud Haddak, Institut National de REcherche sur les Transports et leur Sécurité (INRETS); Alexis Marsan, Ministère de l'intérieur; Yves Rauch, Ministère des transports

Georgia

Population: **4.40 million (2007)**

Median age: **36** years

Life expectancy at birth: **70** years

Income group:[a] **middle**

Gross national income per person: **US$ 2120**   Rank: **44** of 49[b]

Human Development Index:[c] **0.763**   Rank: **42** of 49[b]

Private car ownership per 1000 population:[d] **107.6**

CO_2 emissions (tonnes) per person per year:[a] **0.9**

[a] World Bank data.
[b] Rank among the 49 countries in the WHO European Region participating in the survey.
[c] United Nations Development Programme data.
[d] WHO European Region average: 339.

Institutional framework for road safety

Lead agency: Transport Commission	
Status of the agency	Special body coordinated by the prime minister
Funded in national budget	NA
National road safety strategy	Yes
Measurable targets	Yes
Implementation funded	Yes
Money allocated (in € (year))	No information

Key data

Reported number of road traffic deaths (2007)	737[a] (78% males, 22% females)
Reported number of non-fatal road traffic injuries (2007)	7349[b]
Road traffic deaths involving alcohol	37.0%[c]
Wearing motorcycle helmets	No information
Using seat-belts in cars	
Overall	No information
Front-seat occupants	No information
Rear-seat occupants	No information
Costing study available	No
Annual estimated costs (in € (year))	NA
Study included deaths, injuries or both	NA
Methods used	NA

[a] Ministry of Internal Affairs of Georgia data, defined as died within 20 days of the crash.
[b] Ministry of Internal Affairs of Georgia data.
[c] 2007, Ministry of Internal Affairs of Georgia.

NA: not applicable

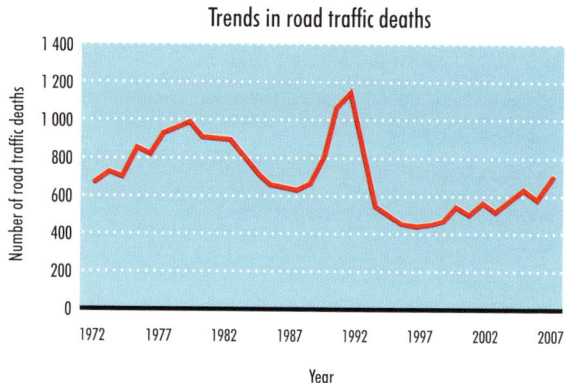

Trends in road traffic deaths

Source: Ministry of Internal Affairs of Georgia

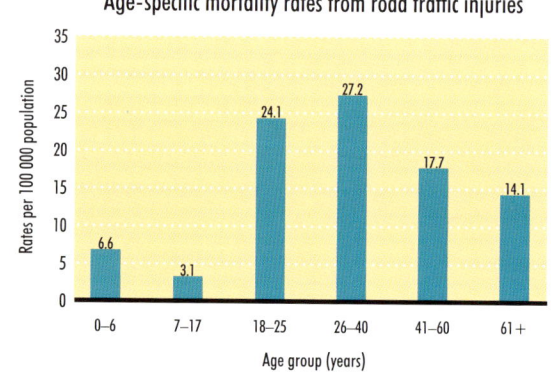

Age-specific mortality rates from road traffic injuries

Source: 2007, Ministry of Internal Affairs of Georgia

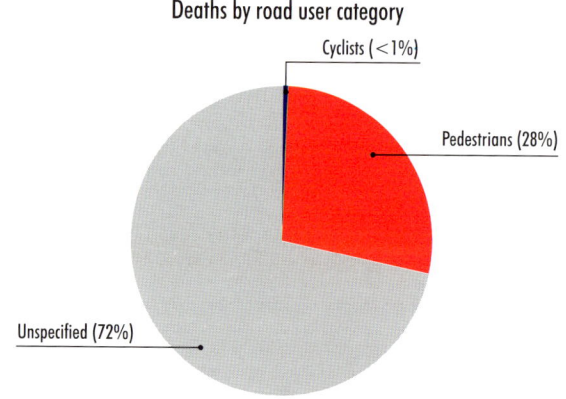

Deaths by road user category
- Cyclists (<1%)
- Pedestrians (28%)
- Unspecified (72%)

Source: 2007, Ministry of Internal Affairs of Georgia

National legislation	
Speed limits set nationally	Yes
Local authorities may set lower limits	Yes
Speed limits differ by vehicle type	Yes
Maximum speed limits (km/h)	
Urban roads	60
Rural roads	60
Highways and motorways	90–110
Enforcement[a]	0 1 2 3 4 5 6 7 **8** 9 10
Drink–driving law	Yes
Drink–driving defined by:	
blood alcohol concentration (BAC) limit	Yes
breath content	Yes
physician certificate	Yes
BAC limit: general population	0.02 g/dl
BAC limit: young or novice drivers	0.02 g/dl
BAC limit: professional and commercial drivers	0.02 g/dl
Mechanisms to enforce drink–driving laws	
Random breath testing	No
Police checkpoints	No
Breath testing of all drivers involved in crashes	Yes
Blood testing of all drivers involved in crashes	Yes
Enforcement[a]	0 1 2 3 4 5 6 7 8 **9** 10
Law requiring motorcycle helmets	Yes
Applies to all riders	Yes
Applies to all engine types	Yes
Exception to the legislation	No
Helmet standards mandated	No
Enforcement[a]	0 1 2 3 4 5 **6** 7 8 9 10
Seat-belt law	Yes
Applies to front-seat occupants	Yes
Applies to rear-seat occupants	No
Enforcement applied to:	front-seat occupants only
Enforcement[a]	0 1 2 3 4 5 6 7 **8** 9 10
Law requiring child restraints in cars	Yes
Enforcement[a]	0 1 2 3 4 5 6 **7** 8 9 10

[a] The enforcement score represents a consensus based on the professional opinion of respondents on a scale of 0 to 10, where 0 is not effective and 10 is highly effective.

Road safety audits	
Formal audits required for major new road construction projects	Yes
Regular audits of existing road infrastructure	Yes

Vehicle standards	
No car manufacturers	

Promoting transport alternatives to cars	
National policies to promote walking or cycling	No
Investment in bicycle lanes	NA
Investment in foot paths	NA
Traffic-calming measures	NA
Investment for increasing cycling	NA
Disincentives for private car use	NA
National policies to promote public transport	No (subnational)
Subsidized pricing of public transport	NA
Improving the frequency and coverage of public transport	NA
Disincentives for private car use	NA

Vehicle regulations	
Compulsory insurance for vehicles	No
Periodic vehicle inspection for:	
cars	No
motorized 2- or 3-wheeled vehicles	No
minibuses and vans	No
lorries	Yes
buses	Yes

Registered motor vehicles	
Total (2008)	567 900
Cars	83%
Motorized 2- and 3-wheelers	<1%
Lorries	10%
Buses	7%

Source: Ministry of Internal Affairs of Georgia

Care after road crashes	
Formal, publicly available prehospital care system	Yes
National universal access telephone number	Yes (03)

Acknowledgements

Authority approving the data for publication: Ministry of Labour, Health and Social Affairs
National data coordinator: Kakha Kheladze, Ministry of Labour, Health and Social Affairs
Respondents: Mamuka Vatsadze, Ministry of Economic Development; Zaza Devdariani, Ministry of Internal Affairs of Georgia; Kakhaber Chikhradze, Tbilisi Ambulance Service 033 and National Medical Centre; Eka Laliashvili, Partnership for Road Safety; Aleqsandre Tudziladze, Georgia Health and Social Projects' Implementation Centre

Germany[a]

- Population: **82.60 million (2007)**
- Median age: **42** years
- Life expectancy at birth: **80** years
- Income group:[b] **high**
- Gross national income per person: **US$ 38 860** Rank: **12** of 49[c]
- Human Development Index:[d] **0.940** Rank: **15** of 49[c]
- Private car ownership per 1000 population:[e] **564.5**
- CO_2 emissions (tonnes) per person per year:[b] **9.8**

[a] Questionnaire completed by the Federal Highway Research Institute BASt (no consensus meeting).
[b] World Bank data.
[c] Rank among the 49 countries in the WHO European Region participating in the survey.
[d] United Nations Development Programme data.
[e] WHO European Region average: 339.

Institutional framework for road safety

Lead agency: Federal Ministry for Traffic, Building and Housing	
Status of the agency	No information
Funded in national budget	Yes
National road safety strategy	Yes
Measurable targets	No
Implementation funded	Yes
Money allocated (in € (year))	No information

Key data

Reported number of road traffic deaths (2007)	4949[a] (73% males, 27% females)
Reported number of non-fatal road traffic injuries (2007)	431 419[b]
Road traffic deaths involving alcohol	12.0%[c]
Wearing motorcycle helmets	97% Drivers; 96% Passengers[d]
Using seat-belts in cars	
Overall	95%[d]
Front-seat occupants	95% Drivers; 96% Passengers[d]
Rear-seat occupants	88%[d]
Costing study available	Yes
Annual estimated costs (in € (2004))	30.90 billion
Study included deaths, injuries or both	Both deaths and injuries
Methods used	Gross output method

[a] Federal Statistical Office data, defined as died within 30 days of the crash.
[b] Federal Statistical Office data.
[c] 2006, Federal Statistical Office.
[d] 2007, Federal Highway Research Institute BASt.

NA: not applicable

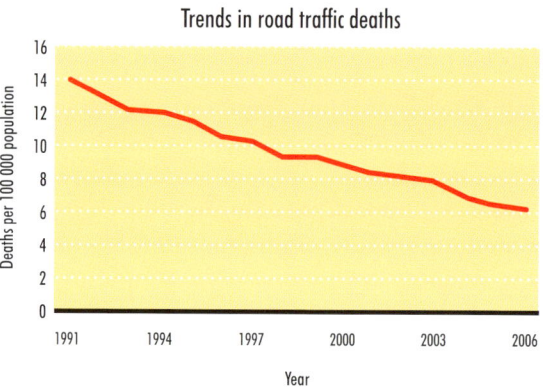

Trends in road traffic deaths

Source: Federal Statistical Office

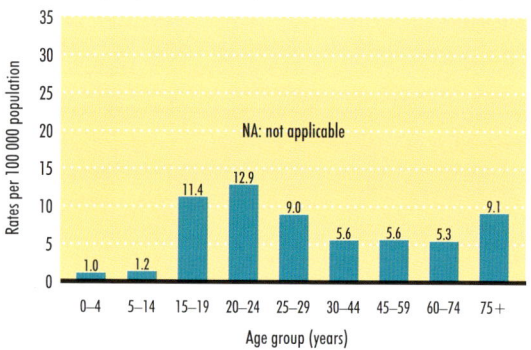

Age-specific mortality rates from road traffic injuries

Source: 2006, Federal Statistical Office

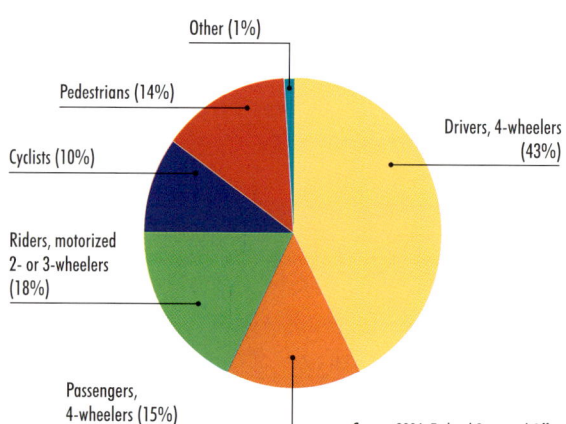

Deaths by road user category

Source: 2006, Federal Statistical Office

National legislation

Speed limits set nationally	Yes
Local authorities may set lower limits	No
Speed limits differ by vehicle type	Yes
Maximum speed limits (km/h)	
Urban roads	50
Rural roads	100
Highways and motorways	130[a]
Enforcement[b]	NA
Drink–driving law	Yes
Drink–driving defined by:	
blood alcohol concentration (BAC) limit	Yes
breath content	Yes
physician certificate	No
BAC limit: general population	0.05 g/dl
BAC limit: young or novice drivers	0.00 g/dl
BAC limit: professional and commercial drivers	0.05 g/dl
Mechanisms to enforce drink–driving laws	
Random breath testing	No
Police checkpoints	Yes
Breath testing of all drivers involved in crashes	Yes
Blood testing of all drivers involved in crashes	Yes
Enforcement[b]	NA
Law requiring motorcycle helmets	Yes
Applies to all riders	Yes
Applies to all engine types	Yes
Exception to the legislation	No
Helmet standards mandated	Yes
Enforcement[b]	NA
Seat-belt law	Yes
Applies to front-seat occupants	Yes
Applies to rear-seat occupants	Yes
Enforcement applied to:	front- and rear-seat occupants
Enforcement[b]	NA
Law requiring child restraints in cars	Yes
Enforcement[b]	NA

[a] Recommended speed limit.
[b] The enforcement score represents a consensus based on the professional opinion of respondents on a scale of 0 to 10, where 0 is not effective and 10 is highly effective.

Road safety audits

Formal audits required for major new road construction projects	No
Regular audits of existing road infrastructure	Yes

Vehicle standards

Car manufacturers required to adhere to standards on	
Fuel consumption	No
Seat-belt installation for all seats	Yes

Promoting transport alternatives to cars

National policies to promote walking or cycling	Yes
Investment in bicycle lanes	Yes
Investment in foot paths	No
Traffic-calming measures	Yes
Investment for increasing cycling	No
Disincentives for private car use	No
National policies to promote public transport	Yes
Subsidized pricing of public transport	No
Improving the frequency and coverage of public transport	No
Disincentives for private car use	No

Vehicle regulations

Compulsory insurance for vehicles	Yes
Periodic vehicle inspection for:	
cars	Yes
motorized 2- or 3-wheeled vehicles	Yes
minibuses and vans	Yes
lorries	Yes
buses	Yes

Registered motor vehicles

Total (2007)	55 511 374
Cars	84%
Motorized 2- and 3-wheelers	7%
Lorries	8%
Buses	<1%
Other	1%

Source: Federal Motor Transport Authority

Care after road crashes

Formal, publicly available prehospital care system	Yes
National universal access telephone number	Yes[a] (112)

[a] Regional access number also available.

Acknowledgements

Authority approving the data for publication: Federal Highway Research Institute BASt
National data coordinator: NA
Respondents: Rosemarie Schleh, Federal Highway Research Institute BASt

Greece

Population: **11.15 million (2007)**

Median age: **40** years

Life expectancy at birth: **80** years

Income group:[a] **high**

Gross national income per person: **US$ 29 630**   Rank: **15 of 49**[b]

Human Development Index:[c] **0.947**   Rank: **12 of 49**[b]

Private car ownership per 1000 population:[d] **455.0**

CO_2 emissions (tonnes) per person per year:[a] **8.7**

[a] World Bank data.
[b] Rank among the 49 countries in the WHO European Region participating in the survey.
[c] United Nations Development Programme data.
[d] WHO European Region average: 339.

Institutional framework for road safety	
Lead agency	No
Status of the agency	NA
Funded in national budget	NA
National road safety strategy	Yes
Measurable targets	Yes
Implementation funded	No
Money allocated (in € (year))	NA

Key data	
Reported number of road traffic deaths (2006)	1657[a] (82% males, 18% females)[b]
Reported number of non-fatal road traffic injuries (2006)	20 675[c]
Road traffic deaths involving alcohol	7.2%[d]
Wearing motorcycle helmets	58% Drivers; 32% Passengers[e]
Using seat-belts in cars	
Overall	No information
Front-seat occupants	75%[e]
Rear-seat occupants	42%[e]
Costing study available	No
Annual estimated costs (in € (year))	NA
Study included deaths, injuries or both	NA
Methods used	NA

[a] National Statistical Service data, defined as died within 30 days of the crash.
[b] Unknown gender <1%.
[c] Police data.
[d] 2006, Road Traffic Police, Port Police Authorities, data apply to drivers involved in fatal crashes only.
[e] 2006, Road Traffic Police, Port Police Authorities, data apply to people involved in reported road traffic crashes only.

NA: not applicable

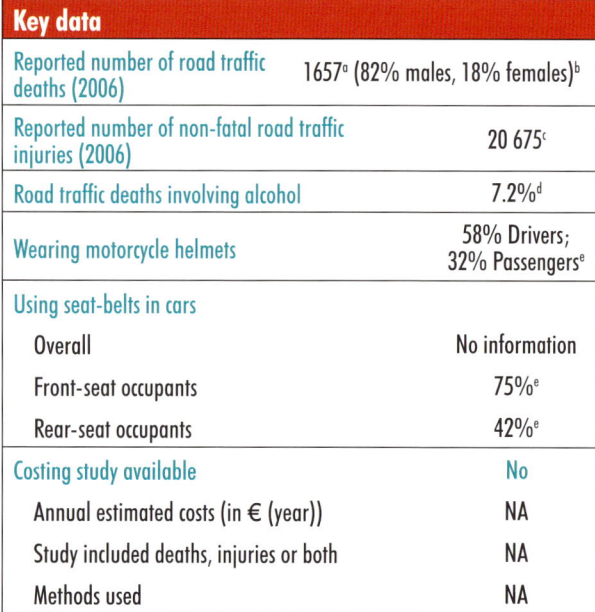

Trends in road traffic deaths

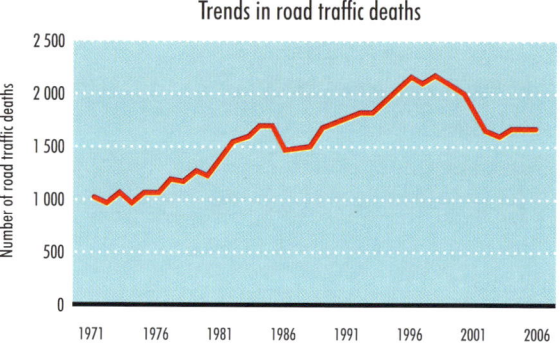

Source: National Statistical Service

Age-specific mortality rates from road traffic injuries

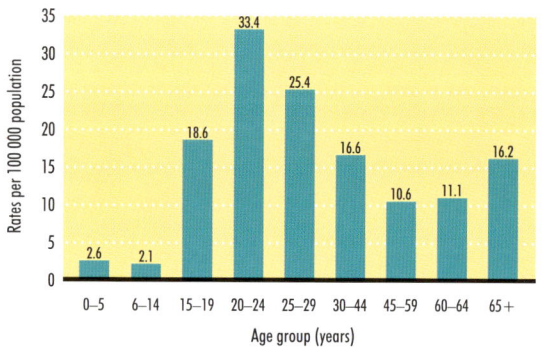

Source: 2006, National Statistical Service

Deaths by road user category

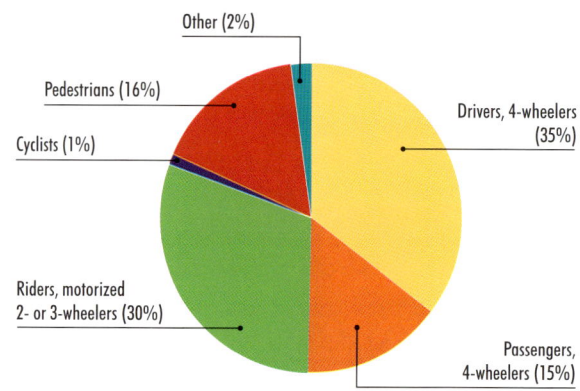

Source: 2006, National Statistical Service

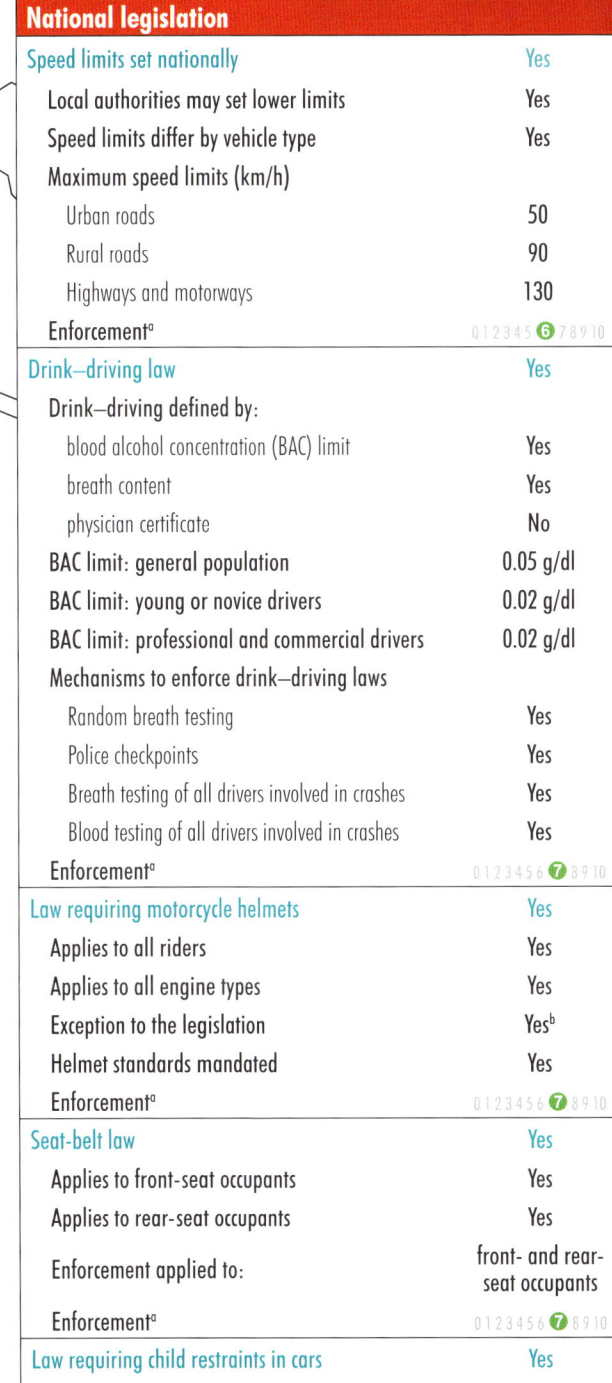

National legislation	
Speed limits set nationally	Yes
Local authorities may set lower limits	Yes
Speed limits differ by vehicle type	Yes
Maximum speed limits (km/h)	
Urban roads	50
Rural roads	90
Highways and motorways	130
Enforcement[a]	0 1 2 3 4 5 **6** 7 8 9 10
Drink–driving law	Yes
Drink–driving defined by:	
blood alcohol concentration (BAC) limit	Yes
breath content	Yes
physician certificate	No
BAC limit: general population	0.05 g/dl
BAC limit: young or novice drivers	0.02 g/dl
BAC limit: professional and commercial drivers	0.02 g/dl
Mechanisms to enforce drink–driving laws	
Random breath testing	Yes
Police checkpoints	Yes
Breath testing of all drivers involved in crashes	Yes
Blood testing of all drivers involved in crashes	Yes
Enforcement[a]	0 1 2 3 4 5 6 **7** 8 9 10
Law requiring motorcycle helmets	Yes
Applies to all riders	Yes
Applies to all engine types	Yes
Exception to the legislation	Yes[b]
Helmet standards mandated	Yes
Enforcement[a]	0 1 2 3 4 5 6 **7** 8 9 10
Seat-belt law	Yes
Applies to front-seat occupants	Yes
Applies to rear-seat occupants	Yes
Enforcement applied to:	front- and rear-seat occupants
Enforcement[a]	0 1 2 3 4 5 6 **7** 8 9 10
Law requiring child restraints in cars	Yes
Enforcement[a]	0 1 2 3 4 5 **6** 7 8 9 10

[a] The enforcement score represents a consensus based on the professional opinion of respondents on a scale of 0 to 10, where 0 is not effective and 10 is highly effective.
[b] Exceptions: medical reasons.

Road safety audits	
Formal audits required for major new road construction projects	Yes
Regular audits of existing road infrastructure	No information

Vehicle standards	
No car manufacturers	

Promoting transport alternatives to cars	
National policies to promote walking or cycling	Yes
Investment in bicycle lanes	No
Investment in foot paths	No
Traffic-calming measures	Yes
Investment for increasing cycling	No
Disincentives for private car use	No
National policies to promote public transport	Yes
Subsidized pricing of public transport	Yes
Improving the frequency and coverage of public transport	Yes
Disincentives for private car use	No

Vehicle regulations	
Compulsory insurance for vehicles	Yes
Periodic vehicle inspection for:	
cars	Yes
motorized 2- or 3-wheeled vehicles	Yes
minibuses and vans	Yes
lorries	Yes
buses	Yes

Registered motor vehicles	
Total (2006)	7 212 236
Cars	65%
Motorized 2- and 3-wheelers	17%
Lorries	17%
Buses	<1%
Other	1%

Source: Ministry of Transport and Communication

Care after road crashes	
Formal, publicly available prehospital care system	Yes
National universal access telephone number	Yes (166)

Acknowledgements

Authority approving the data for publication: Ministry of Health and Social Solidarity
National data coordinator: Dimitrios Efthymiadis, Ministry of Health and Social Solidarity
Respondents: Spyros Panagopoulos, Ministry of Interior, Hellenic Police Headquarters, Road Traffic Police; Vilelmini Paraschou, Ministry of Economy and Finance, National Statistical Service; Vasiliki Mylona-Danelli, Road Safety Institute "Panos Mylonas"; Georgios Kanellaidis, National Technical University of Athens, Metsovo, School of Civil Engineering, Department of Transportation Planning and Engineering; Maria Vaniotou, Ministry of Environment, Land Planning and Public Works, Directorate of Road Works Conservation; Konstantina Kosmidou, Ministry of Transport and Communication, Directorate of Road Safety and Environment, Department of Road Safety

Hungary

Population: **10.03 million (2007)**
Median age: **39** years
Life expectancy at birth: **73** years
Income group:[a] **high**
Gross national income per person: **US$ 11 570**   Rank: **25** of 49[b]
Human Development Index:[c] **0.877**   Rank: **22** of 49[b]
Private car ownership per 1000 population:[d] **300.4**
CO_2 emissions (tonnes) per person per year:[a] **5.7**

[a] World Bank data.
[b] Rank among the 49 countries in the WHO European Region participating in the survey.
[c] United Nations Development Programme data.
[d] WHO European Region average: 339.

Institutional framework for road safety

Lead agency: Interministerial Committee for Road Safety	
Status of the agency	Interministerial
Funded in national budget	Yes
National road safety strategy	**Yes**
Measurable targets	Yes
Implementation funded	Yes
Money allocated (in € (2008))	13.03 million

Key data

Reported number of road traffic deaths (2007)	1232[a] (74% males, 25% females)[b]
Reported number of non-fatal road traffic injuries (2007)	27 452[c]
Road traffic deaths involving alcohol	12.0%[d]
Wearing motorcycle helmets	95%[e]
Using seat-belts in cars	
Overall	69%[f]
Front-seat occupants	71%[f]
Rear-seat occupants	40%[f]
Costing study available	**Yes**
Annual estimated costs (in € (2002))	0.77 million[g]
Study included deaths, injuries or both	Deaths only
Methods used	Willingness to pay

[a] Police data, defined as died within 30 days of the crash.
[b] Unknown gender <1%.
[c] Police data.
[d] 2006, Hungarian Central Statistical Office (KSH).
[e] Estimation by consensus group.
[f] 2007, Observational study.
[g] Costs for one road traffic death.

NA: not applicable

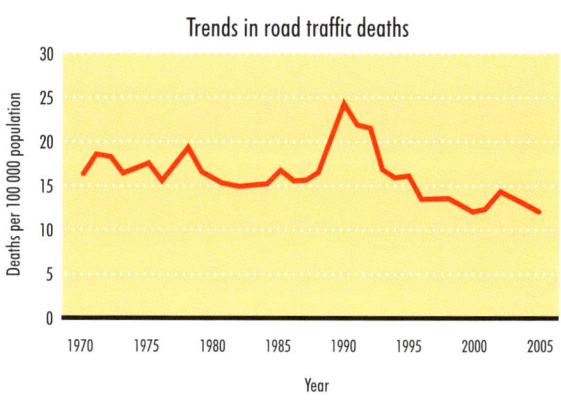

Trends in road traffic deaths

Source: Country questionnaire

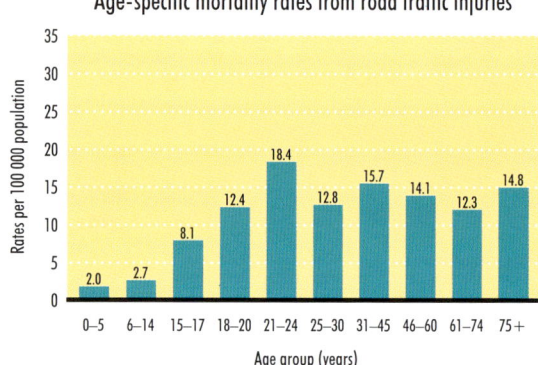

Age-specific mortality rates from road traffic injuries

Source: 2007, Police

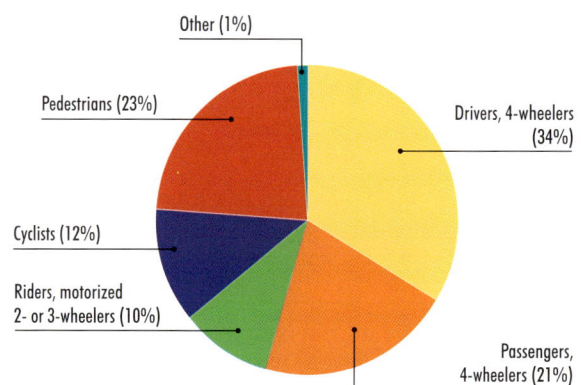

Deaths by road user category

Other (1%)
Pedestrians (23%)
Drivers, 4-wheelers (34%)
Cyclists (12%)
Riders, motorized 2- or 3-wheelers (10%)
Passengers, 4-wheelers (21%)

Source: 2006, *Traffic Accidents 2006*, Hungarian Central Statistical Office (KSH).

National legislation	
Speed limits set nationally	Yes
Local authorities may set lower limits	Yes
Speed limits differ by vehicle type	Yes
Maximum speed limits (km/h)	
Urban roads	50
Rural roads	90
Highways and motorways	130
Enforcement[a]	0 1 2 3 **4** 5 6 7 8 9 10
Drink–driving law	Yes
Drink–driving defined by:	
blood alcohol concentration (BAC) limit	Yes
breath content	Yes
physician certificate	No
BAC limit: general population	0.00 g/dl
BAC limit: young or novice drivers	0.00 g/dl
BAC limit: professional and commercial drivers	0.00 g/dl
Mechanisms to enforce drink–driving laws	
Random breath testing	Yes
Police checkpoints	Yes
Breath testing of all drivers involved in crashes	Yes
Blood testing of all drivers involved in crashes	Yes
Enforcement[a]	0 1 2 3 4 **5** 6 7 8 9 10
Law requiring motorcycle helmets	Yes
Applies to all riders	Yes
Applies to all engine types	Yes
Exception to the legislation	No
Helmet standards mandated	Yes
Enforcement[a]	0 1 2 3 4 5 6 7 8 **9** 10
Seat-belt law	Yes
Applies to front-seat occupants	Yes
Applies to rear-seat occupants	Yes
Enforcement applied to:	front- and rear-seat occupants
Enforcement[a]	0 1 2 3 **4** 5 6 7 8 9 10
Law requiring child restraints in cars	Yes
Enforcement[a]	0 1 2 3 **4** 5 6 7 8 9 10

[a] The enforcement score represents a consensus based on the professional opinion of respondents on a scale of 0 to 10, where 0 is not effective and 10 is highly effective.

Road safety audits	
Formal audits required for major new road construction projects	No
Regular audits of existing road infrastructure	Yes

Vehicle standards	
Car manufacturers required to adhere to standards on	
Fuel consumption	No
Seat-belt installation for all seats	Yes

Promoting transport alternatives to cars	
National policies to promote walking or cycling	Yes
Investment in bicycle lanes	Yes
Investment in foot paths	No
Traffic-calming measures	Yes
Investment for increasing cycling	No
Disincentives for private car use	No
National policies to promote public transport	No (subnational)
Subsidized pricing of public transport	NA
Improving the frequency and coverage of public transport	NA
Disincentives for private car use	NA

Vehicle regulations	
Compulsory insurance for vehicles	Yes
Periodic vehicle inspection for:	
cars	Yes
motorized 2- or 3-wheeled vehicles	Yes
minibuses and vans	Yes
lorries	Yes
buses	Yes

Registered motor vehicles	
Total (2007)	3 625 386
Cars	83%
Motorized 2- and 3-wheelers	4%
Lorries	12%
Buses	<1%
Other	1%

Source: Hungarian Central Statistical Office (KSH)

Care after road crashes	
Formal, publicly available prehospital care system	Yes
National universal access telephone number	Yes (112)

Acknowledgements

Authority approving the data for publication: Ministry of Health
National data coordinator: Mária Bényi, National Centre for Healthcare Audit and Inspection
Respondents: Péter Holló, Institute for Transport Sciences Non Profit Ltd. (KTI); Ákos Probáld, Hungarian Central Statistical Office (KSH); Csaba Kiss, National Committee for Accident Prevention; Kirisztina Tálas, Ministry of Health; Zsófia Szász, National Police Headquarters

Iceland

Population: 0.30 million (2007)
Median age: 35 years
Life expectancy at birth: 81 years
Income group:[a] high
Gross national income per person: US$ 54 100   Rank: 3 of 49[b]
Human Development Index:[c] 0.968   Rank: 1 of 49[b]
Private car ownership per 1000 population:[d] 688.9
CO_2 emissions (tonnes) per person per year:[a] No information

[a] World Bank data.
[b] Rank among the 49 countries in the WHO European Region participating in the survey.
[c] United Nations Development Programme data.
[d] WHO European Region average: 339.

Institutional framework for road safety

Lead agency: The Road Traffic Directorate	
Status of the agency	Government
Funded in national budget	Yes
National road safety strategy	Yes
Measurable targets	Yes
Implementation funded	Yes
Money allocated (in € (2007))	3.49 million

Key data

Reported number of road traffic deaths (2006)	30[a] (67% males, 33% females)
Reported number of non-fatal road traffic injuries (2006)	2092[b]
Road traffic deaths involving alcohol	20.0%[c]
Wearing motorcycle helmets	95%[d]
Using seat-belts in cars	
Overall	80%[e]
Front-seat occupants	88%[e]
Rear-seat occupants	68%[e]
Costing study available	Yes
Annual estimated costs (in € (2005))	369.43 million
Study included deaths, injuries or both	Both deaths and injuries
Methods used	Gross output method

[a] Statistics Iceland Mortality Coding Register data, defined as died within 30 days of the crash.
[b] Icelandic Accident Register data.
[c] 2007, The Road Traffic Directorate.
[d] Estimation by consensus group.
[e] 2007, National telephone survey conducted by Capacent Gallup.

NA: not applicable

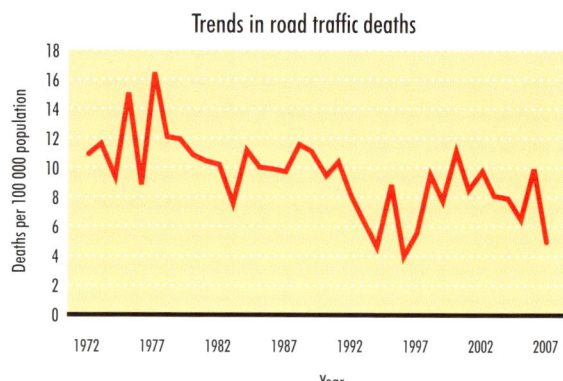

Trends in road traffic deaths

Source: The Road Traffic Directorate

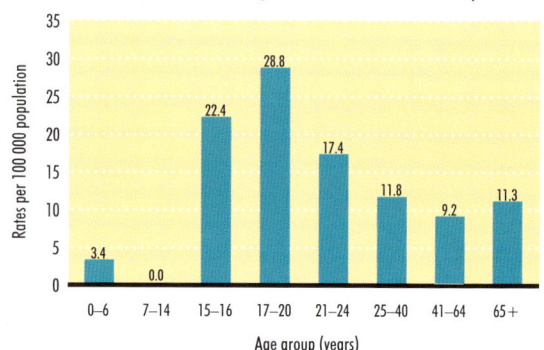

Age-specific mortality rates from road traffic injuries

Source: 2007, *Road Traffic Accidents in Iceland*, The Road Traffic Directorate

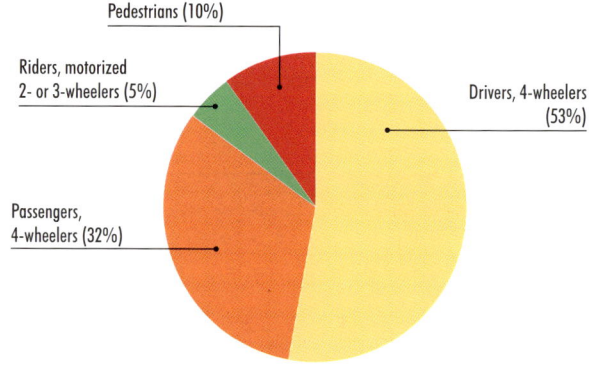

Deaths by road user category

Source: 1998-2007, *Road Traffic Accidents in Iceland*, The Road Traffic Directorate

National legislation

Speed limits set nationally	Yes
Local authorities may set lower limits	Yes
Speed limits differ by vehicle type	Yes
Maximum speed limits (km/h)	
Urban roads	50
Rural roads	80–90
Highways and motorways	NA
Enforcement[a]	0 1 2 3 4 5 6 **7** 8 9 10
Drink–driving law	Yes
Drink–driving defined by:	
blood alcohol concentration (BAC) limit	Yes
breath content	Yes
physician certificate	No
BAC limit: general population	0.05 g/dl
BAC limit: young or novice drivers	0.05 g/dl
BAC limit: professional and commercial drivers	0.05 g/dl
Mechanisms to enforce drink–driving laws	
Random breath testing	Yes
Police checkpoints	Yes
Breath testing of all drivers involved in crashes	No
Blood testing of all drivers involved in crashes	No
Enforcement[a]	0 1 2 3 4 5 6 **7** 8 9 10
Law requiring motorcycle helmets	Yes
Applies to all riders	Yes
Applies to all engine types	Yes
Exception to the legislation	No
Helmet standards mandated	No
Enforcement[a]	0 1 2 3 4 5 6 7 **8** 9 10
Seat-belt law	Yes
Applies to front-seat occupants	Yes
Applies to rear-seat occupants	Yes
Enforcement applied to:	front- and rear-seat occupants
Enforcement[a]	0 1 2 3 4 5 6 7 **8** 9 10
Law requiring child restraints in cars	Yes
Enforcement[a]	0 1 2 3 4 5 6 7 **8** 9 10

[a] The enforcement score represents a consensus based on the professional opinion of respondents on a scale of 0 to 10, where 0 is not effective and 10 is highly effective.

Road safety audits

Formal audits required for major new road construction projects	Yes
Regular audits of existing road infrastructure	No

Vehicle standards

No car manufacturers	

Promoting transport alternatives to cars

National policies to promote walking or cycling	No (subnational)
Investment in bicycle lanes	NA
Investment in foot paths	NA
Traffic-calming measures	NA
Investment for increasing cycling	NA
Disincentives for private car use	NA
National policies to promote public transport	No (subnational)
Subsidized pricing of public transport	NA
Improving the frequency and coverage of public transport	NA
Disincentives for private car use	NA

Vehicle regulations

Compulsory insurance for vehicles	Yes
Periodic vehicle inspection for:	
cars	Yes
motorized 2- or 3-wheeled vehicles	Yes
minibuses and vans	Yes
lorries	Yes
buses	Yes

Registered motor vehicles

Total (2007)	293 299
Cars	71%
Motorized 2- and 3-wheelers	5%
Minibuses, vans, etc. (seating <20 people)	7%
Lorries	3%
Buses	<1%
Other	14%

Source: Ministry of Transport

Care after road crashes

Formal, publicly available prehospital care system	Yes
National universal access telephone number	Yes (112)

Acknowledgements

Authority approving the data for publication: Ministry of Health
National data coordinator: Rósa Thorsteinsdóttir, The Public Health Institute
Respondents: Svanhildur Thorsteinsdóttir, The Directorate of Health (representing the Ministry of Health); Birna Hreiðarsdóttir, Ministry of Transport; Kristján Ó Guðnason, Metropolitan Police; Sigurður Helgason, The Road Traffic Directorate; Brynjólfur Mogensen, Landspitali University Hospital

Ireland

Population: **4.30 million (2007)**

Median age: **34** years

Life expectancy at birth: **80** years

Income group:[a] **high**

Gross national income per person: **US$ 48 140** Rank: **4** of 49[b]

Human Development Index:[c] **0.960** Rank: **3** of 49[b]

Private car ownership per 1000 population:[d] **440.6**

CO_2 emissions (tonnes) per person per year:[a] **10.4**

[a] World Bank data.
[b] Rank among the 49 countries in the WHO European Region participating in the survey.
[c] United Nations Development Programme data.
[d] WHO European Region average: 339.

Institutional framework for road safety

Lead agency:	Road Safety Authority
Status of the agency	Agency under the remit of the Department of Transport
Funded in national budget	Yes
National road safety strategy	**Yes**
Measurable targets	Yes
Implementation funded	No information
Money allocated (in € (year))	NA

Key data

Reported number of road traffic deaths (2006)	365[a] (72% males, 27% females)[b]
Reported number of non-fatal road traffic injuries (2006)	8575[c]
Road traffic deaths involving alcohol	37.0%[d]
Wearing motorcycle helmets	No information
Using seat-belts in cars	
Overall	No information
Front-seat occupants	86%[e]
Rear-seat occupants	63%[e]
Costing study available	**Yes**
Annual estimated costs (in € (2006))	1.33 billion
Study included deaths, injuries or both	Both deaths and injuries
Methods used	No information

[a] Road Safety Authority data, defined as died within 30 days of the crash.
[b] Unknown gender 2%.
[c] Road Safety Authority data.
[d] 2006, Based on Bedford D, McKeown N, Vellinga A, Howell F *Alcohol in Fatal Road Crashes in Ireland in 2003*, Population Health Directorate, Health Service Executive.
[e] 2006, Survey of Seat Belt Wearing, Road Safety Authority.

NA: not applicable

Trends in road traffic deaths

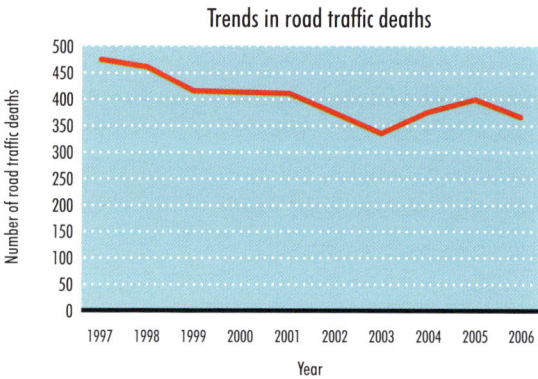

Source: *Road Collision Facts Ireland 2006*, Road Safety Authority

Age-specific mortality rates from road traffic injuries

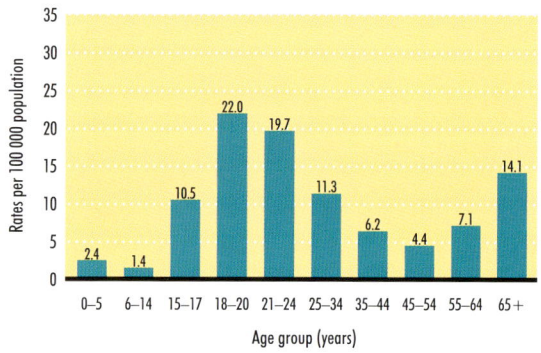

Source: 2006, *Road Collision Facts Ireland 2006*, Road Safety Authority

Deaths by road user category

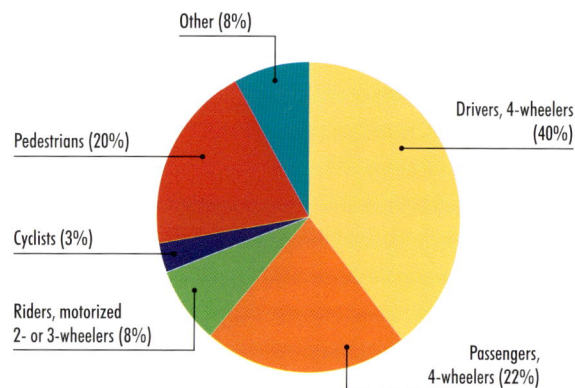

- Drivers, 4-wheelers (40%)
- Passengers, 4-wheelers (22%)
- Riders, motorized 2- or 3-wheelers (8%)
- Cyclists (3%)
- Pedestrians (20%)
- Other (8%)

Source: 2006, *Road Collision Facts Ireland 2006*, Road Safety Authority

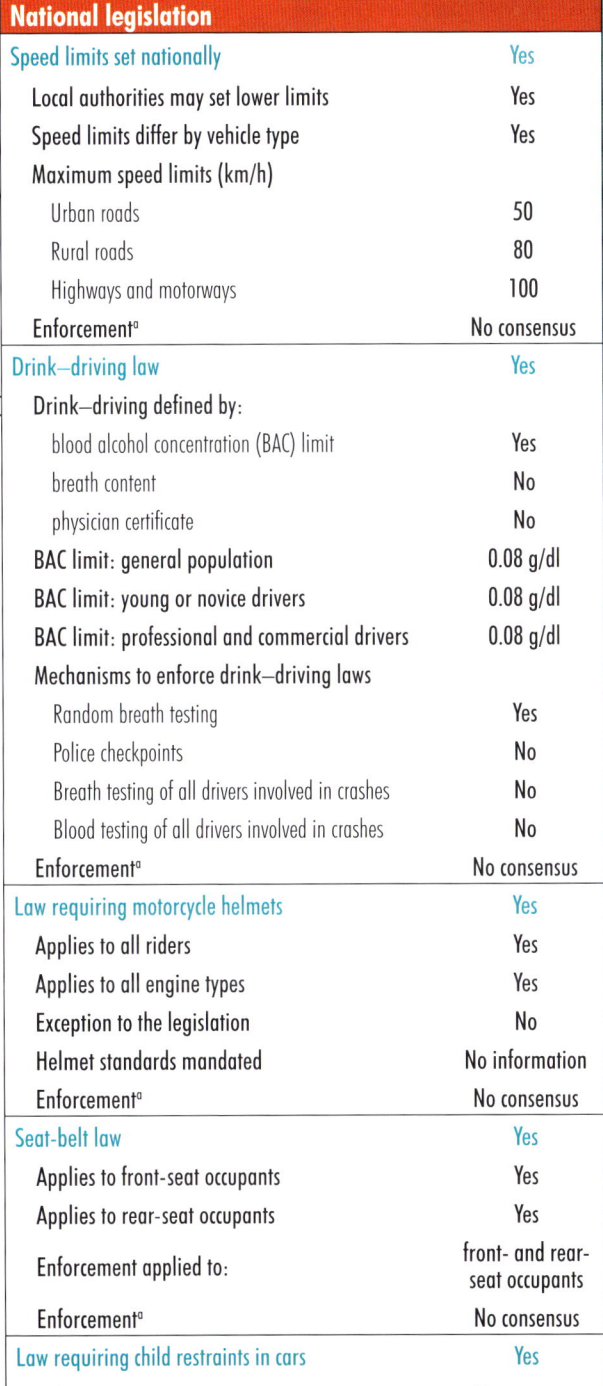

National legislation	
Speed limits set nationally	Yes
Local authorities may set lower limits	Yes
Speed limits differ by vehicle type	Yes
Maximum speed limits (km/h)	
Urban roads	50
Rural roads	80
Highways and motorways	100
Enforcement[a]	No consensus
Drink–driving law	Yes
Drink–driving defined by:	
blood alcohol concentration (BAC) limit	Yes
breath content	No
physician certificate	No
BAC limit: general population	0.08 g/dl
BAC limit: young or novice drivers	0.08 g/dl
BAC limit: professional and commercial drivers	0.08 g/dl
Mechanisms to enforce drink–driving laws	
Random breath testing	Yes
Police checkpoints	No
Breath testing of all drivers involved in crashes	No
Blood testing of all drivers involved in crashes	No
Enforcement[a]	No consensus
Law requiring motorcycle helmets	Yes
Applies to all riders	Yes
Applies to all engine types	Yes
Exception to the legislation	No
Helmet standards mandated	No information
Enforcement[a]	No consensus
Seat-belt law	Yes
Applies to front-seat occupants	Yes
Applies to rear-seat occupants	Yes
Enforcement applied to:	front- and rear-seat occupants
Enforcement[a]	No consensus
Law requiring child restraints in cars	Yes
Enforcement[a]	No consensus

[a] The enforcement score represents a consensus based on the professional opinion of respondents on a scale of 0 to 10, where 0 is not effective and 10 is highly effective.

Road safety audits	
Formal audits required for major new road construction projects	Yes
Regular audits of existing road infrastructure	Yes

Vehicle standards
No car manufacturers

Promoting transport alternatives to cars	
National policies to promote walking or cycling	No
Investment in bicycle lanes	NA
Investment in foot paths	NA
Traffic-calming measures	NA
Investment for increasing cycling	NA
Disincentives for private car use	NA
National policies to promote public transport	Yes[a]
Subsidized pricing of public transport	Yes
Improving the frequency and coverage of public transport	No
Disincentives for private car use	No

[a] Other policies are implemented in addition to those listed.

Vehicle regulations	
Compulsory insurance for vehicles	Yes
Periodic vehicle inspection for:	
cars	Yes
motorized 2- or 3-wheeled vehicles	No
minibuses and vans	Yes
lorries	Yes
buses	Yes

Registered motor vehicles	
Total (2006)	2 444 159
Cars	76%
Motorized 2- and 3-wheelers	2%
Minibuses, vans, etc. (seating <20 people)	16%
Lorries	2%
Buses	<1%
Other	4%

Source: Department of Transport, NVDF Shannon

Care after road crashes	
Formal, publicly available prehospital care system	Yes
National universal access telephone number	Yes (999; 112)

Acknowledgements

Authority approving the data for publication: Department of Transport
National data coordinator: Declan Hayes, Road Safety and Traffic Division
Respondents: Robbie Breen, Department of Health and Children; Gerry O'Malley, Department of Transport, NVDF Shannon; Ann Cody, Department of Transport; Harry Cullen, National Roads Authority; Michael Brosnan, Road Safety Authority; Con O'Donohue, Garda Headquarters

Israel

Population: **6.93 million (2007)**

Median age: **29** years

Life expectancy at birth: **81** years

Income group:[a] **high**

Gross national income per person: **US$ 21 900**   Rank: **18 of 49**[b]

Human Development Index:[c] **0.930**   Rank: **16 of 49**[b]

Private car ownership per 1000 population:[d] **257.1**

CO_2 emissions (tonnes) per person per year:[a] **10.5**

[a] World Bank data.
[b] Rank among the 49 countries in the WHO European Region participating in the survey.
[c] United Nations Development Programme data.
[d] WHO European Region average: 339.

Institutional framework for road safety

Lead agency: National Road Safety Authority	
Status of the agency	National Agency by Act of Knesset (Parliament)
Funded in national budget	Yes
National road safety strategy	**Yes**
Measurable targets	Yes
Implementation funded	Yes
Money allocated (in € (2008))	101.78 million

Key data

Reported number of road traffic deaths (2007)	398[a] (75% males, 25% females)
Reported number of non-fatal road traffic injuries (2007)	2079[b]
Road traffic deaths involving alcohol	7.5%[c]
Wearing motorcycle helmets	95%[d]
Using seat-belts in cars	
Overall	No information
Front-seat occupants	94% Drivers; 88% Passengers[e]
Rear-seat occupants	45%[e]
Costing study available	**Yes**
Annual estimated costs (in € (2005))	1.33 billion
Study included deaths, injuries or both	Both deaths and injuries
Methods used	Gross output method

[a] Police data, defined as died within 30 days of the crash.
[b] Police data.
[c] 2007, Israeli Police.
[d] 2006, National Road Safety Authority, observational study.
[e] 2007, National Road Safety Authority, observational study.

NA: not applicable

Trends in road traffic deaths

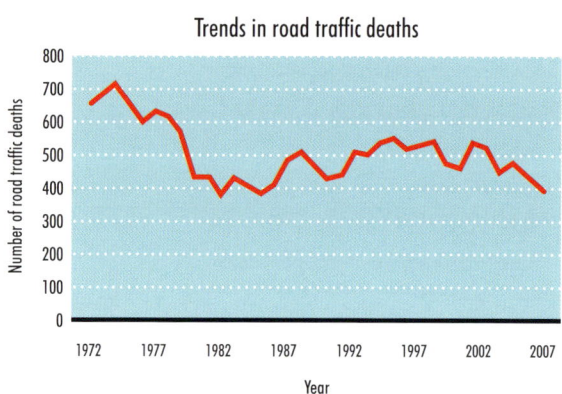

Source: Central Bureau of Statistics, Israeli Police

Age-specific mortality rates from road traffic injuries

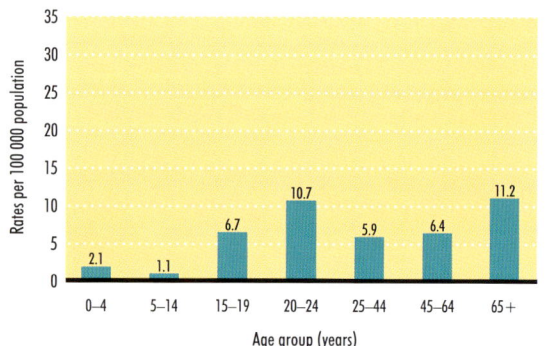

Source: 2007, Central Bureau of Statistics, Israeli Police

Deaths by road user category

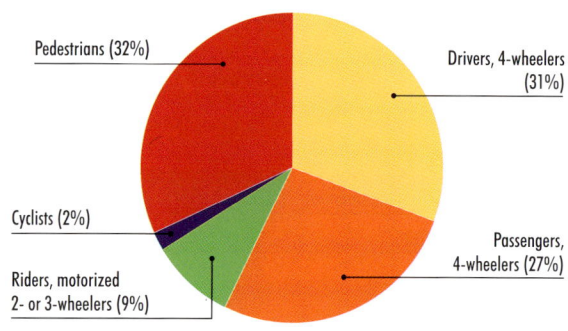

Pedestrians (32%); Drivers, 4-wheelers (31%); Passengers, 4-wheelers (27%); Riders, motorized 2- or 3-wheelers (9%); Cyclists (2%)

Source: Central Bureau of Statistics, Israeli Police

National legislation

Speed limits set nationally	Yes
Local authorities may set lower limits	Yes
Speed limits differ by vehicle type	Yes
Maximum speed limits (km/h)	
Urban roads	50
Rural roads	80–90
Highways and motorways	90–110
Enforcement[a]	5 (0–10)
Drink–driving law	**Yes**
Drink–driving defined by:	
blood alcohol concentration (BAC) limit	Yes
breath content	No
physician certificate	No
BAC limit: general population	0.05 g/dl
BAC limit: young or novice drivers	0.05 g/dl
BAC limit: professional and commercial drivers	0.05 g/dl
Mechanisms to enforce drink–driving laws	
Random breath testing	Yes
Police checkpoints	Yes
Breath testing of all drivers involved in crashes	No
Blood testing of all drivers involved in crashes	No
Enforcement[a]	6 (0–10)
Law requiring motorcycle helmets	**Yes**
Applies to all riders	Yes
Applies to all engine types	Yes
Exception to the legislation	No
Helmet standards mandated	No
Enforcement[a]	9 (0–10)
Seat-belt law	**Yes**
Applies to front-seat occupants	Yes
Applies to rear-seat occupants	Yes
Enforcement applied to:	front- and rear-seat occupants
Enforcement[a]	8 (0–10)
Law requiring child restraints in cars	**Yes**
Enforcement[a]	5 (0–10)

[a] The enforcement score represents a consensus based on the professional opinion of respondents on a scale of 0 to 10, where 0 is not effective and 10 is highly effective.

Road safety audits

Formal audits required for major new road construction projects	Yes
Regular audits of existing road infrastructure	Yes

Vehicle standards

No car manufacturers	

Promoting transport alternatives to cars

National policies to promote walking or cycling	No (subnational)
Investment in bicycle lanes	NA
Investment in foot paths	NA
Traffic-calming measures	NA
Investment for increasing cycling	NA
Disincentives for private car use	NA
National policies to promote public transport	Yes[a]
Subsidized pricing of public transport	Yes
Improving the frequency and coverage of public transport	Yes
Disincentives for private car use	No

[a] Other policies are implemented in addition to those listed.

Vehicle regulations

Compulsory insurance for vehicles	Yes
Periodic vehicle inspection for:	
cars	Yes
motorized 2- or 3-wheeled vehicles	Yes
minibuses and vans	Yes
lorries	Yes
buses	Yes

Registered motor vehicles

Total (2007)	2 283 634
Cars	78%
Motorized 2- and 3-wheelers	4%
Minibuses, vans, etc. (seating <20 people)	14%
Lorries	2%
Buses	1%
Other	1%

Source: Central Bureau of Statistics (based on Ministry of Transport files)

Care after road crashes

Formal, publicly available prehospital care system	Yes
National universal access telephone number	Yes (101)

Acknowledgements

Authority approving the data for publication: Ministry of Health
National data coordinator: Kobi Peleg, National Center Trauma and EM Research; Sarit Levi, National Road Safety Authority (RSA)
Respondents: Rinat Zaig, National Road Safety Authority (RSA); Orit Yalon-Shuqrun, Central Bureau of Statistics (CBS); Tsippy Lotan, Or Yarok (Green Light); Maya Siman-Tov, National Center Trauma and EM Research; Vered Yeshouia, Traffic Department, Israeli Police; Zeev Shadmi, Ministry of Transportation

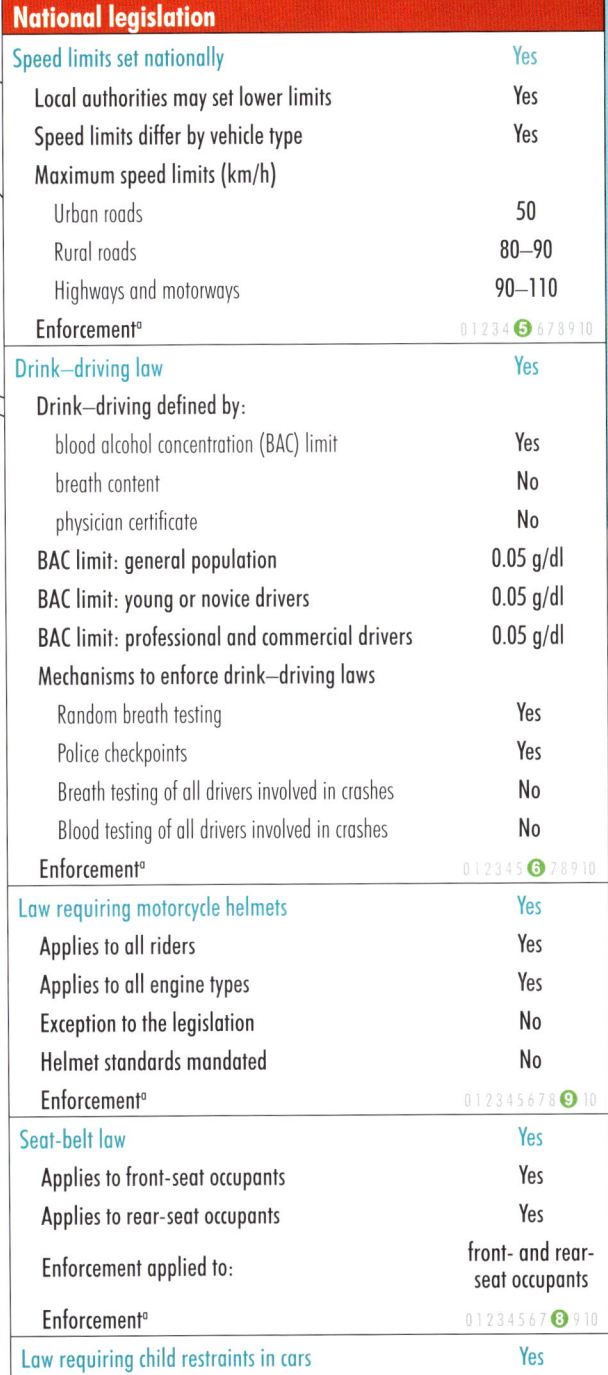

Italy

Population: **58.88 million (2007)**

Median age: **42** years

Life expectancy at birth: **81** years

Income group:[a] **high**

Gross national income per person: **US$ 33 540** Rank: **14** of 49[b]

Human Development Index:[c] **0.945** Rank: **13** of 49[b]

Private car ownership per 1000 population:[d] **610.1**

CO_2 emissions (tonnes) per person per year:[a] **7.7**

[a] World Bank data.
[b] Rank among the 49 countries in the WHO European Region participating in the survey.
[c] United Nations Development Programme data.
[d] WHO European Region average: 339.

Institutional framework for road safety

Lead agency: General Directorate for Road Safety	
Status of the agency	Government
Funded in national budget	Yes
National road safety strategy	Yes
Measurable targets	Yes
Implementation funded	Yes
Money allocated (in € (2008))	53.00 million

Key data

Reported number of road traffic deaths (2006)	5669[a] (77% males, 23% females)
Reported number of non-fatal road traffic injuries (2006)	332 995[b]
Road traffic deaths involving alcohol	No consensus
Wearing motorcycle helmets	60%[c]
Using seat-belts in cars	
Overall	No information
Front-seat occupants	65%[c]
Rear-seat occupants	10%[c]
Costing study available	Yes
Annual estimated costs (in € (2006))	32.24 billion
Study included deaths, injuries or both	Both deaths and injuries
Methods used	Gross output method

[a] National Statistics Office (ISTAT), Automobile Club d'Italia (ACI) data, defined as died within 30 days of the crash.
[b] National Statistics Office (ISTAT), Automobile Club d'Italia (ACI) data.
[c] 2007, Sistema ULISSE – Monitoraggio Nazionale sull'uso dei dispositivi di sicurezza.

NA: not applicable

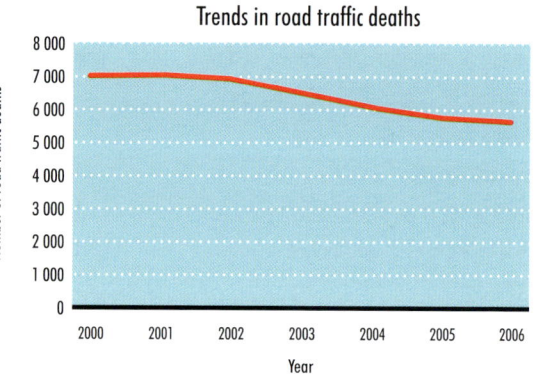

Trends in road traffic deaths

Source: National Statistics Office (ISTAT), Automobile Club d'Italia (ACI)

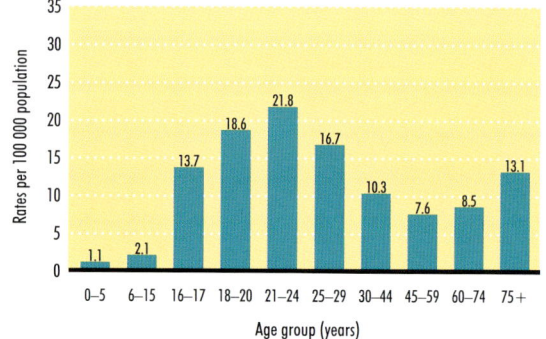

Age-specific mortality rates from road traffic injuries

Source: 2006, National Statistics Office (ISTAT), Automobile Club d'Italia (ACI)

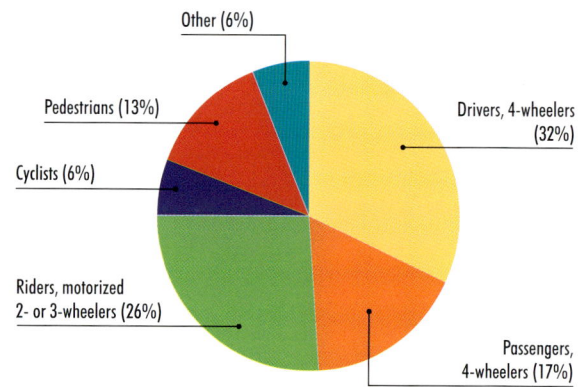

Deaths by road user category

Source: 2006, National Statistics Office (ISTAT), Automobile Club d'Italia (ACI)

National legislation

Speed limits set nationally	Yes
Local authorities may set lower limits	Yes
Speed limits differ by vehicle type	Yes
Maximum speed limits (km/h)	
Urban roads	50
Rural roads	90
Highways and motorways	110–130
Enforcement[a]	0 1 2 3 4 5 6 **7** 8 9 10
Drink–driving law	Yes
Drink–driving defined by:	
blood alcohol concentration (BAC) limit	Yes
breath content	Yes
physician certificate	No
BAC limit: general population	0.05 g/dl
BAC limit: young or novice drivers	0.05 g/dl
BAC limit: professional and commercial drivers	0.05 g/dl
Mechanisms to enforce drink–driving laws	
Random breath testing	Yes
Police checkpoints	Yes
Breath testing of all drivers involved in crashes	Yes
Blood testing of all drivers involved in crashes	Yes
Enforcement[a]	0 1 2 3 4 5 6 **7** 8 9 10
Law requiring motorcycle helmets	Yes
Applies to all riders	Yes
Applies to all engine types	Yes
Exception to the legislation	Yes[b]
Helmet standards mandated	Yes
Enforcement[a]	0 1 2 3 4 5 6 **7** 8 9 10
Seat-belt law	Yes
Applies to front-seat occupants	Yes
Applies to rear-seat occupants	Yes
Enforcement applied to:	front- and rear-seat occupants
Enforcement[a]	0 1 2 3 4 5 6 **7** 8 9 10
Law requiring child restraints in cars	Yes
Enforcement[a]	0 1 2 3 4 5 6 **7** 8 9 10

[a] The enforcement score represents a consensus based on the professional opinion of respondents on a scale of 0 to 10, where 0 is not effective and 10 is highly effective.
[b] Exceptions: 3-, 4-wheelers equipped with a cabin; 2-, 3-wheelers equipped with a crash-proof safety frame or other restraining devices.

Road safety audits

Formal audits required for major new road construction projects	Yes
Regular audits of existing road infrastructure	Yes

Vehicle standards

Car manufacturers required to adhere to standards on	
Fuel consumption	Yes
Seat-belt installation for all seats	Yes

Promoting transport alternatives to cars

National policies to promote walking or cycling	Yes
Investment in bicycle lanes	Yes
Investment in foot paths	No
Traffic-calming measures	No
Investment for increasing cycling	Yes
Disincentives for private car use	No
National policies to promote public transport	Yes
Subsidized pricing of public transport	Yes
Improving the frequency and coverage of public transport	Yes
Disincentives for private car use	Yes

Vehicle regulations

Compulsory insurance for vehicles	Yes
Periodic vehicle inspection for:	
cars	Yes
motorized 2- or 3-wheeled vehicles	Yes
minibuses and vans	Yes
lorries	Yes
buses	Yes

Registered motor vehicles

Total (2008)	43 262 992
Cars	83%
Motorized 2- and 3-wheelers	13%
Lorries	3%
Buses	<1%

Source: Ministry of Transport

Care after road crashes

Formal, publicly available prehospital care system	Yes
National universal access telephone number	Yes (118)

Acknowledgements

Authority approving the data for publication: Ministry of Health
National data coordinator: Maria Giuseppina Lecce, Ministry of Health
Respondents: Vito Disanto, Ministry of Transport; Giandomenico Protospataro, State Police; Raffaella Amato, National Statistics Institute (ISTAT); Alba Rosa Bianchi, Italian National Institute for Occupational Safety and Prevention (ISPESL); Alberto Valenti, Municipal police, Rome

Kazakhstan[a]

Population: **15.42 million (2007)**
Median age: **29** years
Life expectancy at birth: **64** years
Income group:[b] **middle**
Gross national income per person: **US$ 5060**   Rank: **34** of 49[c]
Human Development Index:[d] **0.807**   Rank: **35** of 49[c]
Private car ownership per 1000 population:[e] **157.2**
CO_2 emissions (tonnes) per person per year:[b] **13.3**

[a] Questionnaire completed by National Data Coordinator (no consensus meeting).
[b] World Bank data.
[c] Rank among the 49 countries in the WHO European Region participating in the survey.
[d] United Nations Development Programme data.
[e] WHO European Region average: 339.

Institutional framework for road safety	
Lead agency: Road Police Department	
Status of the agency	Government
Funded in national budget	Yes
National road safety strategy	Yes
Measurable targets	No
Implementation funded	Yes
Money allocated (in € (year))	No information

Trends in road traffic deaths

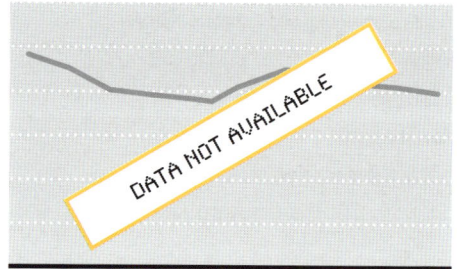

Key data	
Reported number of road traffic deaths (2007)	4365[a] (78% males, 22% females)
Reported number of non-fatal road traffic injuries (2007)	32 988[b]
Road traffic deaths involving alcohol	3.2%[c]
Wearing motorcycle helmets	No information
Using seat-belts in cars	
Overall	No information
Front-seat occupants	No information
Rear-seat occupants	No information
Costing study available	No information
Annual estimated costs (in € (year))	NA
Study included deaths, injuries or both	NA
Methods used	NA

[a] Ministry of Internal Affairs, Health Ministry and Statistics Agency, defined as died within 7 days of the crash.
[b] Health data.
[c] 2007, Ministry of Internal Affairs.

Age-specific mortality rates from road traffic injuries

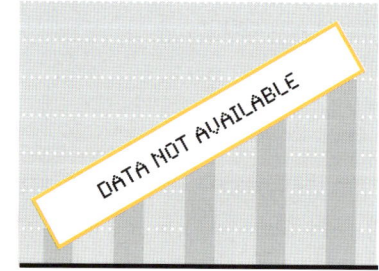

Deaths by road user category

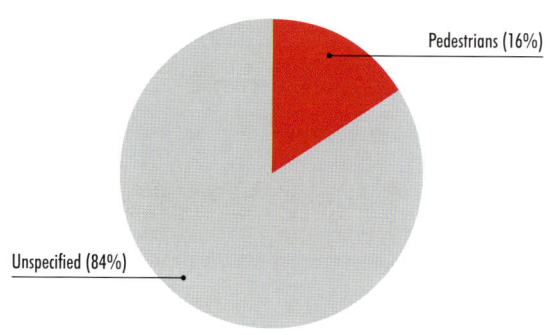

Source: 2007, Ministry of Internal Affairs

NA: not applicable

National legislation

Speed limits set nationally	Yes
Local authorities may set lower limits	No
Speed limits differ by vehicle type	No
Maximum speed limits (km/h)	
Urban roads	60
Rural roads	60
Highways and motorways	120
Enforcement[a]	0 1 2 3 4 **5** 6 7 8 9 10
Drink–driving law	**Yes**
Drink–driving defined by:	
blood alcohol concentration (BAC) limit	No
breath content	No
physician certificate	Yes
BAC limit: general population	None[b]
BAC limit: young or novice drivers	None[b]
BAC limit: professional and commercial drivers	None[b]
Mechanisms to enforce drink–driving laws	
Random breath testing	Yes
Police checkpoints	No
Breath testing of all drivers involved in crashes	Yes
Blood testing of all drivers involved in crashes	Yes
Enforcement[a]	0 1 2 3 4 5 6 7 8 9 **10**
Law requiring motorcycle helmets	**Yes**
Applies to all riders	Yes
Applies to all engine types	No
Exception to the legislation	No information
Helmet standards mandated	No
Enforcement[a]	0 1 2 3 4 **5** 6 7 8 9 10
Seat-belt law	**Yes**
Applies to front-seat occupants	Yes
Applies to rear-seat occupants	Yes
Enforcement applied to:	Driver only
Enforcement[a]	0 1 2 3 4 5 6 **7** 8 9 10
Law requiring child restraints in cars	**Yes**
Enforcement[a]	0 1 2 3 4 5 6 **7** 8 9 10

[a] The enforcement score represents a professional opinion of NDC on a scale of 0 to 10, where 0 is not effective and 10 is highly effective.
[b] Drink-driving not defined by BAC limit.

Road safety audits

Formal audits required for major new road construction projects	Yes
Regular audits of existing road infrastructure	Yes

Vehicle standards

No car manufacturers	

Promoting transport alternatives to cars

National policies to promote walking or cycling	Yes[a]
Investment in bicycle lanes	No
Investment in foot paths	No
Traffic-calming measures	No
Investment for increasing cycling	No
Disincentives for private car use	No
National policies to promote public transport	Yes
Subsidized pricing of public transport	No
Improving the frequency and coverage of public transport	Yes
Disincentives for private car use	Yes

[a] Other policies are implemented in addition to those listed.

Vehicle regulations

Compulsory insurance for vehicles	Yes
Periodic vehicle inspection for:	
cars	Yes
motorized 2- or 3-wheeled vehicles	Yes
minibuses and vans	Yes
lorries	Yes
buses	Yes

Registered motor vehicles

Total (2008)	3 105 954
Cars	79%
Motorized 2- and 3-wheelers	2%
Lorries	13%
Buses	3%
Non-motorized vehicles	4%

Source: Ministry of Internal Affairs

Care after road crashes

Formal, publicly available prehospital care system	Yes
National universal access telephone number	Yes (03)

Acknowledgements

Authority approving the data for publication: Ministry of Health, Traumatology and Orthopedics Scientific Research Institute
National data coordinator: Nurlan Batpenov, Traumatology and Orthopedics Scientific Research Institute
Respondents: Galina Jaxybekova, Traumatology and Orthopedics Scientific Research Institute

Kyrgyzstan

Population: 5.32 million (2007)
Median age: 24 years
Life expectancy at birth: 66 years
Income group:[a] low
Gross national income per person: US$ 590 — Rank: 48 of 49[b]
Human Development Index:[c] 0.694 — Rank: 47 of 49[b]
Private car ownership per 1000 population:[d] No information
CO_2 emissions (tonnes) per person per year:[a] 1.1

[a] World Bank data.
[b] Rank among the 49 countries in the WHO European Region participating in the survey.
[c] United Nations Development Programme data.
[d] WHO European Region average: 339.

Institutional framework for road safety

Lead agency: Commission of Traffic Accident Prevention to the Government of the Kyrgyz Republic	
Status of the agency	Interministerial
Funded in national budget	No
National road safety strategy	Multiple strategies
Measurable targets	NA
Implementation funded	NA
Money allocated (in € (year))	NA

Key data

Reported number of road traffic deaths (2007)	1252[a]
Reported number of non-fatal road traffic injuries (2007)	6223[b]
Road traffic deaths involving alcohol	No information
Wearing motorcycle helmets	No information
Using seat-belts in cars	
Overall	No information
Front-seat occupants	No information
Rear-seat occupants	No information
Costing study available	No
Annual estimated costs (in € (year))	NA
Study included deaths, injuries or both	NA
Methods used	NA

[a] Health and Ministry of Internal Affairs data, defined as died within 1 year of the crash.
[b] Health and Ministry of Internal Affairs data.

NA: not applicable

Trends in road traffic deaths

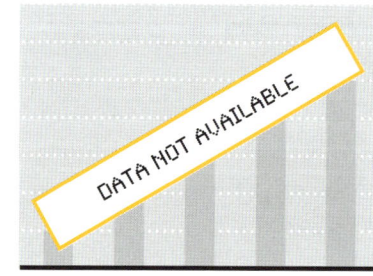

YEAR	NUMBER OF DEATHS
2006	1 051
2007	1 252

Age-specific mortality rates from road traffic injuries

DATA NOT AVAILABLE

Deaths by road user category

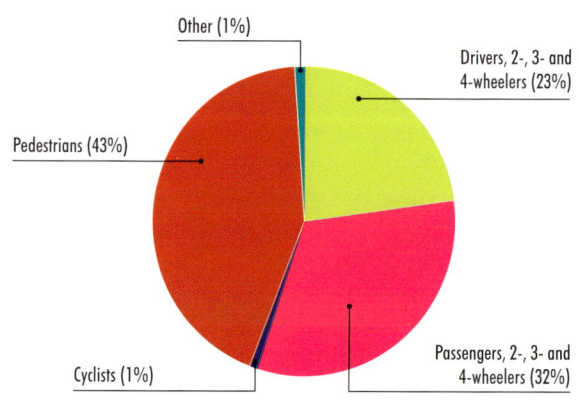

- Other (1%)
- Drivers, 2-, 3- and 4-wheelers (23%)
- Pedestrians (43%)
- Passengers, 2-, 3- and 4-wheelers (32%)
- Cyclists (1%)

Source: 2007, Central Administration of Road Safety to the Ministry of Internal Affairs of the Kyrgyz Republic, Republican Medical Information Center to the Ministry of Public Health of the Kyrgyz Republic

National legislation

Speed limits set nationally	Yes
Local authorities may set lower limits	Yes
Speed limits differ by vehicle type	No information
Maximum speed limits (km/h)	
Urban roads	60
Rural roads	60
Highways and motorways	100
Enforcement[a]	0 1 2 3 4 5 6 **7** 8 9 10
Drink–driving law	Yes
Drink–driving defined by:	
blood alcohol concentration (BAC) limit	No
breath content	Yes
physician certificate	Yes
BAC limit: general population	None[b]
BAC limit: young or novice drivers	None[b]
BAC limit: professional and commercial drivers	None[b]
Mechanisms to enforce drink–driving laws	
Random breath testing	Yes
Police checkpoints	No
Breath testing of all drivers involved in crashes	Yes
Blood testing of all drivers involved in crashes	Yes
Enforcement[a]	0 1 2 3 **4** 5 6 7 8 9 10
Law requiring motorcycle helmets	Yes
Applies to all riders	Yes
Applies to all engine types	Yes
Exception to the legislation	No
Helmet standards mandated	No
Enforcement[a]	0 1 2 3 4 5 6 **7** 8 9 10
Seat-belt law	Yes
Applies to front-seat occupants	Yes
Applies to rear-seat occupants	No
Enforcement applied to:	front-seat occupants only
Enforcement[a]	0 1 2 3 4 **5** 6 7 8 9 10
Law requiring child restraints in cars	No
Enforcement[a]	NA

[a] The enforcement score represents a consensus based on the professional opinion of respondents on a scale of 0 to 10, where 0 is not effective and 10 is highly effective.
[b] Drink–driving not defined by BAC limit.

Promoting transport alternatives to cars

National policies to promote walking or cycling	No
Investment in bicycle lanes	NA
Investment in foot paths	NA
Traffic-calming measures	NA
Investment for increasing cycling	NA
Disincentives for private car use	NA
National policies to promote public transport	Yes
Subsidized pricing of public transport	Yes
Improving the frequency and coverage of public transport	No
Disincentives for private car use	No

Vehicle regulations

Compulsory insurance for vehicles	No
Periodic vehicle inspection for:	
cars	Yes
motorized 2- or 3-wheeled vehicles	Yes
minibuses and vans	Yes
lorries	Yes
buses	Yes

Registered motor vehicles

Total (2007)	318 581
Registered vehicle types: data not available	

Source: Central Administration of Road Safety to the Ministry of Internal Affairs of the Kyrgyz Republic

Care after road crashes

Formal, publicly available prehospital care system	Yes
National universal access telephone number	Yes (103)

Road safety audits

Formal audits required for major new road construction projects	Yes
Regular audits of existing road infrastructure	Yes

Vehicle standards

No car manufacturers	

Acknowledgements

Authority approving the data for publication: Ministry of Health and the Executive Director of Road Safety Under the Kyrgyz Government

National data coordinator: Samatbek Toimatov, Ministry of Public Health of the Kyrgyz Republic

Respondents: Viktor Kustov, Government of the Kyrgyz Republic; Elvira Torobekova, Ministry of Public Health of the Kyrgyz Republic; Zoya Tulegenova, Government of the Kyrgyz Republic; Ludmila Turgasheva, Government of the Kyrgyz Republic; Imanali Sarkulov, Ministry of Internal Affairs of the Kyrgyz Republic; Soolot Begaliev, Ministry of Internal Affairs of the Kyrgyz Republic; Emil Omuraliev, Country WHO office on Coordination and Communications in Kyrgyzstan

Latvia

Population: **2.28 million (2007)**

Median age: **40** years

Life expectancy at birth: **71** years

Income group:[a] **middle**

Gross national income per person: **US$ 9930**   Rank: **27** of 49[b]

Human Development Index:[c] **0.863**   Rank: **27** of 49[b]

Private car ownership per 1000 population:[d] **358.9**

CO_2 emissions (tonnes) per person per year:[a] **3.1**

[a] World Bank data.
[b] Rank among the 49 countries in the WHO European Region participating in the survey.
[c] United Nations Development Programme data.
[d] WHO European Region average: 339.

Institutional framework for road safety

Lead agency: Road Traffic Safety Council	
Status of the agency	Interministerial
Funded in national budget	Yes
National road safety strategy	**Yes**
Measurable targets	Yes
Implementation funded	Yes
Money allocated (in € (2006))	7.33 million

Key data

Reported number of road traffic deaths (2006)	407[a] (76% males, 24% females)
Reported number of non-fatal road traffic injuries (2006)	5404[b]
Road traffic deaths involving alcohol	20.6%[c]
Wearing motorcycle helmets	93% Drivers[d]
Using seat-belts in cars	
Overall	No information
Front-seat occupants	77%[e]
Rear-seat occupants	32%[e]
Costing study available	**Yes**
Annual estimated costs (in € (2006))	191.78 million
Study included deaths, injuries or both	Both deaths and injuries
Methods used	Gross output method

[a] Road Safety Directorate data, defined as died within 30 days of the crash.
[b] Road Safety Directorate data.
[c] 2006, *Statistics of Road Accidents in Latvia*, Road Traffic Safety Directorate.
[d] 2006, Research by Road Traffic Research, LTD, data apply to motorcycles in Riga and Riga region only.
[e] 2006, Observational studies by Road Traffic Research, LTD and Data Serviss, LTD.

NA: not applicable

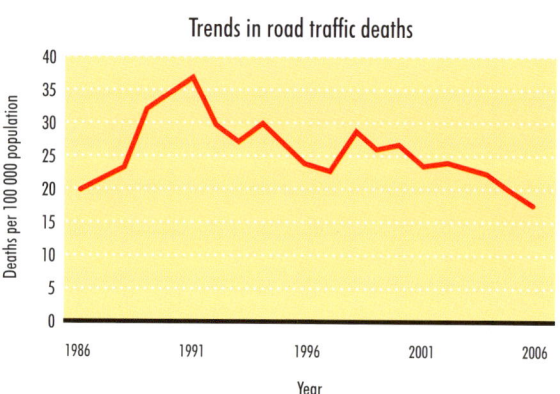

Trends in road traffic deaths

Source: Road Safety Directorate

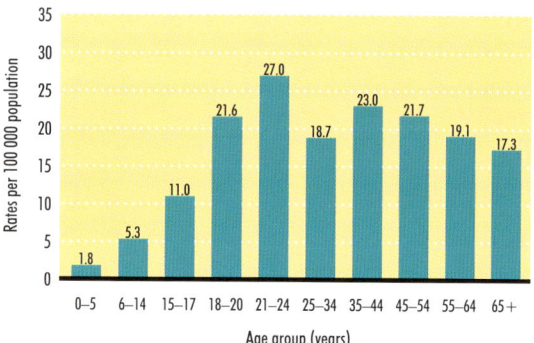

Age-specific mortality rates from road traffic injuries

Source: 2006, *Statistics of Road Traffic Accidents in Latvia 2007*, Road Safety Directorate

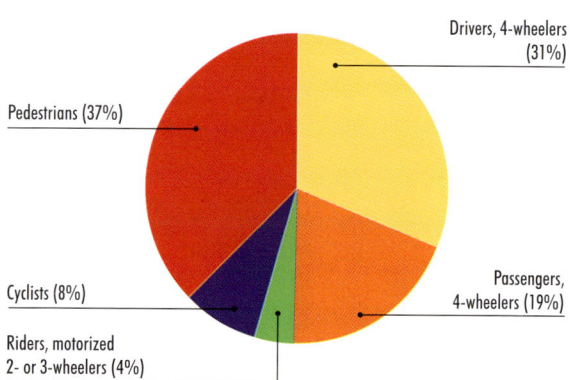

Deaths by road user category

- Drivers, 4-wheelers (31%)
- Passengers, 4-wheelers (19%)
- Riders, motorized 2- or 3-wheelers (4%)
- Cyclists (8%)
- Pedestrians (37%)

Source: 2006, *Statistics of Road Traffic Accidents in Latvia 2007*, Road Safety Directorate

National legislation	
Speed limits set nationally	Yes
Local authorities may set lower limits	Yes
Speed limits differ by vehicle type	Yes
Maximum speed limits (km/h)	
Urban roads	50
Rural roads	90
Highways and motorways	110
Enforcement[a]	0 1 2 3 4 5 6 ⑦ 8 9 10
Drink–driving law	Yes
Drink–driving defined by:	
blood alcohol concentration (BAC) limit	Yes
breath content	No
physician certificate	No
BAC limit: general population	0.05 g/dl
BAC limit: young or novice drivers	0.02 g/dl
BAC limit: professional and commercial drivers	0.05 g/dl
Mechanisms to enforce drink–driving laws	
Random breath testing	Yes
Police checkpoints	No
Breath testing of all drivers involved in crashes	Yes
Blood testing of all drivers involved in crashes	Yes
Enforcement[a]	0 1 2 3 4 5 6 ⑦ 8 9 10
Law requiring motorcycle helmets	Yes
Applies to all riders	Yes
Applies to all engine types	Yes
Exception to the legislation	No
Helmet standards mandated	No
Enforcement[a]	0 1 2 3 4 5 ⑥ 7 8 9 10
Seat-belt law	Yes
Applies to front-seat occupants	Yes
Applies to rear-seat occupants	Yes
Enforcement applied to:	front- and rear-seat occupants
Enforcement[a]	0 1 2 3 4 5 6 ⑦ 8 9 10
Law requiring child restraints in cars	Yes
Enforcement[a]	0 1 2 3 4 5 ⑥ 7 8 9 10

[a] The enforcement score represents a consensus based on the professional opinion of respondents on a scale of 0 to 10, where 0 is not effective and 10 is highly effective.

Road safety audits	
Formal audits required for major new road construction projects	Yes
Regular audits of existing road infrastructure	Yes

Vehicle standards	
No car manufacturers	

Promoting transport alternatives to cars	
National policies to promote walking or cycling	No (subnational)
Investment in bicycle lanes	NA
Investment in foot paths	NA
Traffic-calming measures	NA
Investment for increasing cycling	NA
Disincentives for private car use	NA
National policies to promote public transport	No (subnational)
Subsidized pricing of public transport	NA
Improving the frequency and coverage of public transport	NA
Disincentives for private car use	NA

Vehicle regulations	
Compulsory insurance for vehicles	Yes
Periodic vehicle inspection for:	
cars	Yes
motorized 2- or 3-wheeled vehicles	Yes
minibuses and vans	Yes
lorries	Yes
buses	Yes

Registered motor vehicles	
Total (2006)	1 062 935
Cars	77%
Motorized 2- and 3-wheelers	4%
Lorries	11%
Buses	1%
Other	7%

Source: Road Safety Directorate

Care after road crashes	
Formal, publicly available prehospital care system	Yes
National universal access telephone number	Yes (112)

Acknowledgements

Authority approving the data for publication: Ministry of Health
National data coordinator: Jana Feldmane, Ministry of Health, Head of the Division of Environmental Health
Respondents: Aldis Lama, Road Traffic Directorate; Georgijs Sovetovs, Riga's City Council Department of Transport; Jolanta Skrule, Public Health Agency; Maija Gaide, Health Statistics and Medical Technologies State Agency; Vida Lukasevica, Central Statistical Bureau; Arnis Vilums, State Policy; Anita Villerusa, Riga's Stradina University

Lithuania

Population: **3.39 million (2007)**

Median age: **38** years

Life expectancy at birth: **71** years

Income group:[a] **middle**

Gross national income per person: **US$ 9920**   Rank: **28** of 49[b]

Human Development Index:[c] **0.869**   Rank: **26** of 49[b]

Private car ownership per 1000 population:[d] **467.4**

CO_2 emissions (tonnes) per person per year:[a] **3.9**

[a] World Bank data.
[b] Rank among the 49 countries in the WHO European Region participating in the survey.
[c] United Nations Development Programme data.
[d] WHO European Region average: 339.

Institutional framework for road safety	
Lead agency: State Traffic Safety Commission	
Status of the agency	Interministerial
Funded in national budget	No
National road safety strategy	Yes
Measurable targets	Yes
Implementation funded	Yes
Money allocated (in € (2007))	5.69 million

Key data	
Reported number of road traffic deaths (2006)	759[a] (72% males, 26% females)[b]
Reported number of non-fatal road traffic injuries (2006)	8254[c]
Road traffic deaths involving alcohol	11.7%[d]
Wearing motorcycle helmets	No information
Using seat-belts in cars	
Overall	No information
Front-seat occupants	No information
Rear-seat occupants	No information
Costing study available	Yes
Annual estimated costs (in € (2006))	434.86 million
Study included deaths, injuries or both	Both deaths and injuries
Methods used	No information

[a] Police data, defined as died within 30 days of the crash.
[b] Unknown gender 2%.
[c] Police data.
[d] 2006, Police Department (Ministry of Interior).

NA: not applicable

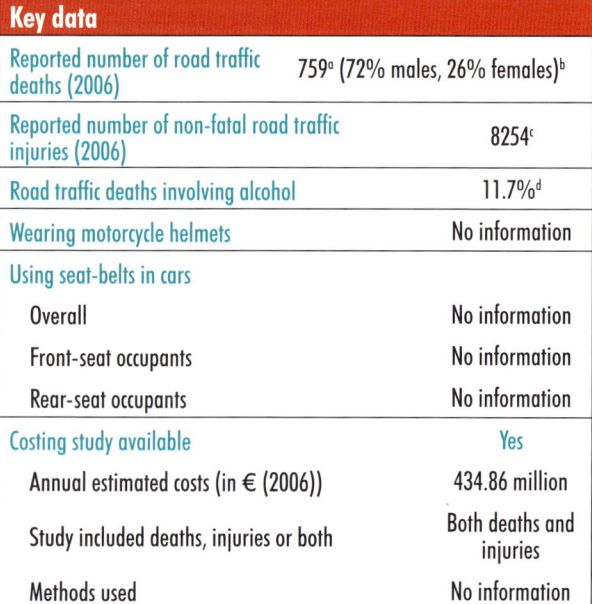

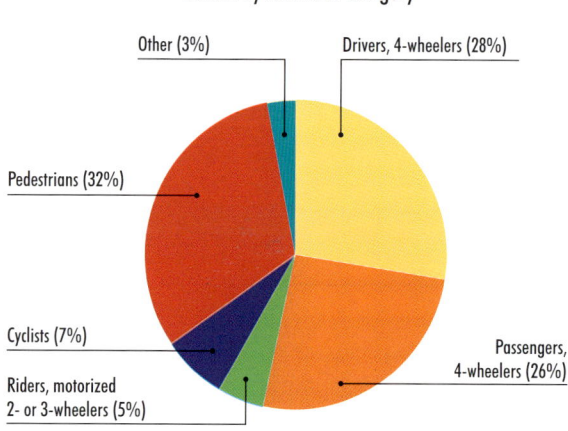

88   EUROPEAN STATUS REPORT ON ROAD SAFETY

National legislation

Speed limits set nationally	Yes
Local authorities may set lower limits	Yes
Speed limits differ by vehicle type	Yes
Maximum speed limits (km/h)	
Urban roads	50
Rural roads	90
Highways and motorways	130
Enforcement[a]	0 1 2 3 4 5 ⑥ 7 8 9 10
Drink–driving law	Yes
Drink–driving defined by:	
blood alcohol concentration (BAC) limit	Yes
breath content	No
physician certificate	No
BAC limit: general population	0.04 g/dl
BAC limit: young or novice drivers	0.02 g/dl
BAC limit: professional and commercial drivers	0.02 g/dl
Mechanisms to enforce drink–driving laws	
Random breath testing	Yes
Police checkpoints	Yes
Breath testing of all drivers involved in crashes	No
Blood testing of all drivers involved in crashes	No
Enforcement[a]	0 1 2 3 4 5 ⑥ 7 8 9 10
Law requiring motorcycle helmets	Yes
Applies to all riders	Yes
Applies to all engine types	Yes
Exception to the legislation	No
Helmet standards mandated	No
Enforcement[a]	0 1 2 3 4 5 ⑥ 7 8 9 10
Seat-belt law	Yes
Applies to front-seat occupants	Yes
Applies to rear-seat occupants	Yes
Enforcement applied to:	front- and rear-seat occupants
Enforcement[a]	0 1 2 3 4 5 ⑥ 7 8 9 10
Law requiring child restraints in cars	Yes
Enforcement[a]	0 1 2 3 4 ⑤ 6 7 8 9 10

[a] The enforcement score represents a consensus based on the professional opinion of respondents on a scale of 0 to 10, where 0 is not effective and 10 is highly effective.

Road safety audits

Formal audits required for major new road construction projects	Yes
Regular audits of existing road infrastructure	Yes

Vehicle standards

No car manufacturers	

Promoting transport alternatives to cars

National policies to promote walking or cycling	Yes
Investment in bicycle lanes	Yes
Investment in foot paths	Yes
Traffic-calming measures	No
Investment for increasing cycling	No
Disincentives for private car use	No
National policies to promote public transport	No (subnational)
Subsidized pricing of public transport	NA
Improving the frequency and coverage of public transport	NA
Disincentives for private car use	NA

Vehicle regulations

Compulsory insurance for vehicles	Yes
Periodic vehicle inspection for:	
cars	Yes
motorized 2- or 3-wheeled vehicles	Yes
minibuses and vans	Yes
lorries	Yes
buses	Yes

Registered motor vehicles

Total (2006)	1 781 686
Cars	89%
Motorized 2- and 3-wheelers	1%
Lorries	8%
Buses	1%
Other	1%

Source: State Enterprise REGITRA

Care after road crashes

Formal, publicly available prehospital care system	Yes
National universal access telephone number	Yes (112)

Acknowledgements

Authority approving the data for publication: Ministry of Health
National data coordinator: Ramunė Meižienė, Ministry of Health
Respondents: Gintaras Aliksandravičius, Lithuanian Police Traffic Supervision Service; Marius Vitėnas, Ministry of Transport and Communications of the Republic of Lithuania; Jelena Selivonec, Lithuanian Statistics; Aušra Želvienė, Lithuanian Health Information Centre; Aida Laukaitienė, State Environmental Health Center

Malta

Population: 0.41 million (2007)
Median age: 38 years
Life expectancy at birth: 79 years
Income group:[a] high
Gross national income per person: US$ 14 575   Rank: 21 of 49[b]
Human Development Index:[c] 0.894   Rank: 21 of 49[b]
Private car ownership per 1000 population:[d] 647.0
CO_2 emissions (tonnes) per person per year:[a] No information

[a] World Bank data.
[b] Rank among the 49 countries in the WHO European Region participating in the survey.
[c] United Nations Development Programme data.
[d] WHO European Region average: 339.

Institutional framework for road safety

Lead agency: Malta Transport Authority	
Status of the agency	Government
Funded in national budget	Yes
National road safety strategy	Multiple strategies
Measurable targets	NA
Implementation funded	NA
Money allocated (in € (year))	NA

Key data

Reported number of road traffic deaths (2007)	14[a] (79% males, 21% females)
Reported number of non-fatal road traffic injuries (2007)	1195[b]
Road traffic deaths involving alcohol	No information
Wearing motorcycle helmets	No information
Using seat-belts in cars	
Overall	No information
Front-seat occupants	96%[c]
Rear-seat occupants	21%[c]
Costing study available	No
Annual estimated costs (in € (year))	NA
Study included deaths, injuries or both	NA
Methods used	NA

[a] Police data, defined as died within 30 days of the crash; Health data, defined by ICD-10 codes.
[b] Police data.
[c] 2006, Malta Transport Authority survey.

NA: not applicable

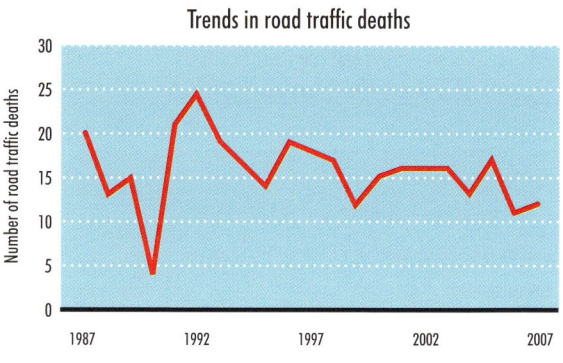

Trends in road traffic deaths

Source: Country questionnaire

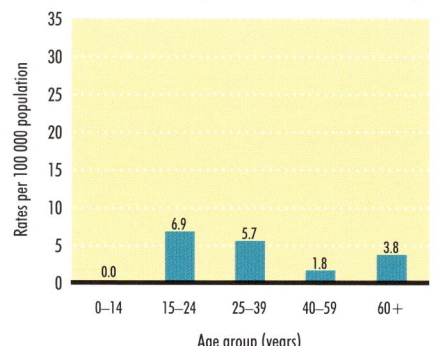

Age-specific mortality rates from road traffic injuries

Source: 2007, National Statistics Office Library and Information Unit

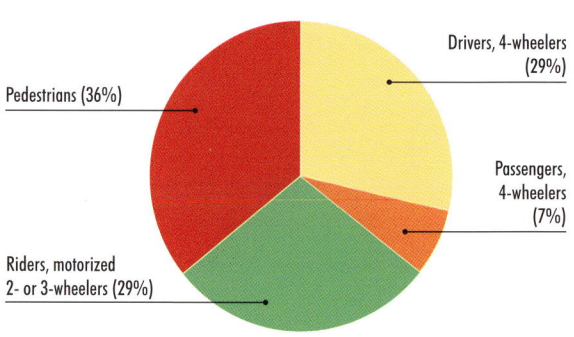

Deaths by road user category

Source: 2007, Malta Police, published by the National Statistics Office

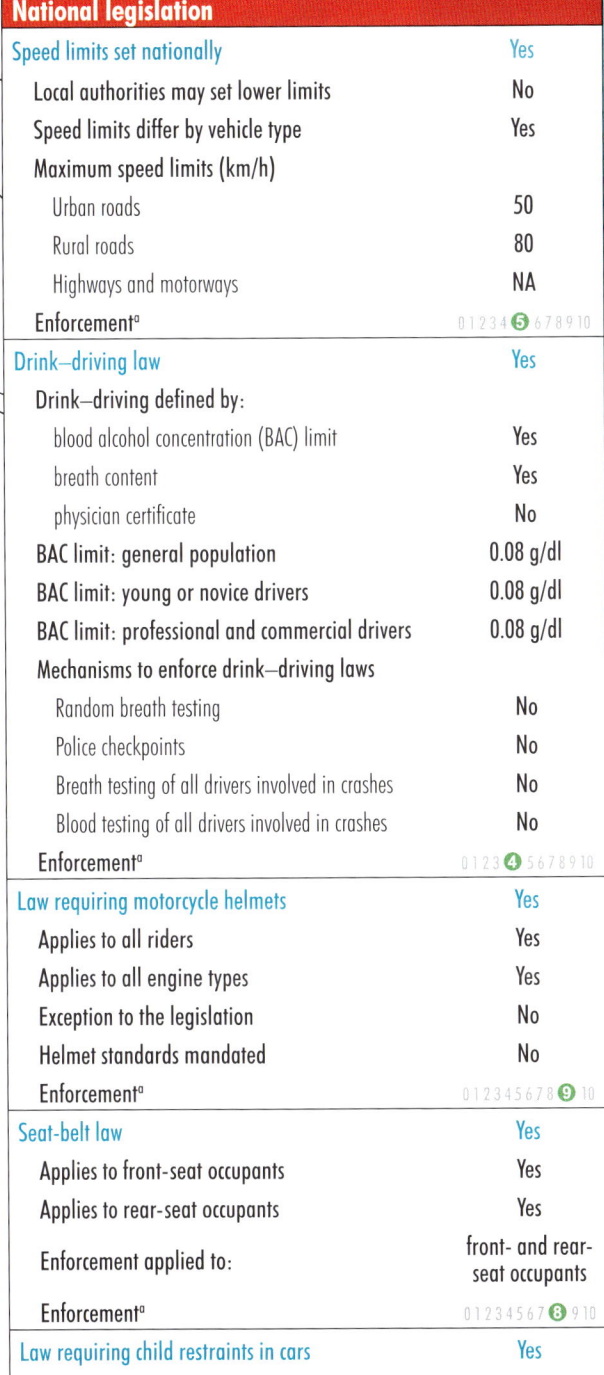

National legislation	
Speed limits set nationally	Yes
Local authorities may set lower limits	No
Speed limits differ by vehicle type	Yes
Maximum speed limits (km/h)	
Urban roads	50
Rural roads	80
Highways and motorways	NA
Enforcement[a]	0 1 2 3 4 ⑤ 6 7 8 9 10
Drink–driving law	Yes
Drink–driving defined by:	
blood alcohol concentration (BAC) limit	Yes
breath content	Yes
physician certificate	No
BAC limit: general population	0.08 g/dl
BAC limit: young or novice drivers	0.08 g/dl
BAC limit: professional and commercial drivers	0.08 g/dl
Mechanisms to enforce drink–driving laws	
Random breath testing	No
Police checkpoints	No
Breath testing of all drivers involved in crashes	No
Blood testing of all drivers involved in crashes	No
Enforcement[a]	0 1 2 3 ④ 5 6 7 8 9 10
Law requiring motorcycle helmets	Yes
Applies to all riders	Yes
Applies to all engine types	Yes
Exception to the legislation	No
Helmet standards mandated	No
Enforcement[a]	0 1 2 3 4 5 6 7 8 ⑨ 10
Seat-belt law	Yes
Applies to front-seat occupants	Yes
Applies to rear-seat occupants	Yes
Enforcement applied to:	front- and rear-seat occupants
Enforcement[a]	0 1 2 3 4 5 6 7 ⑧ 9 10
Law requiring child restraints in cars	Yes
Enforcement[a]	0 1 2 3 4 5 ⑥ 7 8 9 10

[a] The enforcement score represents a consensus based on the professional opinion of respondents on a scale of 0 to 10, where 0 is not effective and 10 is highly effective.

Road safety audits	
Formal audits required for major new road construction projects	No
Regular audits of existing road infrastructure	No

Vehicle standards	
No car manufacturers	

Promoting transport alternatives to cars	
National policies to promote walking or cycling	No
Investment in bicycle lanes	NA
Investment in foot paths	NA
Traffic-calming measures	NA
Investment for increasing cycling	NA
Disincentives for private car use	NA
National policies to promote public transport	Yes
Subsidized pricing of public transport	Yes
Improving the frequency and coverage of public transport	Yes
Disincentives for private car use	Yes

Vehicle regulations	
Compulsory insurance for vehicles	Yes
Periodic vehicle inspection for:	
cars	Yes
motorized 2- or 3-wheeled vehicles	No
minibuses and vans	Yes
lorries	Yes
buses	Yes

Registered motor vehicles	
Total (2007)	346 118
Cars	76%
Motorized 2- and 3-wheelers	6%
Minibuses, vans, etc. (seating <20 people)	<1%
Lorries	17%
Buses	<1%
Other	1%

Source: Malta Transport Authority

Care after road crashes	
Formal, publicly available prehospital care system	Yes
National universal access telephone number	Yes (112)

Acknowledgements

Authority approving the data for publication: Parliamentary Secretary for Health
National data coordinator: Neville Calleja, Department of Health Information and Research; Audrey Galea, Department of Health Information and Research
Respondents: Joseph Galea, National Statistics Office; Therese Ciantar, Malta Transport Authority; Josie Brincat, Malta Police; Maryanne Massa, Deptartment of Health Promotion and Disease Prevention; Kathleen England, Department of Health Information and Research

Montenegro

Population: 0.60 million (2007)
Median age: 35 years
Life expectancy at birth: 74 years
Income group:[a] middle
Gross national income per person: US$ 5180   Rank: 33 of 49[b]
Human Development Index:[c] 0.822   Rank: 31 of 49[b]
Private car ownership per 1000 population:[d] 298.5
CO_2 emissions (tonnes) per person per year:[a] No information

[a] World Bank data.
[b] Rank among the 49 countries in the WHO European Region participating in the survey.
[c] United Nations Development Programme data.
[d] WHO European Region average: 339.

Institutional framework for road safety	
Lead agency:	No
Status of the agency	NA
Funded in national budget	NA
National road safety strategy	No
Measurable targets	NA
Implementation funded	NA
Money allocated (in € (year))	NA

Key data	
Reported number of road traffic deaths (2007)	122[a] (82% males, 18% females)
Reported number of non-fatal road traffic injuries (2007)	2796[b]
Road traffic deaths involving alcohol	No information
Wearing motorcycle helmets	No information
Using seat-belts in cars	
Overall	No information
Front-seat occupants	No information
Rear-seat occupants	No information
Costing study available	No
Annual estimated costs (in € (year))	NA
Study included deaths, injuries or both	NA
Methods used	NA

[a] Police data, defined as died within 30 days of the crash.
[b] Police data.

NA: not applicable

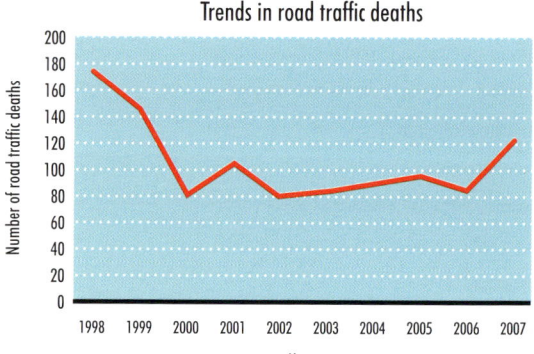

Trends in road traffic deaths

Source: Police Directorate, Department for Road Safety Surveillance and Control

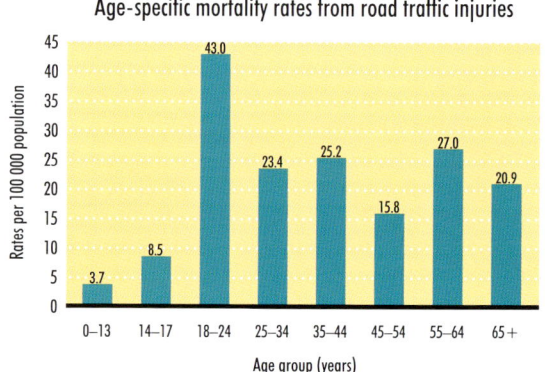

Age-specific mortality rates from road traffic injuries

Source: 2007, Police Directorate, Department for Road Safety Surveillance and Control

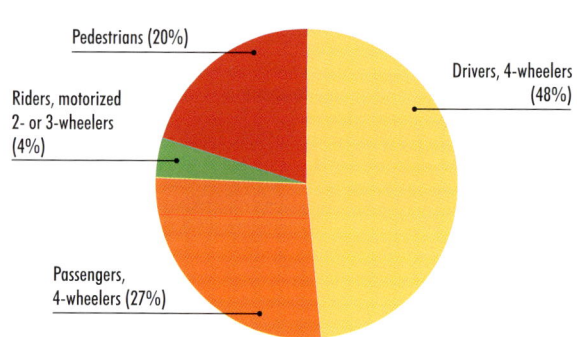

Deaths by road user category

- Pedestrians (20%)
- Riders, motorized 2- or 3-wheelers (4%)
- Passengers, 4-wheelers (27%)
- Drivers, 4-wheelers (48%)

Source: 2007, Police Directorate, Department for Road Safety Surveillance and Control

National legislation	
Speed limits set nationally	Yes
Local authorities may set lower limits	Yes
Speed limits differ by vehicle type	Yes
Maximum speed limits (km/h)	
Urban roads	50
Rural roads	80
Highways and motorways	100
Enforcement[a]	0 1 2 3 4 5 **6** 7 8 9 10
Drink–driving law	Yes
Drink–driving defined by:	
blood alcohol concentration (BAC) limit	Yes
breath content	Yes
physician certificate	Yes
BAC limit: general population	0.05 g/dl
BAC limit: young or novice drivers	0.05 g/dl
BAC limit: professional and commercial drivers	0.00 g/dl
Mechanisms to enforce drink–driving laws	
Random breath testing	Yes
Police checkpoints	No
Breath testing of all drivers involved in crashes	Yes
Blood testing of all drivers involved in crashes	Yes
Enforcement[a]	0 1 2 3 4 5 **6** 7 8 9 10
Law requiring motorcycle helmets	Yes
Applies to all riders	Yes
Applies to all engine types	Yes
Exception to the legislation	No
Helmet standards mandated	No
Enforcement[a]	0 1 2 3 4 5 **6** 7 8 9 10
Seat-belt law	Yes
Applies to front-seat occupants	Yes
Applies to rear-seat occupants	Yes
Enforcement applied to:	front- and rear-seat occupants
Enforcement[a]	0 1 2 3 4 5 **6** 7 8 9 10
Law requiring child restraints in cars	No
Enforcement[a]	NA

[a] The enforcement score represents a consensus based on the professional opinion of respondents on a scale of 0 to 10, where 0 is not effective and 10 is highly effective.

Road safety audits	
Formal audits required for major new road construction projects	Yes
Regular audits of existing road infrastructure	Yes

Vehicle standards	
No car manufacturers	

Promoting transport alternatives to cars	
National policies to promote walking or cycling	No
Investment in bicycle lanes	NA
Investment in foot paths	NA
Traffic-calming measures	NA
Investment for increasing cycling	NA
Disincentives for private car use	NA
National policies to promote public transport	No
Subsidized pricing of public transport	NA
Improving the frequency and coverage of public transport	NA
Disincentives for private car use	NA

Vehicle regulations	
Compulsory insurance for vehicles	Yes
Periodic vehicle inspection for:	
cars	Yes
motorized 2- or 3-wheeled vehicles	Yes
minibuses and vans	Yes
lorries	Yes
buses	Yes

Registered motor vehicles	
Total (2007)	199 014
Cars	90%
Motorized 2- and 3-wheelers	2%
Minibuses, vans, etc. (seating <20 people)	<1%
Lorries	6%
Buses	<1%
Other	2%

Source: Ministry of Interior Affairs and Public Administration

Care after road crashes	
Formal, publicly available prehospital care system	Yes
National universal access telephone number	Yes (124)

Acknowledgements

Authority approving the data for publication: Ministry of Health, Labour and Social Welfare
National data coordinator: Svetlana Stojanovic, Ministry of Health, Labour and Social Welfare
Respondents: Saša Stefanovic, Emergency Medical Department, Podgorica; Dijana Subotic, Ministry of Interior Affairs and Public Administration; Nevenka Tomic, Ministry of Maritime Affairs, Transportation and Telecommunication; Klikovac Dragan, Police Directorate; Sovjetka Veljic, Statistical Office of Montenegro (MONSTAT); Slobodan Tadic, NGO ALPHA Center

Netherlands

Population: 16.42 million (2007)
Median age: 39 years
Life expectancy at birth: 80 years
Income group:[a] high
Gross national income per person: US$ 45 820   Rank: 6 of 49[b]
Human Development Index:[c] 0.958   Rank: 4 of 49[b]
Private car ownership per 1000 population:[d] 440.5
CO_2 emissions (tonnes) per person per year:[a] 8.7

[a] World Bank data.
[b] Rank among the 49 countries in the WHO European Region participating in the survey.
[c] United Nations Development Programme data.
[d] WHO European Region average: 339.

Institutional framework for road safety

Lead agency: Ministry of Transport, Public Works and Water Management, Directorate-General Passenger Transport, Road Safety Division	
Status of the agency	Government
Funded in national budget	Yes
National road safety strategy	**Yes**
Measurable targets	Yes
Implementation funded	Yes
Money allocated (in € (2008))	80.00 million

Key data

Reported number of road traffic deaths (2007)	791[a] (73% males, 27% females)
Reported number of non-fatal road traffic injuries (2007)	16 750[b]
Road traffic deaths involving alcohol	25.0%[c]
Wearing motorcycle helmets	92% Drivers; 72% Passengers[d]
Using seat-belts in cars	
Overall	92%[e]
Front-seat occupants	94%[e]
Rear-seat occupants	73%[e]
Costing study available	**Yes**
Annual estimated costs (in € (2003))	12.30 billion
Study included deaths, injuries or both	Both deaths and injuries
Methods used	Gross output method; Willingness to pay

[a] *Road Safety in the Netherlands: Key Figures 2008*, Ministry of Transport, Water and Public Works, defined as died within 30 days of the crash.
[b] Transport data, data apply to hospitalized subjects.
[c] 2005, Case-control study in Tilburg police district, data apply to drivers only.
[d] *Monitoring Bromfietshelmen 2007*, Grontmij Transport and Infrastructure, data apply to mopeds only.
[e] 2006, *Road Safety in the Netherlands: Key Figures 2008*, Ministry of Transport, Water and Public Work.

NA: not applicable

Trends in road traffic deaths

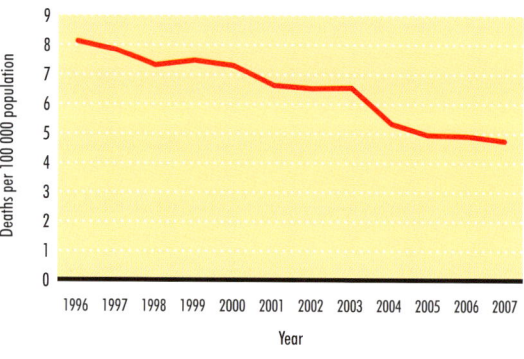

Source: 2007, Statistics Netherlands (CBS), Ministry of Transport

Age-specific mortality rates from road traffic injuries

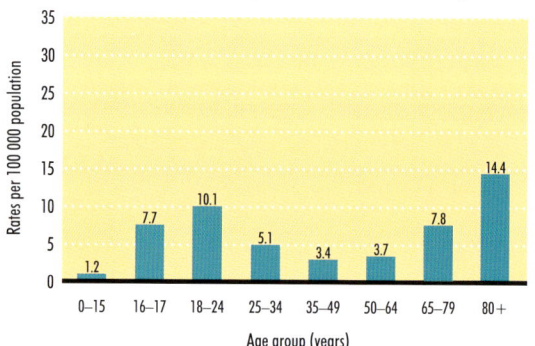

Source: 2007, Ministry of Transport, Public Works and Water Management, Centre for Traffic and Navigation (DVS), Statistics Netherlands (CBS)

Deaths by road user category

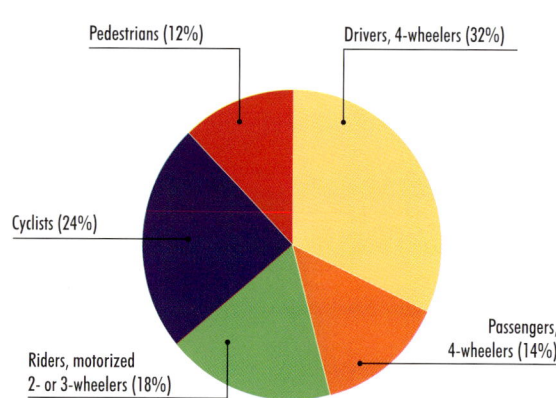

Pedestrians (12%)
Drivers, 4-wheelers (32%)
Cyclists (24%)
Passengers, 4-wheelers (14%)
Riders, motorized 2- or 3-wheelers (18%)

Source: 2007, Institute for Road Safety Research (SWOV), Statistics Netherlands (CBS)

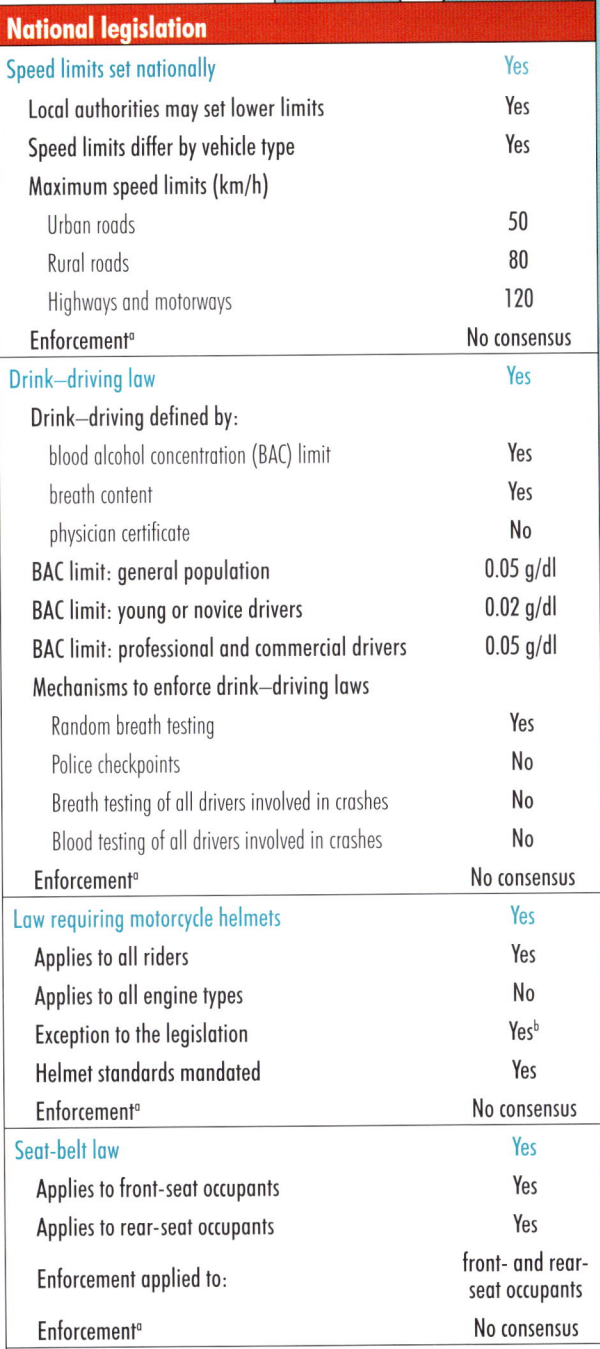

National legislation	
Speed limits set nationally	Yes
Local authorities may set lower limits	Yes
Speed limits differ by vehicle type	Yes
Maximum speed limits (km/h)	
Urban roads	50
Rural roads	80
Highways and motorways	120
Enforcement[a]	No consensus
Drink–driving law	Yes
Drink–driving defined by:	
blood alcohol concentration (BAC) limit	Yes
breath content	Yes
physician certificate	No
BAC limit: general population	0.05 g/dl
BAC limit: young or novice drivers	0.02 g/dl
BAC limit: professional and commercial drivers	0.05 g/dl
Mechanisms to enforce drink–driving laws	
Random breath testing	Yes
Police checkpoints	No
Breath testing of all drivers involved in crashes	No
Blood testing of all drivers involved in crashes	No
Enforcement[a]	No consensus
Law requiring motorcycle helmets	Yes
Applies to all riders	Yes
Applies to all engine types	No
Exception to the legislation	Yes[b]
Helmet standards mandated	Yes
Enforcement[a]	No consensus
Seat-belt law	Yes
Applies to front-seat occupants	Yes
Applies to rear-seat occupants	Yes
Enforcement applied to:	front- and rear-seat occupants
Enforcement[a]	No consensus
Law requiring child restraints in cars	Yes
Enforcement[a]	No consensus

[a] The enforcement score represents a consensus based on the professional opinion of respondents on a scale of 0 to 10, where 0 is not effective and 10 is highly effective.
[b] Exceptions: light moped.

Road safety audits	
Formal audits required for major new road construction projects	No
Regular audits of existing road infrastructure	No

Vehicle standards	
No car manufacturers	

Promoting transport alternatives to cars	
National policies to promote walking or cycling	Yes[a]
Investment in bicycle lanes	Yes
Investment in foot paths	No
Traffic-calming measures	Yes
Investment for increasing cycling	Yes
Disincentives for private car use	No
National policies to promote public transport	Yes
Subsidized pricing of public transport	Yes
Improving the frequency and coverage of public transport	No
Disincentives for private car use	Yes

[a] Other policies are implemented in addition to those listed.

Vehicle regulations	
Compulsory insurance for vehicles	Yes
Periodic vehicle inspection for:	
cars	Yes
motorized 2- or 3-wheeled vehicles	No
minibuses and vans	Yes
lorries	Yes
buses	Yes

Registered motor vehicles	
Total (2007)	8 862 935
Cars	82%
Motorized 2- and 3-wheelers	6%
Lorries	2%
Buses	<1%
Other	10%

Source: Institute for Road Safety Research (SWOV), Statistics Netherlands (CBS)

Care after road crashes	
Formal, publicly available prehospital care system	Yes
National universal access telephone number	Yes (112)

Acknowledgements

Authority approving the data for publication: Institute for Road Safety Research (SWOV); Ministry of Health, Welfare and Sport; Bureau of Traffic Law Enforcement; Ministry of Transport, Water Mangement and Public Works
National data coordinator: Martijn Vis, Institute for Road Safety Research (SWOV)
Respondents: Niels Bos, Institute for Road Safety Research (SWOV); Peter van Vilet, Ministry of Transport, Public Works and Water Management, Centre for Traffic and Navigation (DVS); Harry Derriks, KiM Netherlands Institute for Transport Policy Analysis; Loek Hesemans, Ministry of Health, Welfare and Sport, Nutrition, Health Protection and Prevention Department; B. Van Bruggen, Public Prosecutors Office

Norway

Population: **4.70 million (2007)**

Median age: **38** years

Life expectancy at birth: **80** years

Income group:[a] **high**

Gross national income per person: **US$ 76 450**   Rank: **1** of 49[b]

Human Development Index:[c] **0.968**   Rank: **2** of 49[b]

Private car ownership per 1000 population:[d] **442.7**

CO_2 emissions (tonnes) per person per year:[a] **19.1**

[a] World Bank data.
[b] Rank among the 49 countries in the WHO European Region participating in the survey.
[c] United Nations Development Programme data.
[d] WHO European Region average: 339.

Institutional framework for road safety

Lead agency: Ministry of Transport and Communications	
Status of the agency	Government
Funded in national budget	Yes
National road safety strategy	Yes
Measurable targets	Yes
Implementation funded	Yes
Money allocated (in € (2007))	103.42 million

Key data

Reported number of road traffic deaths (2007)	233[a] (70% males, 30% females)
Reported number of non-fatal road traffic injuries (2007)	11 755[b]
Road traffic deaths involving alcohol	20.0–30.0%[c]
Wearing motorcycle helmets	100%[c]
Using seat-belts in cars	
Overall	88%[c]
Front-seat occupants	93%[c]
Rear-seat occupants	85%[c]
Costing study available	Yes
Annual estimated costs (in € (2008))	3.75 billion
Study included deaths, injuries or both	Both deaths and injuries
Methods used	Gross output method

[a] Statistics Norway data, defined as died within 30 days of the crash.
[b] Statistics Norway data.
[c] 2007, Norwegian Public Roads Administration.

NA: not applicable

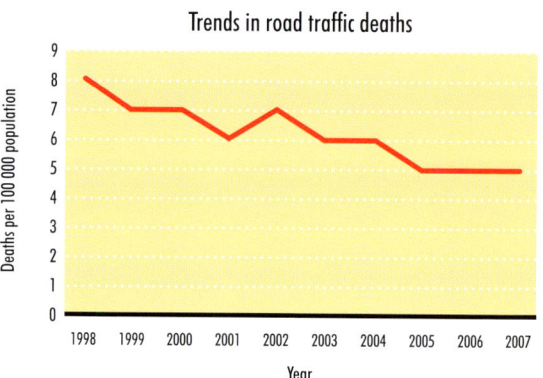

Trends in road traffic deaths

Source: Statistics Norway

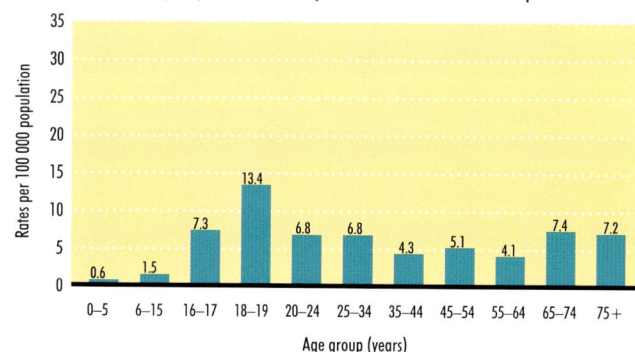

Age-specific mortality rates from road traffic injuries

Source: 2007, Statistics Norway

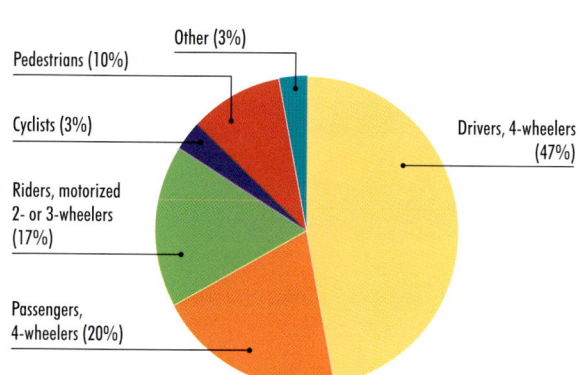

Deaths by road user category

- Pedestrians (10%)
- Other (3%)
- Cyclists (3%)
- Riders, motorized 2- or 3-wheelers (17%)
- Passengers, 4-wheelers (20%)
- Drivers, 4-wheelers (47%)

Source: 2007, Statistics Norway

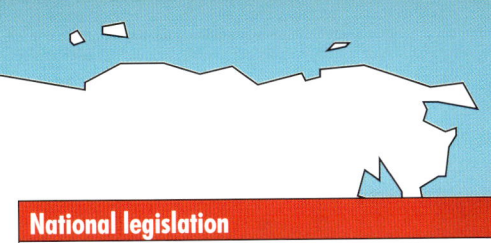

National legislation	
Speed limits set nationally	Yes
Local authorities may set lower limits	Yes
Speed limits differ by vehicle type	Yes
Maximum speed limits (km/h)	
Urban roads	50
Rural roads	80
Highways and motorways	80
Enforcement[a]	0 1 2 3 4 5 **6** 7 8 9 10
Drink–driving law	Yes
Drink–driving defined by:	
blood alcohol concentration (BAC) limit	Yes
breath content	Yes
physician certificate	No
BAC limit: general population	0.02 g/dl
BAC limit: young or novice drivers	0.02 g/dl
BAC limit: professional and commercial drivers	0.02 g/dl
Mechanisms to enforce drink–driving laws	
Random breath testing	Yes
Police checkpoints	Yes
Breath testing of all drivers involved in crashes	No
Blood testing of all drivers involved in crashes	No
Enforcement[a]	0 1 2 3 **4** 5 6 7 8 9 10
Law requiring motorcycle helmets	Yes
Applies to all riders	Yes
Applies to all engine types	Yes
Exception to the legislation	No
Helmet standards mandated	Yes
Enforcement[a]	0 1 2 3 4 5 6 7 8 **9** 10
Seat-belt law	Yes
Applies to front-seat occupants	Yes
Applies to rear-seat occupants	Yes
Enforcement applied to:	front- and rear-seat occupants
Enforcement[a]	0 1 2 3 4 5 **6** 7 8 9 10
Law requiring child restraints in cars	Yes
Enforcement[a]	0 1 2 3 4 5 6 7 8 **9** 10

[a] The enforcement score represents a consensus based on the professional opinion of respondents on a scale of 0 to 10, where 0 is not effective and 10 is highly effective.

Road safety audits	
Formal audits required for major new road construction projects	Yes
Regular audits of existing road infrastructure	Yes

Vehicle standards	
Car manufacturers required to adhere to standards on	
Fuel consumption	No
Seat-belt installation for all seats	Yes

Promoting transport alternatives to cars	
National policies to promote walking or cycling	Yes
Investment in bicycle lanes	Yes
Investment in foot paths	Yes
Traffic-calming measures	Yes
Investment for increasing cycling	No
Disincentives for private car use	No
National policies to promote public transport	Yes
Subsidized pricing of public transport	Yes
Improving the frequency and coverage of public transport	Yes
Disincentives for private car use	No

Vehicle regulations	
Compulsory insurance for vehicles	Yes
Periodic vehicle inspection for:	
cars	Yes
motorized 2- or 3-wheeled vehicles	No
minibuses and vans	Yes
lorries	Yes
buses	Yes

Registered motor vehicles	
Total (2007)	2 599 712
Cars	80%
Minibuses, vans, etc. (seating <20 people)	16%
Lorries	3%
Buses	1%

Source: Norwegian Public Roads Administration

Care after road crashes	
Formal, publicly available prehospital care system	Yes
National universal access telephone number	Yes (113)

Acknowledgements

Authority approving the data for publication: Ministry of Health and Care Services
National data coordinator: Jakob Linhave, Norwegian Directorate of Health; Signe Vind, Norwegian Directorate of Health
Respondents: Marthe Lillehagen, Ministry of Transport and Communications; Finn Harald Amundsen, Norwegian Public Roads Administration; Jan Guttormsen, National Police Directorate; Kristin Øyen, Trygg Trafikk

Poland

Population: **38.08 million (2007)**

Median age: **37** years

Life expectancy at birth: **75** years

Income group:[a] **middle**

Gross national income per person: **US$ 9840**   Rank: **29** of 49[b]

Human Development Index:[c] **0.875**   Rank: **23** of 49[b]

Private car ownership per 1000 population:[d] **354.6**

CO_2 emissions (tonnes) per person per year:[a] **8.0**

[a] World Bank data.
[b] Rank among the 49 countries in the WHO European Region participating in the survey.
[c] United Nations Development Programme data.
[d] WHO European Region average: 339.

Institutional framework for road safety

Lead agency: The National Road Safety Council	
Status of the agency	Government
Funded in national budget	Yes
National road safety strategy	**Yes**
Measurable targets	Yes
Implementation funded	Yes
Money allocated (in € (2005–2007))	1.87 billion

Key data

Reported number of road traffic deaths (2007)	5583[a] (76% males, 24% females)
Reported number of non-fatal road traffic injuries (2007)	63 244[b]
Road traffic deaths involving alcohol	14.0%[c]
Wearing motorcycle helmets	No information
Using seat-belts in cars	
Overall	65%[d]
Front-seat occupants	74%[d]
Rear-seat occupants	45%[d]
Costing study available	**Yes**
Annual estimated costs (in € (2006))	4.32 billion
Study included deaths, injuries or both	Both deaths and injuries
Methods used	Gross output method

[a] Police data, defined as died within 30 days of the crash.
[b] Police data.
[c] 2007, Police.
[d] 2006, National Road Safety Council observational study.

NA: not applicable

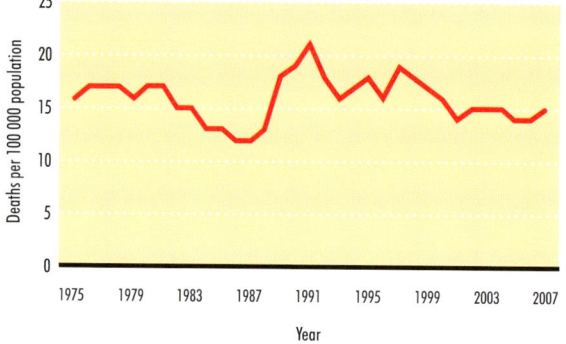

Trends in road traffic deaths

Source: Country questionnaire

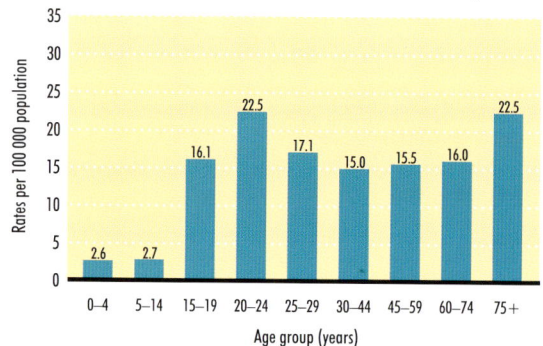

Age-specific mortality rates from road traffic injuries

Source: 2007, Police, Motor Transport Institute

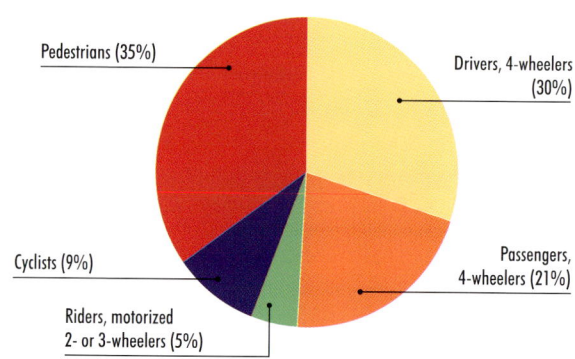

Deaths by road user category

Pedestrians (35%), Drivers, 4-wheelers (30%), Passengers, 4-wheelers (21%), Riders, motorized 2- or 3-wheelers (5%), Cyclists (9%)

Source: 2007, Police, Motor Transport Institute

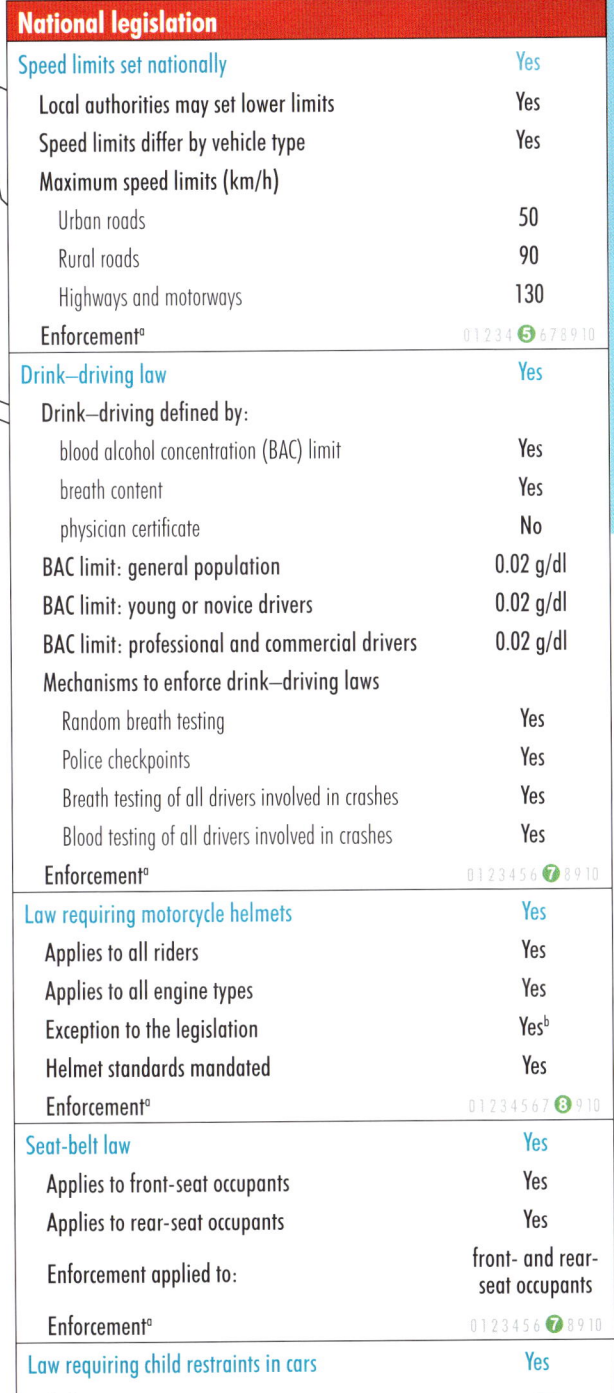

National legislation	
Speed limits set nationally	Yes
Local authorities may set lower limits	Yes
Speed limits differ by vehicle type	Yes
Maximum speed limits (km/h)	
Urban roads	50
Rural roads	90
Highways and motorways	130
Enforcement[a]	0 1 2 3 4 **5** 6 7 8 9 10
Drink–driving law	Yes
Drink–driving defined by:	
blood alcohol concentration (BAC) limit	Yes
breath content	Yes
physician certificate	No
BAC limit: general population	0.02 g/dl
BAC limit: young or novice drivers	0.02 g/dl
BAC limit: professional and commercial drivers	0.02 g/dl
Mechanisms to enforce drink–driving laws	
Random breath testing	Yes
Police checkpoints	Yes
Breath testing of all drivers involved in crashes	Yes
Blood testing of all drivers involved in crashes	Yes
Enforcement[a]	0 1 2 3 4 5 6 **7** 8 9 10
Law requiring motorcycle helmets	Yes
Applies to all riders	Yes
Applies to all engine types	Yes
Exception to the legislation	Yes[b]
Helmet standards mandated	Yes
Enforcement[a]	0 1 2 3 4 5 6 7 **8** 9 10
Seat-belt law	Yes
Applies to front-seat occupants	Yes
Applies to rear-seat occupants	Yes
Enforcement applied to:	front- and rear-seat occupants
Enforcement[a]	0 1 2 3 4 5 6 **7** 8 9 10
Law requiring child restraints in cars	Yes
Enforcement[a]	0 1 2 3 4 5 **6** 7 8 9 10

[a] The enforcement score represents a consensus based on the professional opinion of respondents on a scale of 0 to 10, where 0 is not effective and 10 is highly effective.
[b] Exceptions: bikes equiped with safety belts (motorcycle with overhead "cabin").

Road safety audits	
Formal audits required for major new road construction projects	Yes
Regular audits of existing road infrastructure	Yes

Vehicle standards	
Car manufacturers required to adhere to standards on	
Fuel consumption	No
Seat-belt installation for all seats	Yes

Promoting transport alternatives to cars	
National policies to promote walking or cycling	Yes
Investment in bicycle lanes	Yes
Investment in foot paths	Yes
Traffic-calming measures	Yes
Investment for increasing cycling	No
Disincentives for private car use	No
National policies to promote public transport	No (subnational)
Subsidized pricing of public transport	NA
Improving the frequency and coverage of public transport	NA
Disincentives for private car use	NA

Vehicle regulations	
Compulsory insurance for vehicles	Yes
Periodic vehicle inspection for:	
cars	Yes
motorized 2- or 3-wheeled vehicles	Yes
minibuses and vans	Yes
lorries	Yes
buses	Yes

Registered motor vehicles	
Total (2006)	18 035 047
Cars	75%
Motorized 2- and 3-wheelers	4%
Lorries	13%
Buses	1%
Other	7%

Source: Central Statistical Office

Care after road crashes	
Formal, publicly available prehospital care system	Yes
National universal access telephone number	Yes (112)

Acknowledgements

Authority approving the data for publication: Ministry of Infrastructure
National data coordinator: Barbara Król, National Road Safety Council, Ministry of Infrastructure
Respondents: Jacek Zalewski, The National Headquarters of Police; Robert Trajan vel Trojanowski, General Directorate for National Roads and Motorways; Andrzej Grzegorczyk, National Road Safety Council, Ministry of Infrastructure; Ryszard Krystek, Technical University of Gdansk; Maria Dabrowska-Loranc, Motor Transport Institute; Anna Zielinska, Motor Transport Institute

Portugal

Population: **10.62 million (2007)**

Median age: **39** years

Life expectancy at birth: **79** years

Income group:[a] **high**

Gross national income per person: **US$ 18 950**   Rank: **20** of 49[b]

Human Development Index:[c] **0.900**   Rank: **19** of 49[b]

Private car ownership per 1000 population:[d] **496.5**

CO_2 emissions (tonnes) per person per year:[a] **5.6**

[a] World Bank data.
[b] Rank among the 49 countries in the WHO European Region participating in the survey.
[c] United Nations Development Programme data.
[d] WHO European Region average: 339.

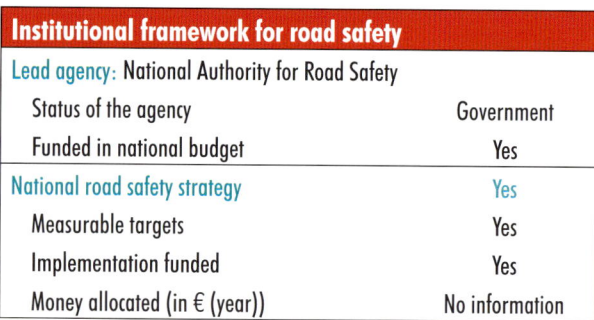

Institutional framework for road safety	
Lead agency: National Authority for Road Safety	
Status of the agency	Government
Funded in national budget	Yes
National road safety strategy	**Yes**
Measurable targets	Yes
Implementation funded	Yes
Money allocated (in € (year))	No information

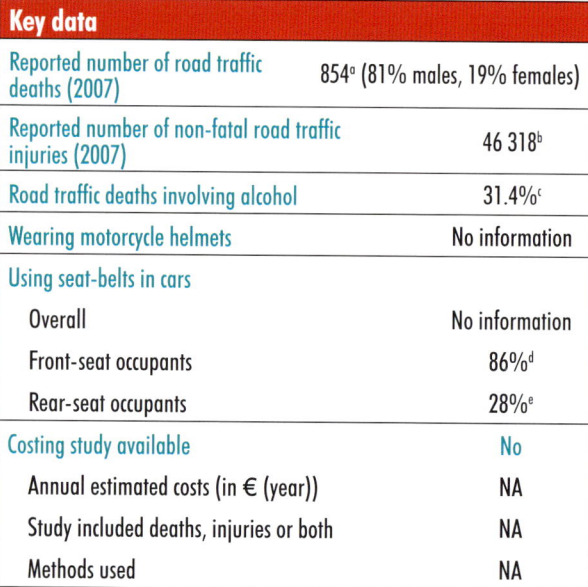

Key data	
Reported number of road traffic deaths (2007)	854[a] (81% males, 19% females)
Reported number of non-fatal road traffic injuries (2007)	46 318[b]
Road traffic deaths involving alcohol	31.4%[c]
Wearing motorcycle helmets	No information
Using seat-belts in cars	
Overall	No information
Front-seat occupants	86%[d]
Rear-seat occupants	28%[e]
Costing study available	**No**
Annual estimated costs (in € (year))	NA
Study included deaths, injuries or both	NA
Methods used	NA

[a] National Authority for Road Safety data, defined as died at crash scene or on the way to health services.
[b] National Authority for Road Safety data.
[c] 2007, National Institute of Legal Medicine.
[d] 2004, Portuguese Association of Road Safety Prevention (PRP), data apply to urban roads only (93% on motorways (2005)).
[e] 2004, Portuguese Association of Road Safety Prevention (PRP), data apply to urban roads only (64% on motorways (2005)).

NA: not applicable

Trends in road traffic deaths

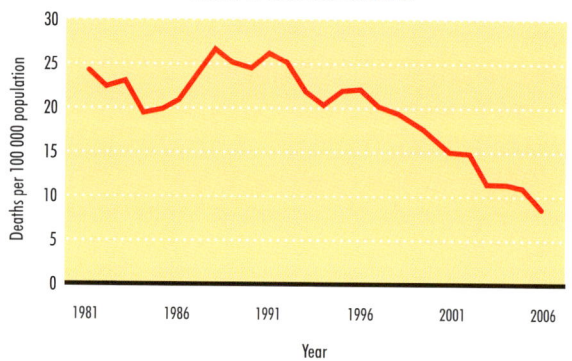

Source: The National Statistics Institute (INE)

Age-specific mortality rates from road traffic injuries

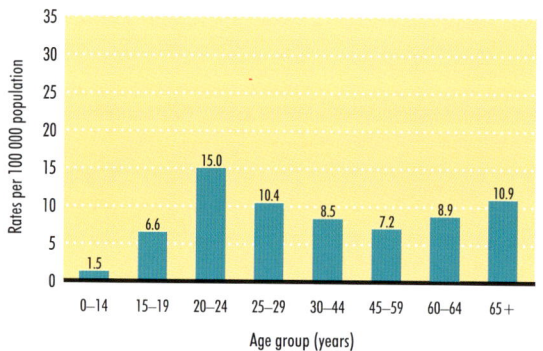

Source: 2007, Annual Report, National Authority for Road Safety

Deaths by road user category

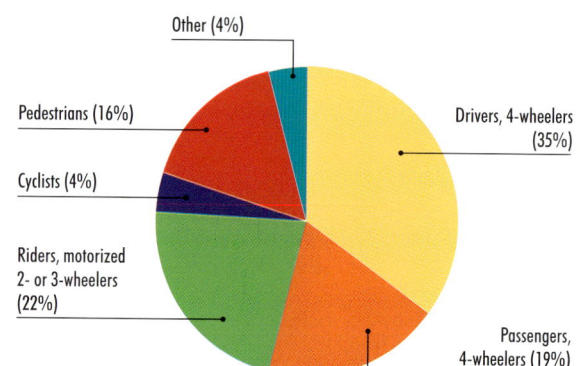

Source: 2007, National Authority for Road Safety

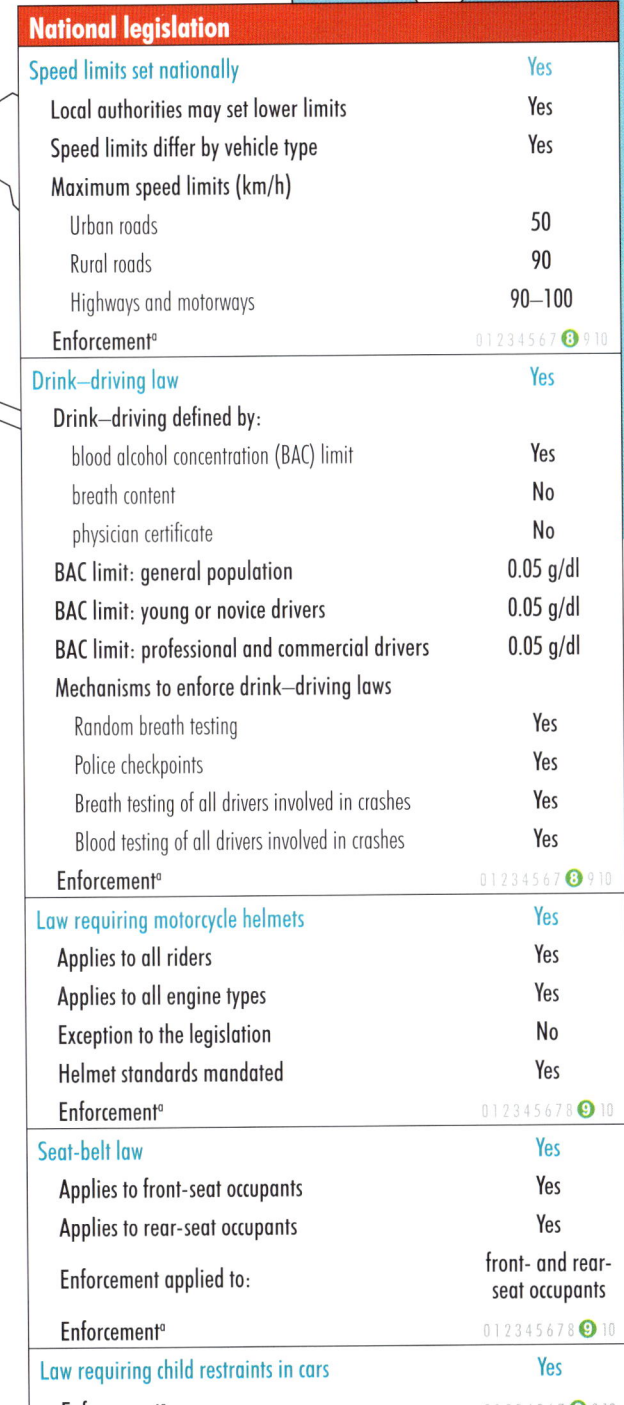

National legislation

Speed limits set nationally	Yes
Local authorities may set lower limits	Yes
Speed limits differ by vehicle type	Yes
Maximum speed limits (km/h)	
Urban roads	50
Rural roads	90
Highways and motorways	90–100
Enforcement[a]	0 1 2 3 4 5 6 7 **8** 9 10
Drink–driving law	Yes
Drink–driving defined by:	
blood alcohol concentration (BAC) limit	Yes
breath content	No
physician certificate	No
BAC limit: general population	0.05 g/dl
BAC limit: young or novice drivers	0.05 g/dl
BAC limit: professional and commercial drivers	0.05 g/dl
Mechanisms to enforce drink–driving laws	
Random breath testing	Yes
Police checkpoints	Yes
Breath testing of all drivers involved in crashes	Yes
Blood testing of all drivers involved in crashes	Yes
Enforcement[a]	0 1 2 3 4 5 6 7 **8** 9 10
Law requiring motorcycle helmets	Yes
Applies to all riders	Yes
Applies to all engine types	Yes
Exception to the legislation	No
Helmet standards mandated	Yes
Enforcement[a]	0 1 2 3 4 5 6 7 8 **9** 10
Seat-belt law	Yes
Applies to front-seat occupants	Yes
Applies to rear-seat occupants	Yes
Enforcement applied to:	front- and rear-seat occupants
Enforcement[a]	0 1 2 3 4 5 6 7 8 **9** 10
Law requiring child restraints in cars	Yes
Enforcement[a]	0 1 2 3 4 5 6 7 **8** 9 10

[a] The enforcement score represents a consensus based on the professional opinion of respondents on a scale of 0 to 10, where 0 is not effective and 10 is highly effective.

Road safety audits

Formal audits required for major new road construction projects	No
Regular audits of existing road infrastructure	No

Vehicle standards

Car manufacturers required to adhere to standards on	
Fuel consumption	No
Seat-belt installation for all seats	Yes

Promoting transport alternatives to cars

National policies to promote walking or cycling	No (subnational)
Investment in bicycle lanes	NA
Investment in foot paths	NA
Traffic-calming measures	NA
Investment for increasing cycling	NA
Disincentives for private car use	NA
National policies to promote public transport	Yes[a]
Subsidized pricing of public transport	Yes
Improving the frequency and coverage of public transport	Yes
Disincentives for private car use	Yes

[a] Other policies are implemented in addition to those listed.

Vehicle regulations

Compulsory insurance for vehicles	Yes
Periodic vehicle inspection for:	
cars	Yes
motorized 2- or 3-wheeled vehicles	No
minibuses and vans	Yes
lorries	Yes
buses	Yes

Registered motor vehicles

Total (2006)	5 948 269
Cars	88%
Motorized 2- and 3-wheelers	9%
Lorries	2%
Buses	<1%

Source: The Automobile Association of Portugal

Care after road crashes

Formal, publicly available prehospital care system	Yes
National universal access telephone number	Yes (112)

Acknowledgements

Authority approving the data for publication: Ministry of Health
National data coordinator: Gregória Paixão von Amann, Directorate-General of Health
Respondents: Ana Coroado, National Authority for Road Safety; Victor Lourenço, Public Security Police; Luís Filipe Branco, Republican National Guard; Angelina Afonso, National Statistic Institute; José Lisboa Santos, Institute of Road Infrastructure; Maria da Conceição Jorge Proença, Public Institute for Mobility and for Inland Transport; Samuel Bonito Martins, Saint Mary's Hospital (Hospital St. Maria); Rodolfo Manuel Martins Soares, Portuguese League Against Trauma

Republic of Moldova

Population: **3.79 million (2007)**

Median age: **33** years

Life expectancy at birth: **68** years

Income group:[a] **middle**

Gross national income per person: **US$ 1260**   Rank: **45 of 49**[b]

Human Development Index:[c] **0.719**   Rank: **45 of 49**[b]

Private car ownership per 1000 population:[d] **87.3**

CO_2 emissions (tonnes) per person per year:[a] **2.0**

[a] World Bank data.
[b] Rank among the 49 countries in the WHO European Region participating in the survey.
[c] United Nations Development Programme data.
[d] WHO European Region average: 339.

Institutional framework for road safety

Lead agency: National Traffic Safety Board	
Status of the agency	Interministerial
Funded in national budget	No
National road safety strategy	**Yes**
Measurable targets	Yes
Implementation funded	Yes
Money allocated (in € (year))	No information

Key data

Reported number of road traffic deaths (2007)	589[a] (74% males, 26% females)
Reported number of non-fatal road traffic injuries (2007)	2985[b]
Road traffic deaths involving alcohol	17.0%[c]
Wearing motorcycle helmets	No information
Using seat-belts in cars	
Overall	No information
Front-seat occupants	No information
Rear-seat occupants	No information
Costing study available	**No**
Annual estimated costs (in € (year))	NA
Study included deaths, injuries or both	NA
Methods used	NA

[a] National Bureau for Statistic (compiles Police and Health data), defined as died within 1 year of the crash.
[b] National Bureau for Statistic data.
[c] 2007, Traffic police database (traffic deaths with alcohol detected/number of road traffic deaths per year).

NA: not applicable

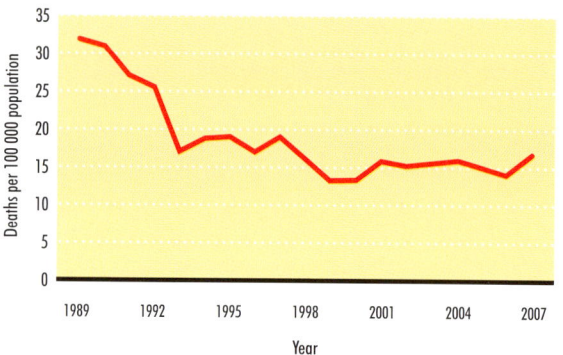

Trends in road traffic deaths

Source: Country questionnaire

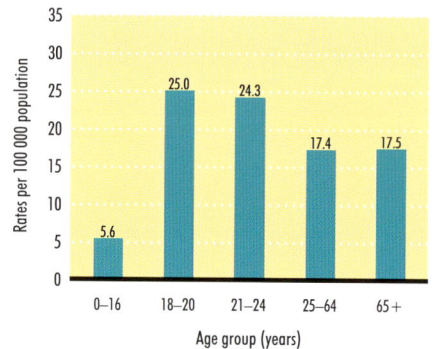

Age-specific mortality rates from road traffic injuries

Source: 2007, National Bureau for Statistic

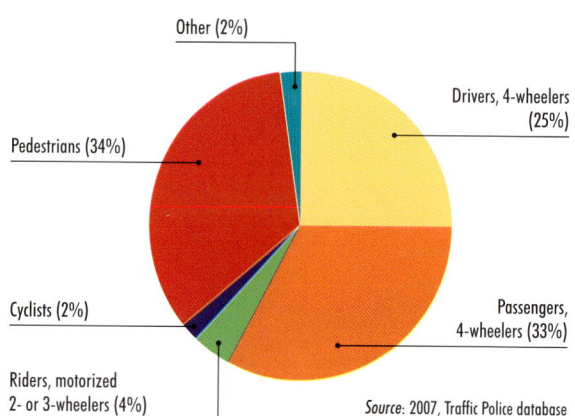

Deaths by road user category

Source: 2007, Traffic Police database

National legislation

Speed limits set nationally	Yes
Local authorities may set lower limits	No
Speed limits differ by vehicle type	Yes
Maximum speed limits (km/h)	
Urban roads	60
Rural roads	60
Highways and motorways	90
Enforcement[a]	No consensus
Drink–driving law	**Yes**
Drink–driving defined by:	
blood alcohol concentration (BAC) limit	Yes
breath content	Yes
physician certificate	Yes
BAC limit: general population	0.05 g/dl
BAC limit: young or novice drivers	0.05 g/dl
BAC limit: professional and commercial drivers	0.05 g/dl
Mechanisms to enforce drink–driving laws	
Random breath testing	Yes
Police checkpoints	Yes
Breath testing of all drivers involved in crashes	Yes
Blood testing of all drivers involved in crashes	Yes
Enforcement[a]	0 1 **2** 3 4 5 6 7 8 9 10
Law requiring motorcycle helmets	**Yes**
Applies to all riders	Yes
Applies to all engine types	No
Exception to the legislation	No
Helmet standards mandated	No
Enforcement[a]	0 **1** 2 3 4 5 6 7 8 9 10
Seat-belt law	**Yes**
Applies to front-seat occupants	Yes
Applies to rear-seat occupants	Yes
Enforcement applied to:	front- and rear-seat occupants
Enforcement[a]	No consensus
Law requiring child restraints in cars	**No**
Enforcement[a]	NA

[a] The enforcement score represents a consensus based on the professional opinion of respondents on a scale of 0 to 10, where 0 is not effective and 10 is highly effective.

Road safety audits

Formal audits required for major new road construction projects	Yes
Regular audits of existing road infrastructure	Yes

Vehicle standards

No car manufacturers	

Promoting transport alternatives to cars

National policies to promote walking or cycling	No
Investment in bicycle lanes	NA
Investment in foot paths	NA
Traffic-calming measures	NA
Investment for increasing cycling	NA
Disincentives for private car use	NA
National policies to promote public transport	No
Subsidized pricing of public transport	NA
Improving the frequency and coverage of public transport	NA
Disincentives for private car use	NA

Vehicle regulations

Compulsory insurance for vehicles	Yes
Periodic vehicle inspection for:	
cars	Yes
motorized 2- or 3-wheeled vehicles	Yes
minibuses and vans	Yes
lorries	Yes
buses	Yes

Registered motor vehicles

Total (2007)	448 202
Cars	74%
Motorized 2- and 3-wheelers	6%
Minibuses, vans, etc. (seating <20 people)	3%
Lorries	16%
Buses	1%

Source: Traffic Police database

Care after road crashes

Formal, publicly available prehospital care system	Yes
National universal access telephone number	Yes (903)

Acknowledgements

Authority approving the data for publication: Ministry of Health

National data coordinator: Filip Gornea, State Medical and Pharmaceutical University "Nicolae Testemutanu"

Respondents: Iurie Untilov, Ministry of Internal Affairs; Petru Crudu, National Center of Health Management; Nicolae Mihul, Republican Clinic Hospital of Orthopedic and Traumatology; Gheorghe Ceban, National Center of the Emergency Medicine

Romania

Population: **21.44 million (2007)**

Median age: **37** years

Life expectancy at birth: **73** years

Income group:[a] **middle**

Gross national income per person: **US$ 6150** Rank: **32** of **49**[b]

Human Development Index:[c] **0.825** Rank: **30** of **49**[b]

Private car ownership per 1000 population:[d] **170.1**

CO_2 emissions (tonnes) per person per year:[a] **4.2**

[a] World Bank data.
[b] Rank among the 49 countries in the WHO European Region participating in the survey.
[c] United Nations Development Programme data.
[d] WHO European Region average: 339.

Institutional framework for road safety

Lead agency: Interministerial Council for Road Safety	
Status of the agency	Interministerial
Funded in national budget	Yes
National road safety strategy	**Yes**[a]
Measurable targets	NA
Implementation funded	NA
Money allocated (in € (year))	NA

[a] Not formally endorsed by the government.

Key data

Reported number of road traffic deaths (2007)	2712[a] (86% males, 14% females)
Reported number of non-fatal road traffic injuries (2007)	29 832[b]
Road traffic deaths involving alcohol	1.5%[c]
Wearing motorcycle helmets	90% Drivers; 65% Passengers[d]
Using seat-belts in cars	
Overall	50%[c]
Front-seat occupants	80%[c]
Rear-seat occupants	20%[c]
Costing study available	**Yes**
Annual estimated costs (in €(2007))	1.20 billion
Study included deaths, injuries or both	Both deaths and injuries
Methods used	No information

[a] Police data, defined as died within 30 days of the crash.
[b] Police data.
[c] 2007, National Road Traffic Police Directorate.
[d] 2007–2008, Road Traffic Police, unofficial estimation for motorcycle riders.

NA: not applicable

Trends in road traffic deaths

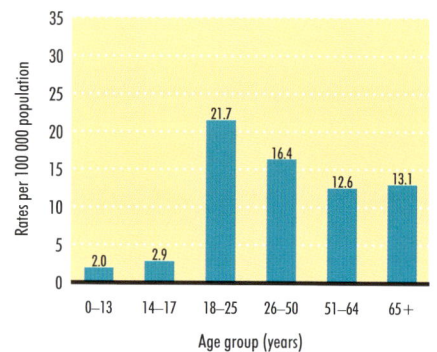

Source: National Road Traffic Police Directorate

Age-specific mortality rates from road traffic injuries

Source: 2007, Ministry of Interior and Administrative Reform, Road Traffic Police

Deaths by road user category

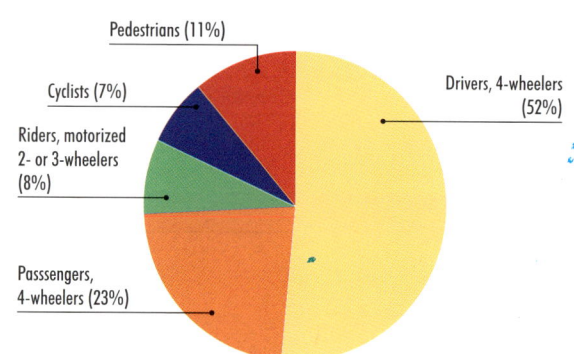

Source: 2007, National Road Traffic Police Directorate

National legislation

Speed limits set nationally	Yes
Local authorities may set lower limits	Yes
Speed limits differ by vehicle type	Yes
Maximum speed limits (km/h)	
Urban roads	50
Rural roads	50
Highways and motorways	90
Enforcement[a]	0 1 2 3 4 **5** 6 7 8 9 10
Drink–driving law	Yes
Drink–driving defined by:	
blood alcohol concentration (BAC) limit	Yes
breath content	Yes
physician certificate	Yes
BAC limit: general population	0.00 g/dl
BAC limit: young or novice drivers	0.00 g/dl
BAC limit: professional and commercial drivers	0.00 g/dl
Mechanisms to enforce drink–driving laws	
Random breath testing	Yes
Police checkpoints	Yes
Breath testing of all drivers involved in crashes	Yes
Blood testing of all drivers involved in crashes	Yes
Enforcement[a]	0 1 2 3 4 5 6 7 **8** 9 10
Law requiring motorcycle helmets	Yes
Applies to all riders	Yes
Applies to all engine types	Yes
Exception to the legislation	No
Helmet standards mandated	Yes
Enforcement[a]	0 1 2 3 4 5 **6** 7 8 9 10
Seat-belt law	Yes
Applies to front-seat occupants	Yes
Applies to rear-seat occupants	Yes
Enforcement applied to:	front- and rear-seat occupants
Enforcement[a]	0 1 2 3 4 **5** 6 7 8 9 10
Law requiring child restraints in cars	Yes
Enforcement[a]	0 1 2 **3** 4 5 6 7 8 9 10

[a] The enforcement score represents a consensus based on the professional opinion of respondents on a scale of 0 to 10, where 0 is not effective and 10 is highly effective.

Road safety audits

Formal audits required for major new road construction projects	Yes
Regular audits of existing road infrastructure	Yes

Vehicle standards

Car manufacturers required to adhere to standards on	
Fuel consumption	Yes
Seat-belt installation for all seats	Yes

Promoting transport alternatives to cars

National policies to promote walking or cycling	Yes
Investment in bicycle lanes	Yes
Investment in foot paths	Yes
Traffic-calming measures	Yes
Investment for increasing cycling	No
Disincentives for private car use	Yes
National policies to promote public transport	Yes
Subsidized pricing of public transport	Yes
Improving the frequency and coverage of public transport	No
Disincentives for private car use	Yes

Vehicle regulations

Compulsory insurance for vehicles	Yes
Periodic vehicle inspection for:	
cars	Yes
motorized 2- or 3-wheeled vehicles	Yes
minibuses and vans	Yes
lorries	Yes
buses	Yes

Registered motor vehicles

Total (2008)	4 611 362
Cars	79%
Motorized 2- and 3-wheelers	1%
Minibuses, vans, etc. (seating <20 people)	11%
Lorries	3%
Buses	<1%
Non-motorized vehicles	4%
Other	2%

Source: Directorate for Driving Licenses and Vehicle Registration

Care after road crashes

Formal, publicly available prehospital care system	Yes
National universal access telephone number	Yes (112)

Acknowledgements
Authority approving the data for publication: Ministry of Health
National data coordinator: Raed Arafat, Ministry of Health
Respondents: Gino Theodor Bosman, Traffic Police Directorate, Ministry of Interior; Cristian Constantinescu, Ministry Of Transportation

105

Russian Federation

Population: 142.50 million (2007)

Median age: 37 years

Life expectancy at birth: 66 years

Income group:[a] middle

Gross national income per person: US$ 7560　　**Rank:** 31 of 49[b]

Human Development Index:[c] 0.806　　**Rank:** 37 of 49[b]

Private car ownership per 1000 population:[d] 195.5

CO_2 emissions (tonnes) per person per year:[a] 10.6

[a] World Bank data.
[b] Rank among the 49 countries in the WHO European Region participating in the survey.
[c] United Nations Development Programme data.
[d] WHO European Region average: 339.

Institutional framework for road safety

Lead agency: The Commission of the Government of Russian Federation for Road Safety	
Status of the agency	Interministerial
Funded in national budget	No
National road safety strategy	**Yes**
Measurable targets	Yes
Implementation funded	Yes
Money allocated (in € (2007))	245.73 million

Key data

Reported number of road traffic deaths (2007)	33 308[a] (74% males, 26% females)
Reported number of non-fatal road traffic injuries (2007)	292 206[b]
Road traffic deaths involving alcohol	9.7%[c]
Wearing motorcycle helmets	No information
Using seat-belts in cars	
Overall	No information
Front-seat occupants	33%[c]
Rear-seat occupants	No information
Costing study available	**Yes**
Annual estimated costs (in € 2007))	8.03 billion
Study included deaths, injuries or both	Both deaths and injuries
Methods used	Direct costing

[a] Ministry of Internal Affairs data, defined as died within 7 days of the crash.
[b] Ministry of Internal Affairs data.
[c] 2007, The Road Safety Department of the Ministry of Internal Affairs.

NA: not applicable

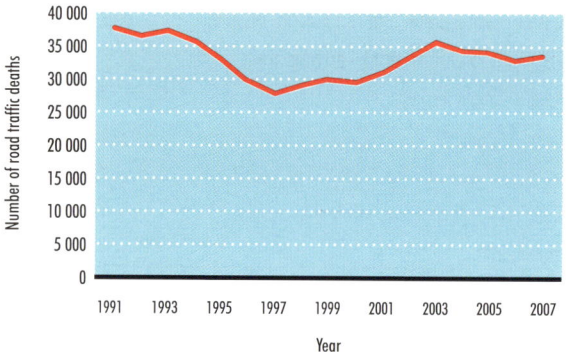

Trends in road traffic deaths

Source: The Road Safety Department of the Ministry of Internal Affairs

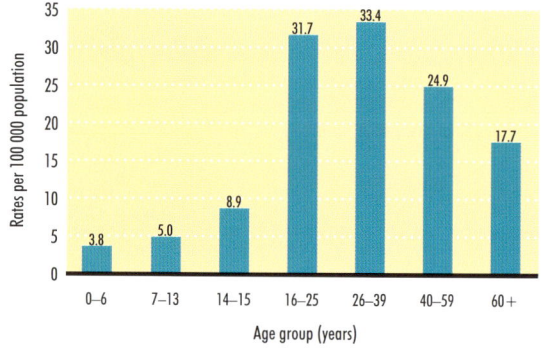

Age-specific mortality rates from road traffic injuries

Source: 2007, The Road Safety Department of the Ministry of Internal Affairs

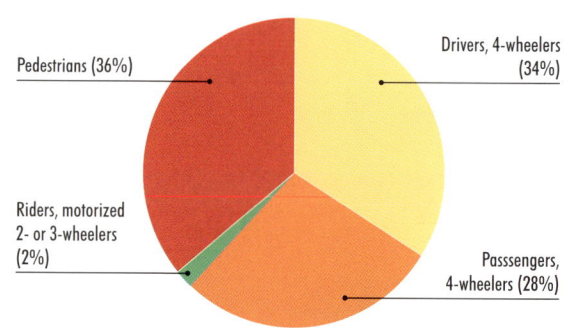

Deaths by road user category

Source: 2007, The Road Safety Department of the Ministry of Internal Affairs

National legislation	
Speed limits set nationally	Yes
Local authorities may set lower limits	Yes
Speed limits differ by vehicle type	Yes
Maximum speed limits (km/h)	
Urban roads	60
Rural roads	90[a]
Highways and motorways	110[b]
Enforcement[c]	0 1 2 3 4 5 **6** 7 8 9 10
Drink–driving law	Yes
Drink–driving defined by:	
blood alcohol concentration (BAC) limit	Yes
breath content	Yes
physician certificate	No
BAC limit: general population	0.03 g/dl
BAC limit: young or novice drivers	0.03 g/dl
BAC limit: professional and commercial drivers	0.03 g/dl
Mechanisms to enforce drink–driving laws	
Random breath testing	Yes
Police checkpoints	No
Breath testing of all drivers involved in crashes	Yes
Blood testing of all drivers involved in crashes	Yes
Enforcement[c]	0 1 2 3 4 5 **6** 7 8 9 10
Law requiring motorcycle helmets	Yes
Applies to all riders	Yes
Applies to all engine types	Yes
Exception to the legislation	No
Helmet standards mandated	Yes
Enforcement[c]	0 1 2 3 4 5 **6** 7 8 9 10
Seat-belt law	Yes
Applies to front-seat occupants	Yes
Applies to rear-seat occupants	Yes
Enforcement applied to:	front- and rear-seat occupants
Enforcement[c]	0 1 2 3 4 5 6 **7** 8 9 10
Law requiring child restraints in cars	Yes
Enforcement[c]	0 1 2 3 4 5 6 7 **8** 9 10

[a] On roads out of populated regions and sites.
[b] On roads marked by special symbols.
[c] The enforcement score represents a consensus based on the professional opinion of respondents on a scale of 0 to 10, where 0 is not effective and 10 is highly effective.

Road safety audits	
Formal audits required for major new road construction projects	Yes
Regular audits of existing road infrastructure	Yes

Vehicle standards	
Car manufacturers required to adhere to standards on	
Fuel consumption	Yes
Seat-belt installation for all seats	Yes

Promoting transport alternatives to cars	
National policies to promote walking or cycling	No
Investment in bicycle lanes	NA
Investment in foot paths	NA
Traffic-calming measures	NA
Investment for increasing cycling	NA
Disincentives for private car use	NA
National policies to promote public transport	No
Subsidized pricing of public transport	NA
Improving the frequency and coverage of public transport	NA
Disincentives for private car use	NA

Vehicle regulations	
Compulsory insurance for vehicles	Yes
Periodic vehicle inspection for:	
cars	Yes
motorized 2- or 3-wheeled vehicles	Yes
minibuses and vans	Yes
lorries	Yes
buses	Yes

Registered motor vehicles	
Total (2007)	38 695 996
Cars	72%
Motorized 2- and 3-wheelers	8%
Lorries	13%
Buses	2%
Other	5%

Source: Ministry of Internal Affairs

Care after road crashes	
Formal, publicly available prehospital care system	Yes
National universal access telephone number	Yes (03)

Acknowledgements

Authority approving the data for publication: Ministry of Internal Affairs
National data coordinator: Gennady Kipor, All-Russian Centre for Disaster Medicine
Respondents: Boris Grebenuk, Head Quarters of All-Russian Service for Disaster Medicine; Aleksei Koldin, All-Russian Centre for Disaster Medicine (Representative of Health and Social Development Ministry); Leonid Borisenko, Agency of Health and Social Development of Russian Federation; Aleksei Voitenkov, Ministry of Internal Affairs of Russian Federation; Andrei Fonski, Ministry of Transport of Russian Federation; Alexandr Gordienko, Ministry of Transport of Russian Federation

San Marino

Population: 0.03 million (2007)
Median age: No information
Life expectancy at birth: 82 years
Income group:[a] high
Gross national income per person: US$ 41 044   Rank: 10 of 49[b]
Human Development Index:[c] No information   Rank: NA
Private car ownership per 1000 population:[d] No information
CO_2 emissions (tonnes) per person per year:[a] No information

[a] World Bank data.
[b] Rank among the 49 countries in the WHO European Region participating in the survey.
[c] United Nations Development Programme data.
[d] WHO European Region average: 339.

Institutional framework for road safety

Lead agency:	Yes
Status of the agency	Interministerial
Funded in national budget	No
National road safety strategy	Multiple strategies
Measurable targets	NA
Implementation funded	NA
Money allocated (in € (year))	NA

Key data

Reported number of road traffic deaths (2007)	1[a] (80% males, 20% females)[b]
Reported number of non-fatal road traffic injuries (2007)	431[c]
Road traffic deaths involving alcohol	No information
Wearing motorcycle helmets	No information
Using seat-belts in cars	
Overall	No information
Front-seat occupants	No information
Rear-seat occupants	No information
Costing study available	No
Annual estimated costs (in € (year))	NA
Study included deaths, injuries or both	NA
Methods used	NA

[a] Health data, defined as died within 30 days of the crash.
[b] 2004–2007, data apply to 5 deaths.
[c] Health data.

NA: not applicable

Trends in road traffic deaths

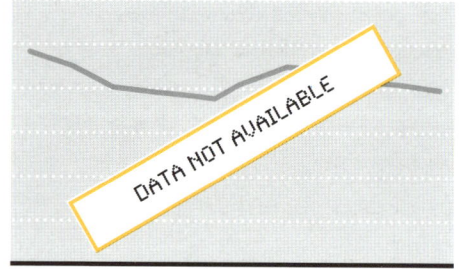

Age-specific mortality rates from road traffic injuries

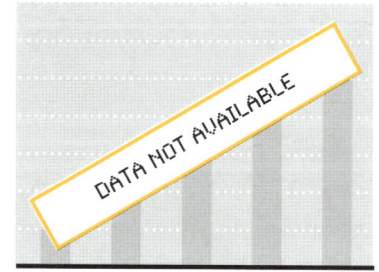

Deaths by road user category

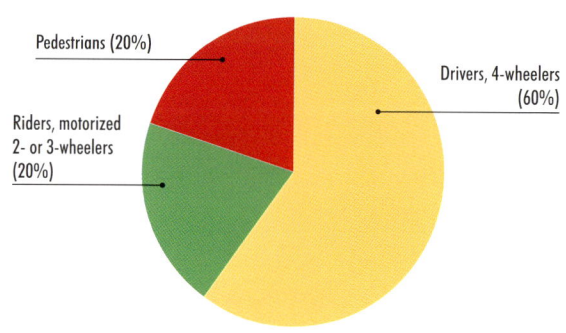

Source: 2004–2007 (5 deaths), Emergency Service

National legislation	
Speed limits set nationally	Yes
Local authorities may set lower limits	No
Speed limits differ by vehicle type	Yes
Maximum speed limits (km/h)	
Urban roads	50
Rural roads	70
Highways and motorways	70
Enforcement[a]	0 1 2 3 4 **5** 6 7 8 9 10
Drink–driving law	Yes
Drink–driving defined by:	
blood alcohol concentration (BAC) limit	Yes
breath content	No
physician certificate	No
BAC limit: general population	0.05 g/dl
BAC limit: young or novice drivers	0.05 g/dl
BAC limit: professional and commercial drivers	0.05 g/dl
Mechanisms to enforce drink–driving laws	
Random breath testing	No
Police checkpoints	Yes
Breath testing of all drivers involved in crashes	No
Blood testing of all drivers involved in crashes	Yes
Enforcement[a]	0 1 2 3 4 5 **6** 7 8 9 10
Law requiring motorcycle helmets	Yes
Applies to all riders	Yes
Applies to all engine types	Yes
Exception to the legislation	No
Helmet standards mandated	Yes
Enforcement[a]	0 1 2 3 4 5 6 7 8 **9** 10
Seat-belt law	Yes
Applies to front-seat occupants	Yes
Applies to rear-seat occupants	Yes
Enforcement applied to:	front- and rear-seat occupants
Enforcement[a]	0 1 2 3 4 5 **6** 7 8 9 10
Law requiring child restraints in cars	Yes
Enforcement[a]	0 1 2 3 4 5 **6** 7 8 9 10

[a] The enforcement score represents a consensus based on the professional opinion of respondents on a scale of 0 to 10, where 0 is not effective and 10 is highly effective.

Road safety audits	
Formal audits required for major new road construction projects	No
Regular audits of existing road infrastructure	Yes

Vehicle standards	
No car manufacturers	

Promoting transport alternatives to cars	
National policies to promote walking or cycling	No
Investment in bicycle lanes	NA
Investment in foot paths	NA
Traffic-calming measures	NA
Investment for increasing cycling	NA
Disincentives for private car use	NA
National policies to promote public transport	Yes
Subsidized pricing of public transport	Yes
Improving the frequency and coverage of public transport	No
Disincentives for private car use	No

Vehicle regulations	
Compulsory insurance for vehicles	Yes
Periodic vehicle inspection for:	
cars	Yes
motorized 2- or 3-wheeled vehicles	Yes
minibuses and vans	Yes
lorries	Yes
buses	Yes

Registered motor vehicles	
Total (2007)	51 590
Cars	66%
Motorized 2- and 3-wheelers	22%
Lorries	7%
Buses	<1%
Other	5%

Source: Economic Programmation Office

Care after road crashes	
Formal, publicly available prehospital care system	Yes
National universal access telephone number	Yes (118)

Acknowledgements
Authority approving the data for publication: Secretariat of State for Health and Social Security
National data coordinator: Andrea Gualtieri, Health Authority
Respondents: Eleonora Liberotti, Internal Affaires Department; Vladimiro Selva, Territorial Environment Department; Eva Guidi, Justice and Information Department; Dennis Guerra, Foreign Affair Department; Federica Renzi, Finances and Economy Department; Marco Podeschi, Labor and Cooperation Department

Serbia

Population: **9.86 million (2007)**

Median age: **37** years

Life expectancy at birth: **73** years

Income group:[a] **middle**

Gross national income per person: **US$ 4730**   Rank: **35** of 49[b]

Human Development Index:[c] **0.821**   Rank: **32** of 49[b]

Private car ownership per 1000 population:[d] **154.0**

CO_2 emissions (tonnes) per person per year:[a] **6.6**

[a] World Bank data.
[b] Rank among the 49 countries in the WHO European Region participating in the survey.
[c] United Nations Development Programme data.
[d] WHO European Region average: 339.

Institutional framework for road safety	
Lead agency:	No
Status of the agency	NA
Funded in national budget	NA
National road safety strategy	Multiple strategies
Measurable targets	NA
Implementation funded	NA
Money allocated (in € (year))	NA

Key data	
Reported number of road traffic deaths (2007)	962[a] (78% males, 22% females)
Reported number of non-fatal road traffic injuries (2007)	22 201[b]
Road traffic deaths involving alcohol	6.0%[c]
Wearing motorcycle helmets	No information
Using seat-belts in cars	
Overall	40–50%[d]
Front-seat occupants	50–60%[d]
Rear-seat occupants	4–5%[d]
Costing study available	No
Annual estimated costs (in € (year))	NA
Study included deaths, injuries or both	NA
Methods used	NA

[a] Police data, defined as died within 30 days of the crash.
[b] Police data.
[c] 2007, Statistics of the Serbian Ministry of the Interior.
[d] 2006, Pilot research of the Academy for Crime Prevention and Police Affairs, observational study.

NA: not applicable

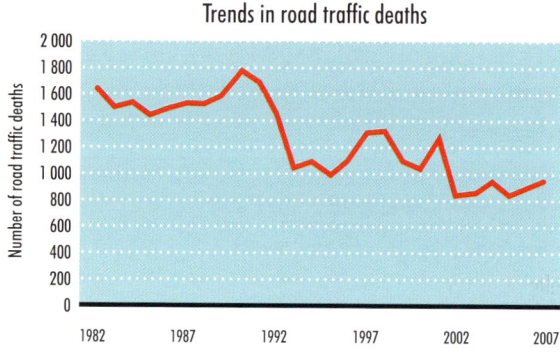

Trends in road traffic deaths

Source: Statistics of the Serbian Ministry of the Interior (data from 1999 to 2007 exclude Kosovo)

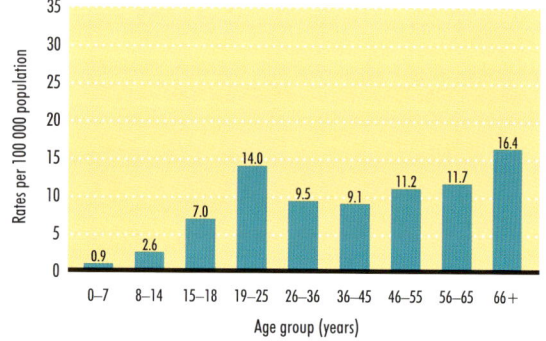

Age-specific mortality rates from road traffic injuries

Source: 2007, Statistics of the Serbian Ministry of the Interior

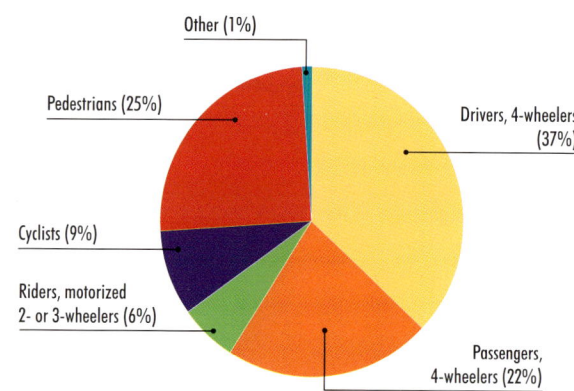

Deaths by road user category

Source: 2007, Statistics of the Serbian Ministry of the Interior

National legislation

Speed limits set nationally	Yes
Local authorities may set lower limits	Yes
Speed limits differ by vehicle type	Yes
Maximum speed limits (km/h)	
Urban roads	60
Rural roads	80
Highways and motorways	120
Enforcement[a]	4 / 10
Drink–driving law	**Yes**
Drink–driving defined by:	
blood alcohol concentration (BAC) limit	Yes
breath content	Yes
physician certificate	Yes
BAC limit: general population	0.05 g/dl
BAC limit: young or novice drivers	0.05 g/dl
BAC limit: professional and commercial drivers	0.00 g/dl
Mechanisms to enforce drink–driving laws	
Random breath testing	Yes
Police checkpoints	Yes
Breath testing of all drivers involved in crashes	Yes
Blood testing of all drivers involved in crashes	Yes
Enforcement[a]	7 / 10
Law requiring motorcycle helmets	**Yes**
Applies to all riders	Yes
Applies to all engine types	Yes
Exception to the legislation	No
Helmet standards mandated	No
Enforcement[a]	3 / 10
Seat-belt law	**Yes**
Applies to front-seat occupants	Yes
Applies to rear-seat occupants	Yes
Enforcement applied to:	front-seat occupants only
Enforcement[a]	4 / 10
Law requiring child restraints in cars	**No (subnational)**
Enforcement[a]	NA

[a] The enforcement score represents a consensus based on the professional opinion of respondents on a scale of 0 to 10, where 0 is not effective and 10 is highly effective.

Road safety audits

Formal audits required for major new road construction projects	Yes
Regular audits of existing road infrastructure	Yes

Vehicle standards

Car manufacturers required to adhere to standards on	
Fuel consumption	No
Seat-belt installation for all seats	Yes

Promoting transport alternatives to cars

National policies to promote walking or cycling	No
Investment in bicycle lanes	NA
Investment in foot paths	NA
Traffic-calming measures	NA
Investment for increasing cycling	NA
Disincentives for private car use	NA
National policies to promote public transport	Yes
Subsidized pricing of public transport	Yes
Improving the frequency and coverage of public transport	Yes
Disincentives for private car use	Yes

Vehicle regulations

Compulsory insurance for vehicles	Yes
Periodic vehicle inspection for:	
cars	Yes
motorized 2- or 3-wheeled vehicles	Yes
minibuses and vans	Yes
lorries	Yes
buses	Yes

Registered motor vehicles

Total (2007)	2 235 389
Cars	68%
Motorized 2- and 3-wheelers	1%
Minibuses, vans, etc. (seating <20 people)	1%
Lorries	8%
Buses	<1%
Other	22%

Source: Statistics of the Serbian Ministry of the Interior

Care after road crashes

Formal, publicly available prehospital care system	Yes
National universal access telephone number	Yes[a] (94)

[a] Regional access number also available.

Acknowledgements

Authority approving the data for publication: Ministry of Health and Ministry of Infrastructure

National data coordinator: Milena Paunovic, Institute of Public Health of Belgrade

Respondents: Jovica Vasiljevic, Ministry of the Interior, Directorate for Traffic Police; Demir Hadzic, Ministry for Infrastructure; Krsto Lipovac, Academy for Crime Prevention and Police Affairs; Ivana Radojicic, Institute for Emergency Medicine of Belgrade; Svetlana Trtica, Institute of Public Health of Belgrade

Slovakia

Population: **5.39 million (2007)**

Median age: **36** years

Life expectancy at birth: **74** years

Income group:[a] **high**

Gross national income per person: **US$ 11 730** Rank: **24** of 49[b]

Human Development Index:[c] **0.872** Rank: **24** of 49[b]

Private car ownership per 1000 population:[d] **272.1**

CO_2 emissions (tonnes) per person per year:[a] **6.7**

[a] World Bank data.
[b] Rank among the 49 countries in the WHO European Region participating in the survey.
[c] United Nations Development Programme data.
[d] WHO European Region average: 339.

Institutional framework for road safety

Lead agency: Road Safety Council	
Status of the agency	Government
Funded in national budget	Yes
National road safety strategy	**Yes**
Measurable targets	Yes
Implementation funded	Yes
Money allocated (in € (2008))	0.96 million

Key data

Reported number of road traffic deaths (2007)	627[a] (76% males, 24% females)
Reported number of non-fatal road traffic injuries (2007)	11 310[b]
Road traffic deaths involving alcohol	4.3%[c]
Wearing motorcycle helmets	No information
Using seat-belts in cars	
Overall	No information
Front-seat occupants	No information
Rear-seat occupants	No information
Costing study available	**Yes**
Annual estimated costs (in € (2007))	297.96 million
Study included deaths, injuries or both	Both deaths and injuries
Methods used	Gross output method

[a] Police data, defined as died within 24 hours of the crash.
[b] Police data.
[c] 2007, Vehicle Register in the Slovak Republic, Ministry of Interior.

NA: not applicable

Trends in road traffic deaths

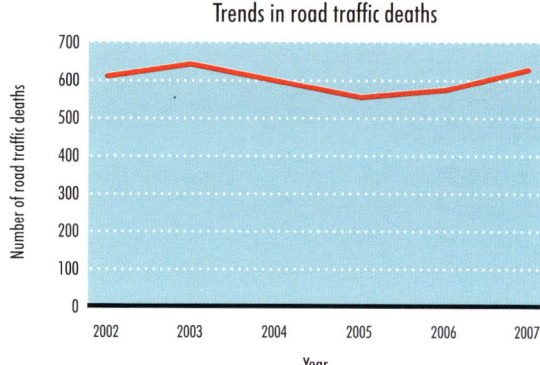

Source: Statistical-Evidence System of Road Traffic Accidents, Ministry of Interior (SR)

Age-specific mortality rates from road traffic injuries

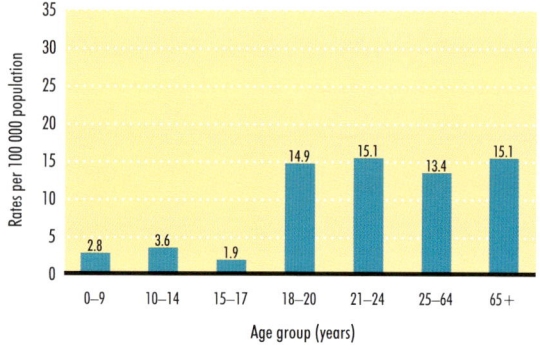

Source: 2007, Statistical Review of Road Traffic Accidents, Department of Traffic Police

Deaths by road user category

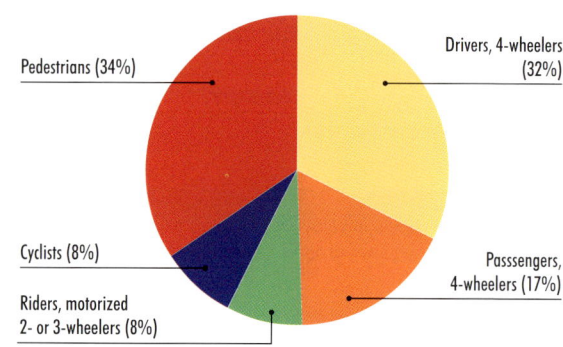

Pedestrians (34%)
Drivers, 4-wheelers (32%)
Passsengers, 4-wheelers (17%)
Riders, motorized 2- or 3-wheelers (8%)
Cyclists (8%)

Source: 2007, Statistical-Evidence System of Road Traffic Accidents, Ministry of Interior

National legislation	
Speed limits set nationally	Yes
Local authorities may set lower limits	Yes
Speed limits differ by vehicle type	Yes
Maximum speed limits (km/h)	
Urban roads	60
Rural roads	90
Highways and motorways	130
Enforcement[a]	0 1 2 3 4 5 6 **7** 8 9 10
Drink–driving law	Yes
Drink–driving defined by:	
blood alcohol concentration (BAC) limit	Yes
breath content	Yes
physician certificate	No
BAC limit: general population	0.00 g/dl
BAC limit: young or novice drivers	0.00 g/dl
BAC limit: professional and commercial drivers	0.00 g/dl
Mechanisms to enforce drink–driving laws	
Random breath testing	Yes
Police checkpoints	Yes
Breath testing of all drivers involved in crashes	Yes
Blood testing of all drivers involved in crashes	Yes
Enforcement[a]	0 1 2 3 4 5 6 7 8 **9** 10
Law requiring motorcycle helmets	Yes
Applies to all riders	Yes
Applies to all engine types	Yes
Exception to the legislation	No
Helmet standards mandated	Yes
Enforcement[a]	0 1 2 3 4 5 6 7 **8** 9 10
Seat-belt law	Yes
Applies to front-seat occupants	Yes
Applies to rear-seat occupants	Yes
Enforcement applied to:	front- and rear-seat occupants
Enforcement[a]	0 1 2 3 4 5 6 7 **8** 9 10
Law requiring child restraints in cars	Yes
Enforcement[a]	0 1 2 3 4 5 6 7 8 **9** 10

[a] The enforcement score represents a consensus based on the professional opinion of respondents on a scale of 0 to 10, where 0 is not effective and 10 is highly effective.

Road safety audits	
Formal audits required for major new road construction projects	Yes
Regular audits of existing road infrastructure	Yes

Vehicle standards	
Car manufacturers required to adhere to standards on	
Fuel consumption	Yes
Seat-belt installation for all seats	Yes

Promoting transport alternatives to cars	
National policies to promote walking or cycling	No
Investment in bicycle lanes	NA
Investment in foot paths	NA
Traffic-calming measures	NA
Investment for increasing cycling	NA
Disincentives for private car use	NA
National policies to promote public transport	No
Subsidized pricing of public transport	NA
Improving the frequency and coverage of public transport	NA
Disincentives for private car use	NA

Vehicle regulations	
Compulsory insurance for vehicles	Yes
Periodic vehicle inspection for:	
cars	Yes
motorized 2- or 3-wheeled vehicles	Yes
minibuses and vans	Yes
lorries	Yes
buses	Yes

Registered motor vehicles	
Total (2007)	2 039 745
Cars	72%
Motorized 2- and 3-wheelers	3%
Minibuses, vans, etc. (seating <20 people)	1%
Lorries	11%
Buses	<1%
Other	12%

Source: Vehicle Register in the Slovak Republic, Home Office of the Slovak Republic

Care after road crashes	
Formal, publicly available prehospital care system	Yes
National universal access telephone number	Yes[a] (112)

[a] Regional access number also available.

Acknowledgements

Authority approving the data for publication: Ministry of Health
National data coordinator: Martin Smrek, University Children's Hospital Bratislava
Respondents: Adam Hochel, Ministry of Heath; Katarina Halzlova, Public Health Authority; Alena Petrikova, Presidium of the Police Force, Ministry of Interior; Stefan Pristas, Ministry of Transportation; Hruskovic Samuel, Rescue Team Slovakia; Darina Sedlakova, WHO Country Office in Slovak Republic

Slovenia

Population: 2.00 million (2007)

Median age: 41 years

Life expectancy at birth: 78 years

Income group:[a] high

Gross national income per person: US$ 20 960   Rank: 19 of 49[b]

Human Development Index:[c] 0.923   Rank: 17 of 49[b]

Private car ownership per 1000 population:[d] 509.9

CO_2 emissions (tonnes) per person per year:[a] 8.1

[a] World Bank data.
[b] Rank among the 49 countries in the WHO European Region participating in the survey.
[c] United Nations Development Programme data.
[d] WHO European Region average: 339.

Institutional framework for road safety

Lead agency: Interministerial Working Group on Road Traffic Safety	
Status of the agency	Interministerial
Funded in national budget	Yes
National road safety strategy	Yes
Measurable targets	Yes
Implementation funded	Yes
Money allocated (in € (2008))	2.20 million

Key data

Reported number of road traffic deaths (2007)	293[a] (79% males, 21% females)
Reported number of non-fatal road traffic injuries (2007)	16 449[b]
Road traffic deaths involving alcohol	38.4%[c]
Wearing motorcycle helmets	No information
Using seat-belts in cars	
Overall	80%[d]
Front-seat occupants	85%[d]
Rear-seat occupants	51%[d]
Costing study available	No
Annual estimated costs (in € (year))	NA
Study included deaths, injuries or both	NA
Methods used	NA

[a] Police data, defined as died within 30 days of the crash.
[b] Police data.
[c] 2007, Ministry of Interior, Police.
[d] 2007, Ministry of Transport, Slovenian Roads Agency, observational study.

NA: not applicable

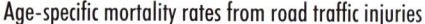

Trends in road traffic deaths

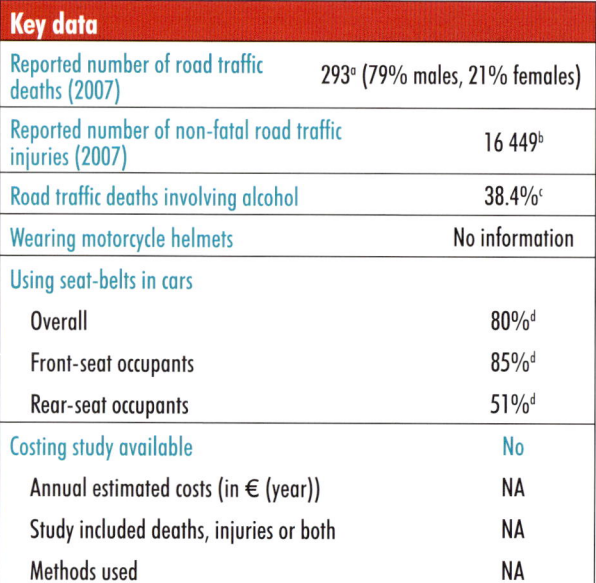

Source: Statistical Office of the Republic of Slovenia

Age-specific mortality rates from road traffic injuries

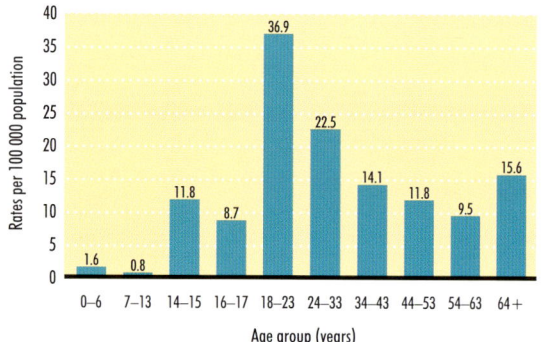

Source: 2007, Ministry of Interior, Police

Deaths by road user category

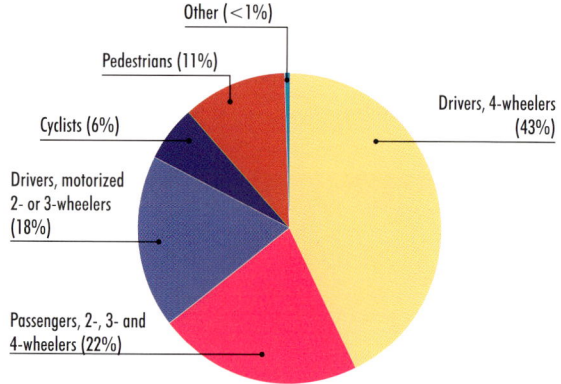

Source: 2008, Ministry of Interior, Police

National legislation	
Speed limits set nationally	Yes
Local authorities may set lower limits	Yes
Speed limits differ by vehicle type	Yes
Maximum speed limits (km/h)	
Urban roads	50
Rural roads	90
Highways and motorways	130
Enforcement[a]	0 1 2 3 4 5 6 ⑦ 8 9 10
Drink–driving law	Yes
Drink–driving defined by:	
blood alcohol concentration (BAC) limit	Yes
breath content	Yes
physician certificate	No
BAC limit: general population	0.05 g/dl
BAC limit: young or novice drivers	0.00 g/dl
BAC limit: professional and commercial drivers	0.00 g/dl
Mechanisms to enforce drink–driving laws	
Random breath testing	Yes
Police checkpoints	Yes
Breath testing of all drivers involved in crashes	Yes
Blood testing of all drivers involved in crashes	Yes
Enforcement[a]	0 1 2 3 4 5 ⑥ 7 8 9 10
Law requiring motorcycle helmets	Yes
Applies to all riders	Yes
Applies to all engine types	No
Exception to the legislation	No
Helmet standards mandated	Yes
Enforcement[a]	0 1 2 3 4 5 6 ⑦ 8 9 10
Seat-belt law	Yes
Applies to front-seat occupants	Yes
Applies to rear-seat occupants	Yes
Enforcement applied to:	front- and rear-seat occupants
Enforcement[a]	0 1 2 3 4 5 6 ⑦ 8 9 10
Law requiring child restraints in cars	Yes
Enforcement[a]	0 1 2 3 4 5 ⑥ 7 8 9 10

[a] The enforcement score represents a consensus based on the professional opinion of respondents on a scale of 0 to 10, where 0 is not effective and 10 is highly effective.

Road safety audits	
Formal audits required for major new road construction projects	No
Regular audits of existing road infrastructure	No

Vehicle standards	
Car manufacturers required to adhere to standards on	
Fuel consumption	No
Seat-belt installation for all seats	Yes

Promoting transport alternatives to cars	
National policies to promote walking or cycling	Yes
Investment in bicycle lanes	Yes
Investment in foot paths	Yes
Traffic-calming measures	Yes
Investment for increasing cycling	Yes
Disincentives for private car use	No
National policies to promote public transport	Yes[a]
Subsidized pricing of public transport	Yes
Improving the frequency and coverage of public transport	Yes
Disincentives for private car use	No

[a] Other policies are implemented in addition to those listed.

Vehicle regulations	
Compulsory insurance for vehicles	Yes
Periodic vehicle inspection for:	
cars	Yes
motorized 2- or 3-wheeled vehicles	Yes
minibuses and vans	Yes
lorries	Yes
buses	Yes

Registered motor vehicles	
Total (2007)	1 286 903
Cars	79%
Motorized 2- and 3-wheelers	6%
Lorries	6%
Buses	<1%
Other	9%

Source: Ministry of Interior

Care after road crashes	
Formal, publicly available prehospital care system	Yes
National universal access telephone number	Yes(112)

Acknowledgements

Authority approving the data for publication: Ministry of Health
National data coordinator: Matej Košir, Ministry of Health
Respondents: Vesna Marinko, Ministry of Transport, Transport Directorate; Bojan Žlender, Ministry of Transport, Slovenian Roads Agency, Road Safety Council; Boštjan Smolej, Ministry of Interior, General Police Directorate, Traffic Police Division; Mateja Rok-Simon, Institute of Public Health of the Republic of Slovenia; Robert Štaba, Zavod Varna pot (Safe Journey Institute)

Spain

Population: 44.28 million (2007)

Median age: 39 years

Life expectancy at birth: 81 years

Income group:[a] high

Gross national income per person: US$ 29 450   Rank: 16 of 49[b]

Human Development Index:[c] 0.949   Rank: 10 of 49[b]

Private car ownership per 1000 population:[d] 480.0

CO_2 emissions (tonnes) per person per year:[a] 7.7

[a] World Bank data.
[b] Rank among the 49 countries in the WHO European Region participating in the survey.
[c] United Nations Development Programme data.
[d] WHO European Region average: 339.

Institutional framework for road safety

Lead agency: General Directorate of Traffic	
Status of the agency	Government
Funded in national budget	Yes
National road safety strategy	**Yes**
Measurable targets	Yes
Implementation funded	Yes
Money allocated (in € (2008))	881.03 million

Key data

Reported number of road traffic deaths (2006)	4104[a] (78% males, 22% females)
Reported number of non-fatal road traffic injuries (2006)	143 450[b]
Road traffic deaths involving alcohol	No information
Wearing motorcycle helmets	98% Drivers; 92% Passengers[c]
Using seat-belts in cars	
Overall	84%[c]
Front-seat occupants	89%[c]
Rear-seat occupants	69%[c]
Costing study available	**Yes**
Annual estimated costs (in € (2007))	6.28 billion
Study included deaths, injuries or both	Both deaths and injuries
Methods used	Gross output method; Willingness to pay

[a] General Directorate of Traffic data, defined as died within 30 days of the crash.
[b] General Directorate of Traffic data.
[c] 2007, General Directorate of Traffic, observational study.

NA: not applicable

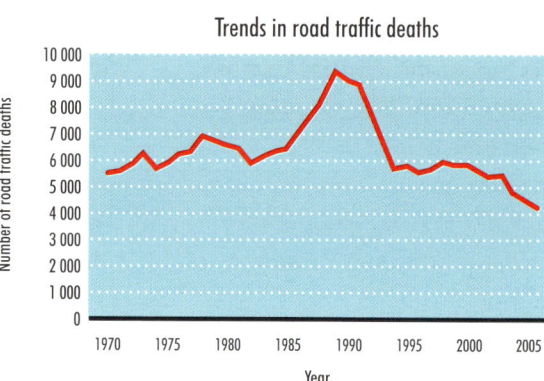

Trends in road traffic deaths

Source: General Directorate of Traffic database

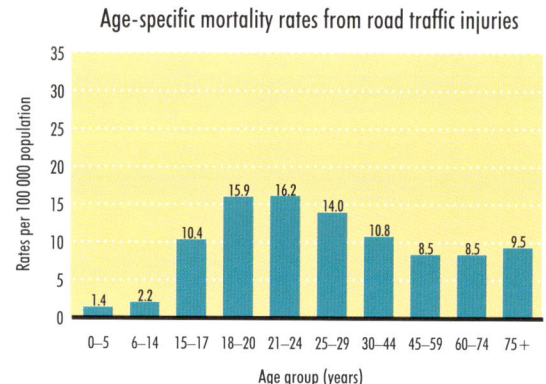

Age-specific mortality rates from road traffic injuries

Source: 2006, General Directorate of Traffic database

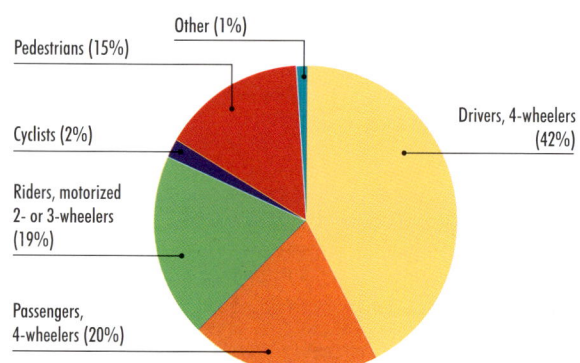

Deaths by road user category

- Drivers, 4-wheelers (42%)
- Passengers, 4-wheelers (20%)
- Riders, motorized 2- or 3-wheelers (19%)
- Cyclists (2%)
- Pedestrians (15%)
- Other (1%)

Source: 2006, General Directorate of Traffic database

EUROPEAN STATUS REPORT ON ROAD SAFETY

National legislation	
Speed limits set nationally	Yes
Local authorities may set lower limits	Yes
Speed limits differ by vehicle type	Yes
Maximum speed limits (km/h)	
Urban roads	50
Rural roads	70
Highways and motorways	90
Enforcement[a]	0 1 2 3 4 **5** 6 7 8 9 10
Drink–driving law	Yes
Drink–driving defined by:	
blood alcohol concentration (BAC) limit	Yes
breath content	Yes
physician certificate	No
BAC limit: general population	0.02 g/dl
BAC limit: young or novice drivers	0.02 g/dl
BAC limit: professional and commercial drivers	0.02 g/dl
Mechanisms to enforce drink–driving laws	
Random breath testing	Yes
Police checkpoints	Yes
Breath testing of all drivers involved in crashes	No
Blood testing of all drivers involved in crashes	No
Enforcement[a]	0 1 2 3 4 5 **6** 7 8 9 10
Law requiring motorcycle helmets	Yes
Applies to all riders	Yes
Applies to all engine types	Yes
Exception to the legislation	Yes[b]
Helmet standards mandated	Yes
Enforcement[a]	0 **1** 2 3 4 5 6 7 8 9 10
Seat-belt law	Yes
Applies to front-seat occupants	Yes
Applies to rear-seat occupants	Yes
Enforcement applied to:	front- and rear-seat occupants
Enforcement[a]	0 1 2 **3** 4 5 6 7 8 9 10
Law requiring child restraints in cars	Yes
Enforcement[a]	0 1 **2** 3 4 5 6 7 8 9 10

[a] The enforcement score represents a consensus based on the professional opinion of respondents on a scale of 0 to 10, where 0 is not effective and 10 is highly effective.
[b] Exceptions: medical reasons.

Road safety audits	
Formal audits required for major new road construction projects	No
Regular audits of existing road infrastructure	No

Vehicle standards	
Car manufacturers required to adhere to standards on	
Fuel consumption	Yes
Seat-belt installation for all seats	Yes

Promoting transport alternatives to cars	
National policies to promote walking or cycling	Yes
Investment in bicycle lanes	Yes
Investment in foot paths	Yes
Traffic-calming measures	Yes
Investment for increasing cycling	No
Disincentives for private car use	Yes
National policies to promote public transport	Yes
Subsidized pricing of public transport	Yes
Improving the frequency and coverage of public transport	Yes
Disincentives for private car use	Yes

Vehicle regulations	
Compulsory insurance for vehicles	Yes
Periodic vehicle inspection for:	
cars	Yes
motorized 2- or 3-wheeled vehicles	Yes
minibuses and vans	Yes
lorries	Yes
buses	Yes

Registered motor vehicles	
Total (2007)	5 500 000
Cars	77%
Motorized 2- and 3-wheelers	8%
Lorries	9%
Buses	<1%
Other	6%

Source: Statistics Sweden (SCB)

Care after road crashes	
Formal, publicly available prehospital care system	Yes
National universal access telephone number	Yes (112)

Acknowledgements

Authority approving the data for publication: Swedish Road Administration
National data coordinator: Thomas Lekander, Swedish Road Administration (SRA)
Respondents: Bengt Svensson, National Police Board; Åsa Ersson, Swedish Road Administration (SRA); Ulf Björnstig, University Hospital in Umeå; Johan Lindberg, The Swedish Association of Local Authorities and Regions; Gunnar Ågren, Swedish National Institute of Public Health; Lars Darin, Ministry of Enterprise and Communications

Switzerland

Population: **7.48 million (2007)**

Median age: **40** years

Life expectancy at birth: **82** years

Income group:[a] **high**

Gross national income per person: **US$ 59 880** Rank: **2** of 49[b]

Human Development Index:[c] **0.955** Rank: **7** of 49[b]

Private car ownership per 1000 population:[d] **515.3**

CO_2 emissions (tonnes) per person per year:[a] **5.5**

[a] World Bank data.
[b] Rank among the 49 countries in the WHO European Region participating in the survey.
[c] United Nations Development Programme data.
[d] WHO European Region average: 339.

Institutional framework for road safety

Lead agency: Federal Roads Agency	
Status of the agency	Government
Funded in national budget	Yes
National road safety strategy	Yes[a]
Measurable targets	NA
Implementation funded	NA
Money allocated (in € (year))	NA

[a] Not formally endorsed by government

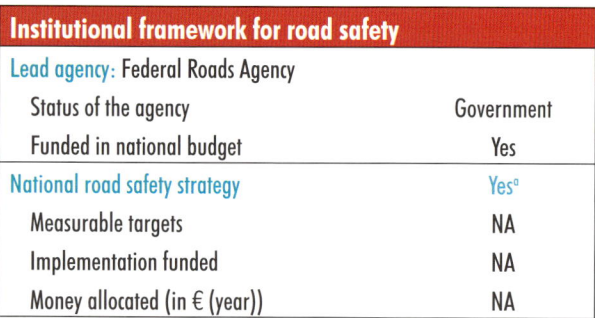

Key data

Reported number of road traffic deaths (2006)	370[a] (76% males, 24% females)
Reported number of non-fatal road traffic injuries (2006)	26 718[b]
Road traffic deaths involving alcohol	16.0%[c]
Wearing motorcycle helmets	100%[d]
Using seat-belts in cars	
Overall	No information
Front-seat occupants	86%[e]
Rear-seat occupants	61%[e]
Costing study available	Yes
Annual estimated costs (in € (2003))	9.06 billion
Study included deaths, injuries or both	Both deaths and injuries
Methods used	Gross output method

[a] Police data, defined as died within 30 days of the crash.
[b] Swiss Council for Accident Prevention data.
[c] 2007, Swiss Council for Accident Prevention.
[d] 2006, Sinus-Report 2007, Swiss Council of Accident Prevention, data apply to motorcycle drivers only.
[e] 2006, Swiss Council for Accident Prevention.

NA: not applicable

Trends in road traffic deaths

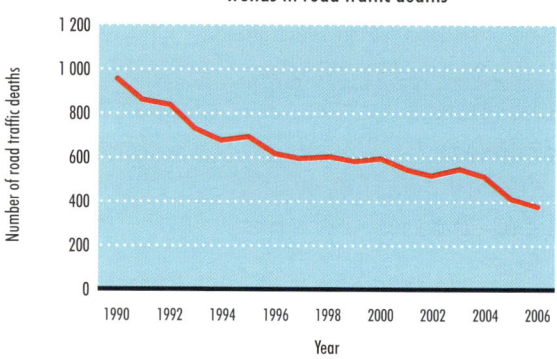

Source: Unfallgeschehen in der Schweiz, bfu-Statistik 2007, Swiss Council of Accident Prevention

Age-specific mortality rates from road traffic injuries

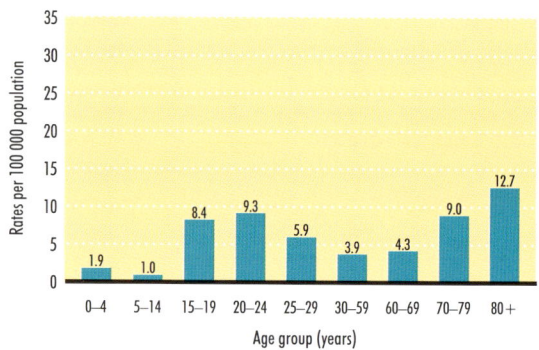

Source: 2006, Unfallgeschehen in der Schweiz, bfu-Statistik 2007, Swiss Council of Accident Prevention

Deaths by road user category

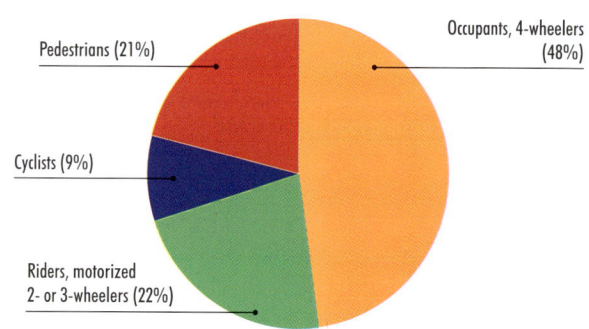

Source: 2006, Unfallgeschehen in der Schweiz, bfu-Statistik 2007, Swiss Council of Accident Prevention

National legislation

Speed limits set nationally	Yes
Local authorities may set lower limits	Yes
Speed limits differ by vehicle type	Yes
Maximum speed limits (km/h)	
Urban roads	50
Rural roads	80
Highways and motorways	120
Enforcement[a]	0 1 2 3 4 5 6 **7** 8 9 10
Drink–driving law	Yes
Drink–driving defined by:	
blood alcohol concentration (BAC) limit	Yes
breath content	No
physician certificate	No
BAC limit: general population	0.05 g/dl
BAC limit: young or novice drivers	0.05 g/dl
BAC limit: professional and commercial drivers	0.05 g/dl
Mechanisms to enforce drink–driving laws	
Random breath testing	Yes
Police checkpoints	Yes
Breath testing of all drivers involved in crashes	Yes
Blood testing of all drivers involved in crashes	Yes
Enforcement[a]	0 1 2 3 4 5 **6** 7 8 9 10
Law requiring motorcycle helmets	Yes
Applies to all riders	Yes
Applies to all engine types	Yes
Exception to the legislation	Yes[b]
Helmet standards mandated	Yes
Enforcement[a]	0 1 2 3 4 5 6 7 8 **9** 10
Seat-belt law	Yes
Applies to front-seat occupants	Yes
Applies to rear-seat occupants	Yes
Enforcement applied to:	front- and rear-seat occupants
Enforcement[a]	0 1 2 3 4 5 6 **7** 8 9 10
Law requiring child restraints in cars	Yes
Enforcement[a]	0 1 2 3 4 5 6 7 **8** 9 10

[a] The enforcement score represents a consensus based on the professional opinion of respondents on a scale of 0 to 10, where 0 is not effective and 10 is highly effective.
[b] Exceptions: low-speed duties, such as mail delivery.

Promoting transport alternatives to cars

National policies to promote walking or cycling	No (subnational)
Investment in bicycle lanes	NA
Investment in foot paths	NA
Traffic-calming measures	NA
Investment for increasing cycling	NA
Disincentives for private car use	NA
National policies to promote public transport	Yes
Subsidized pricing of public transport	Yes
Improving the frequency and coverage of public transport	No
Disincentives for private car use	No

Vehicle regulations

Compulsory insurance for vehicles	Yes
Periodic vehicle inspection for:	
cars	Yes
motorized 2- or 3-wheeled vehicles	Yes
minibuses and vans	Yes
lorries	Yes
buses	Yes

Registered motor vehicles

Total (2007)	5 356 000
Cars	72%
Motorized 2- and 3-wheelers	14%
Lorries	10%
Buses	1%
Other	3%

Source: Federal Office for Statistics

Care after road crashes

Formal, publicly available prehospital care system	Yes
National universal access telephone number	Yes 144)

Road safety audits

Formal audits required for major new road construction projects	Yes
Regular audits of existing road infrastructure	Yes

Vehicle standards

No car manufacturers

Acknowledgements

Authority approving the data for publication: Federal Office of Public Health
National data coordinator: Bertrand Graz, University Institute of Social and Preventive Medicine (IUMSP), Lausanne
Respondents: Christoph Jahn, Federal Roads Office; Lukas Matti, Federal Health Office; Brigitte Buhmann, Swiss Council for Accident Prevention

Tajikistan

Population: **6.74 million (2007)**

Median age: **20** years

Life expectancy at birth: **64** years

Income group:[a] **low**

Gross national income per person: **US$ 460**   Rank: **49** of 49[b]

Human Development Index:[c] **0.684**   Rank: **48** of 49[b]

Private car ownership per 1000 population:[d] **28.8**

CO_2 emissions (tonnes) per person per year:[a] **0.8**

[a] World Bank data.
[b] Rank among the 49 countries in the WHO European Region participating in the survey.
[c] United Nations Development Programme data.
[d] WHO European Region average: 339.

Institutional framework for road safety

Lead agency: Department of the State Automobile Inspection (Ministry of Internal Affairs)	
Status of the agency	Government
Funded in national budget	Yes
National road safety strategy	Multiple strategies
Measurable targets	NA
Implementation funded	NA
Money allocated (in € (year))	NA

Key data

Reported number of road traffic deaths (2007)	464[a] (78% males, 22% females)
Reported number of non-fatal road traffic injuries (2007)	2048[b]
Road traffic deaths involving alcohol	5.0%[c]
Wearing motorcycle helmets	No information
Using seat-belts in cars	
Overall	No information
Front-seat occupants	No information
Rear-seat occupants	No information
Costing study available	No
Annual estimated costs (in € (year))	NA
Study included deaths, injuries or both	NA
Methods used	NA

[a] Department of the State Automobile Inspection of the Ministry of Internal Affairs data, defined as died within 30 days of the crash.
[b] Department of the State Automobile Inspection of the Ministry of Internal Affairs data.
[c] 2007, Department of the State Automobile Inspection of the Ministry of Internal Affairs.

NA: not applicable

Trends in road traffic deaths

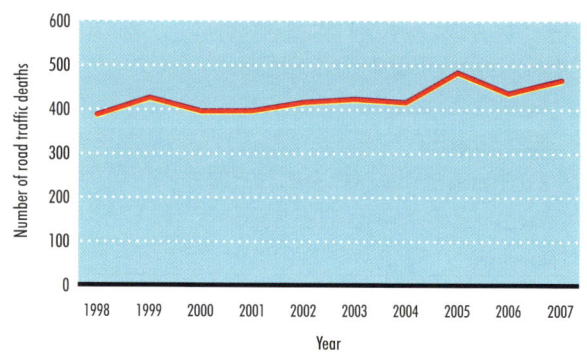

Source: Department of the State Automobile Inspection of the Ministry of Internal Affairs

Age-specific mortality rates from road traffic injuries

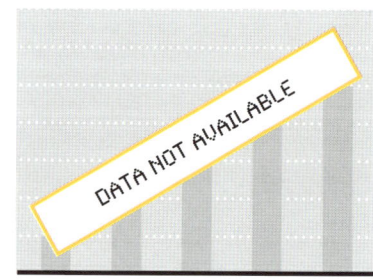

Deaths by road user category

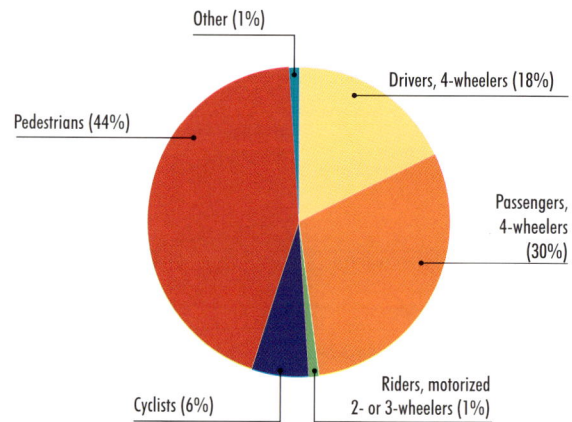

Source: 2007, Department of the State Automobile Inspection of the Ministry of Internal Affairs

National legislation	
Speed limits set nationally	Yes
Local authorities may set lower limits	Yes
Speed limits differ by vehicle type	Yes
Maximum speed limits (km/h)	
Urban roads	50
Rural roads	90
Highways and motorways	100
Enforcement[a]	0 1 2 3 4 5 6 7 **8** 9 10
Drink–driving law	Yes
Drink–driving defined by:	
blood alcohol concentration (BAC) limit	Yes
breath content	Yes
physician certificate	No
BAC limit: general population	0.05 g/dl
BAC limit: young or novice drivers	0.03 g/dl
BAC limit: professional and commercial drivers	0.03 g/dl
Mechanisms to enforce drink–driving laws	
Random breath testing	Yes
Police checkpoints	No
Breath testing of all drivers involved in crashes	Yes
Blood testing of all drivers involved in crashes	Yes
Enforcement[a]	0 1 2 3 4 5 6 **7** 8 9 10
Law requiring motorcycle helmets	Yes
Applies to all riders	Yes
Applies to all engine types	Yes
Exception to the legislation	Yes[b]
Helmet standards mandated	Yes
Enforcement[a]	0 1 2 3 4 5 6 7 **8** 9 10
Seat-belt law	Yes
Applies to front-seat occupants	Yes
Applies to rear-seat occupants	Yes
Enforcement applied to:	front- and rear-seat occupants
Enforcement[a]	0 1 2 3 4 5 6 7 **8** 9 10
Law requiring child restraints in cars	Yes
Enforcement[a]	0 1 2 3 4 5 6 **7** 8 9 10

[a] The enforcement score represents a consensus based on the professional opinion of respondents on a scale of 0 to 10, where 0 is not effective and 10 is highly effective.
[b] Exceptions: serious medical conditions.

Road safety audits	
Formal audits required for major new road construction projects	Yes
Regular audits of existing road infrastructure	Yes

Vehicle standards	
Car manufacturers required to adhere to standards on	
Fuel consumption	Yes
Seat-belt installation for all seats	Yes

Promoting transport alternatives to cars	
National policies to promote walking or cycling	No (subnational)
Investment in bicycle lanes	NA
Investment in foot paths	NA
Traffic-calming measures	NA
Investment for increasing cycling	NA
Disincentives for private car use	NA
National policies to promote public transport	Yes[a]
Subsidized pricing of public transport	Yes
Improving the frequency and coverage of public transport	Yes
Disincentives for private car use	No

[a] Other policies are implemented in addition to those listed.

Vehicle regulations	
Compulsory insurance for vehicles	Yes
Periodic vehicle inspection for:	
cars	Yes
motorized 2- or 3-wheeled vehicles	Yes
minibuses and vans	Yes
lorries	Yes
buses	Yes

Registered motor vehicles	
Total (2006)	31 441 152
Cars	67%
Motorized 2- and 3-wheelers	14%
Minibuses, vans, etc. (seating <20 people)	8%
Lorries	9%
Buses	<1%
Other	3%

Source: General Directorate of Traffic database

Care after road crashes	
Formal, publicly available prehospital care system	Yes
National universal access telephone number	Yes(112)

Acknowledgements

Authority approving the data for publication: Ministry of Health and Consumer Affairs
National data coordinator: Vicenta Lizarbe
Respondents: Pilar Zori Bertolin, Geneneral Directorate of Traffic; Catherine Pérez, Public Health Agency Barcelona; María Seguí-Gómez, Faculty of Medicine, Navarra University; Teodoro Casillas Martin, Agrupación de Tráfico, Guardia Civil; María Librada Escribano, Public Health Directorate. Ministry of Health and Consumer Affairs; María Antonia Astorga, Public Health Directorate, Ministry of Health and Consumer Affair

Sweden

Population: 9.12 million (2007)

Median age: 40 years

Life expectancy at birth: 81 years

Income group:[a] high

Gross national income per person: US$ 46 060   Rank: 5 of 49[b]

Human Development Index:[c] 0.958   Rank: 5 of 49[b]

Private car ownership per 1000 population:[d] 464.4

CO_2 emissions (tonnes) per person per year:[a] 5.9

[a] World Bank data.
[b] Rank among the 49 countries in the WHO European Region participating in the survey.
[c] United Nations Development Programme data.
[d] WHO European Region average: 339.

Institutional framework for road safety

Lead agency: Swedish Road Administration	
Status of the agency	Government
Funded in national budget	Yes
National road safety strategy	Yes
Measurable targets	Yes
Implementation funded	Yes
Money allocated (in € (year))	No information

Key data

Reported number of road traffic deaths (2007)	471[a] (75% males, 25% females)
Reported number of non-fatal road traffic injuries (2006)	26 636[b]
Road traffic deaths involving alcohol	20.0%[c]
Wearing motorcycle helmets	95%[d]
Using seat-belts in cars	
Overall	94%[e]
Front-seat occupants	96%[e]
Rear-seat occupants	90%[e]
Costing study available	Yes
Annual estimated costs (in € (2006))	3.25 billion
Study included deaths, injuries or both	Both deaths and injuries
Methods used	Willingness to pay

[a] Transport data, defined as died within 30 days of the crash.
[b] Police data.
[c] 2006, Estimate based on autopsies of drivers killed in crashes.
[d] 2007, Estimate provided by consensus group.
[e] 2006, Swedish Road and Transport Research Institute observationa studies.

NA: not applicable

Trends in road traffic deaths

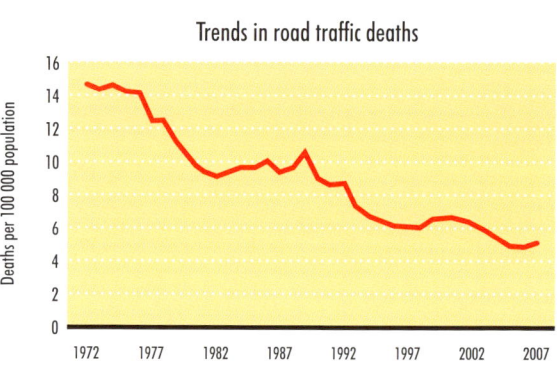

Source: *Road Traffic Injuries 2007 (Vägtrafikskador 2007)*, Swedish Institute for Transport and Communication Analyses

Age-specific mortality rates from road traffic injuries

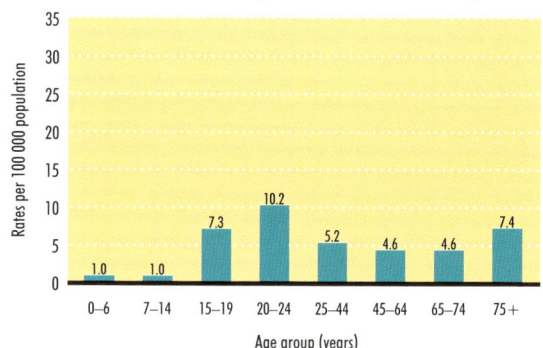

Source: 2006, Swedish Institute for Transport and Communication Analyses

Deaths by road user category

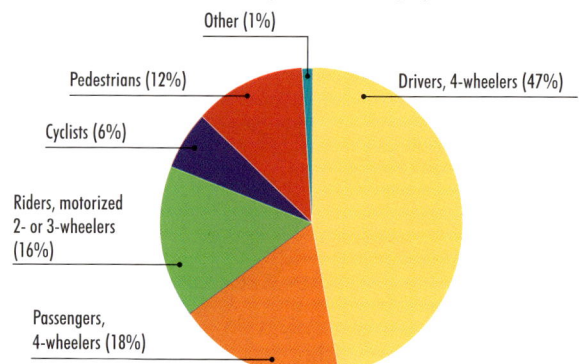

Source: 2006, *Road Traffic Injuries 2006 (Vägtrafikskador 2006)*, Swedish Institute for Transport and Communication Analyses

National legislation	
Speed limits set nationally	Yes
Local authorities may set lower limits	Yes
Speed limits differ by vehicle type	Yes
Maximum speed limits (km/h)	
Urban roads	60
Rural roads	90
Highways and motorways	110
Enforcement[a]	0 1 2 3 4 5 6 7 **8** 9 10
Drink–driving law	Yes
Drink–driving defined by:	
blood alcohol concentration (BAC) limit	Yes
breath content	Yes
physician certificate	Yes
BAC limit: general population	0.03 g/dl
BAC limit: young or novice drivers	0.03 g/dl
BAC limit: professional and commercial drivers	0.03 g/dl
Mechanisms to enforce drink–driving laws	
Random breath testing	Yes
Police checkpoints	Yes
Breath testing of all drivers involved in crashes	Yes
Blood testing of all drivers involved in crashes	Yes
Enforcement[a]	0 1 2 3 4 5 6 7 8 **9** 10
Law requiring motorcycle helmets	Yes
Applies to all riders	Yes
Applies to all engine types	No
Exception to the legislation	No
Helmet standards mandated	No
Enforcement[a]	0 1 2 3 4 5 **6** 7 8 9 10
Seat-belt law	Yes
Applies to front-seat occupants	Yes
Applies to rear-seat occupants	Yes
Enforcement applied to:	front- and rear-seat occupants
Enforcement[a]	0 1 2 **3** 4 5 6 7 8 9 10
Law requiring child restraints in cars	Yes
Enforcement[a]	0 **1** 2 3 4 5 6 7 8 9 10

[a] The enforcement score represents a consensus based on the professional opinion of respondents on a scale of 0 to 10, where 0 is not effective and 10 is highly effective.

Road safety audits	
Formal audits required for major new road construction projects	Yes
Regular audits of existing road infrastructure	Yes

Vehicle standards	
No car manufacturers	

Promoting transport alternatives to cars	
National policies to promote walking or cycling	No
Investment in bicycle lanes	NA
Investment in foot paths	NA
Traffic-calming measures	NA
Investment for increasing cycling	NA
Disincentives for private car use	NA
National policies to promote public transport	No (subnational)
Subsidized pricing of public transport	NA
Improving the frequency and coverage of public transport	NA
Disincentives for private car use	NA

Vehicle regulations	
Compulsory insurance for vehicles	Yes
Periodic vehicle inspection for:	
cars	Yes
motorized 2- or 3-wheeled vehicles	Yes
minibuses and vans	Yes
lorries	Yes
buses	Yes

Registered motor vehicles	
Total (2007)	268 018
Cars	72%
Motorized 2- and 3-wheelers	4%
Minibuses, vans, etc. (seating <20 people)	7%
Lorries	15%
Buses	2%

Source: Department of the State Automobile Inspection of the Ministry Internal Affairs

Care after road crashes	
Formal, publicly available prehospital care system	Yes
National universal access telephone number	Yes (03)

Acknowledgements

Authority approving the data for publication: Ministry of Health
National data coordinator: Abduvali Razzakov, Tajik State Medical University
Respondents: Kurbonkhon Saidov, Ministry of Transport and Communication; Nazarali Rahmatulloev, Department of the State Automobile Inspection of the Ministry Internal Affairs; Hasan Nazarov, Khatlon District Clinic Hospital; Shuhratjon Ziyoboev, Khudjand Clinic Hospital No.1; Shodi Jamshedov, Department on Health Protection of the Badakhshan Avtonomy District

The former Yugoslav Republic of Macedonia

Population: **2.0 million (2007)**

Median age: **35** years

Life expectancy at birth: **73** years

Income group:[a] **middle**

Gross national income per person: **US$ 3460**   Rank: **39** of **49**[b]

Human Development Index:[c] **0.808**   Rank: **34** of **49**[b]

Private car ownership per 1000 population:[d] **109.9**

CO_2 emissions (tonnes) per person per year:[a] **5.1**

[a] World Bank data.
[b] Rank among the 49 countries in the WHO European Region participating in the survey.
[c] United Nations Development Programme data.
[d] WHO European Region average: 339.

Institutional framework for road safety

Lead agency: Republic's Council for Road Traffic Safety	
Status of the agency	Directly under the Parliament
Funded in national budget	Yes
National road safety strategy	**No**
Measurable targets	NA
Implementation funded	NA
Money allocated (in € (year))	NA

Key data

Reported number of road traffic deaths (2006)	140[a] (83% males, 17% females)
Reported number of non-fatal road traffic injuries (2007)	6133[b]
Road traffic deaths involving alcohol	4.6%[c]
Wearing motorcycle helmets	1%[d]
Using seat-belts in cars	
Overall	16%[e]
Front-seat occupants	No information
Rear-seat occupants	No information
Costing study available	**Yes**
Annual estimated costs (in € (2002))	28.25 million
Study included deaths, injuries or both	Both deaths and injuroes
Methods used	Gross output method

[a] State Statistical Office data, defined as died within 30 days of the crash.
[b] Police data.
[c] 2007, Ministry of Interior, Sector for Analysis, Research and Documentation.
[d] 2007, Ministry of Interior, Sector for Information Technology, data apply to motorcycle riders involved in a crash.
[e] 2002, PhD thesis by F.G. Tozija, *Socio-medical Aspects of Traffic-related Traumatism in Children and Youth in the Republic of Macedonia*, Medical Faculty, Skopje (survey of injured drivers and passengers treated in hospital).

NA: not applicable

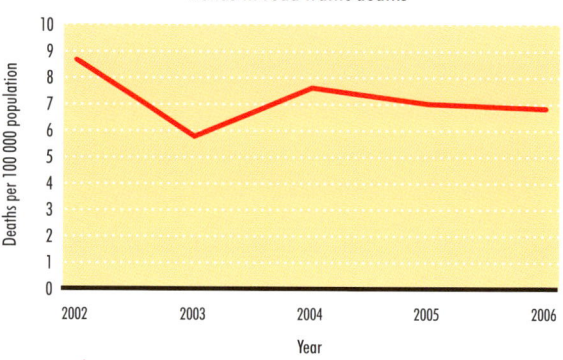

Trends in road traffic deaths

Source: State Statistical Office

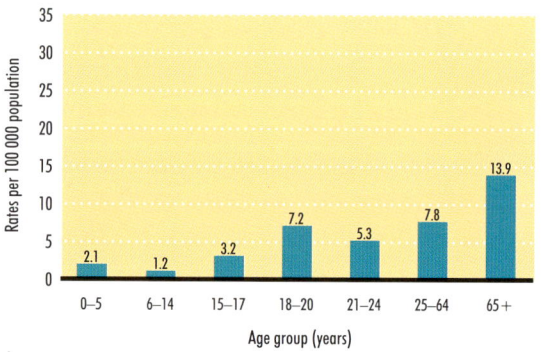

Age-specific mortality rates from road traffic injuries

Source: 2006, State Statistical Office

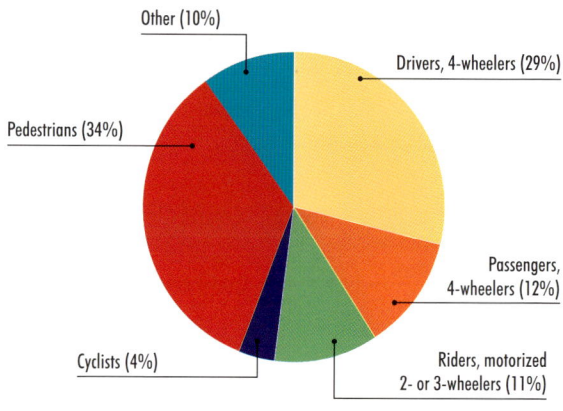

Deaths by road user category

Source: 2006, State Statistical Office

National legislation

Speed limits set nationally	Yes
Local authorities may set lower limits	No
Speed limits differ by vehicle type	Yes
Maximum speed limits (km/h)	
Urban roads	60
Rural roads	80
Highways and motorways	120
Enforcement[a]	0 1 2 3 **4** 5 6 7 8 9 10
Drink–driving law	Yes
Drink–driving defined by:	
blood alcohol concentration (BAC) limit	Yes
breath content	No
physician certificate	No
BAC limit: general population	0.05 g/dl
BAC limit: young or novice drivers	0.00 g/dl
BAC limit: professional and commercial drivers	0.00 g/dl
Mechanisms to enforce drink–driving laws	
Random breath testing	No
Police checkpoints	Yes
Breath testing of all drivers involved in crashes	Yes
Blood testing of all drivers involved in crashes	Yes
Enforcement[a]	0 1 2 3 4 5 **6** 7 8 9 10
Law requiring motorcycle helmets	Yes
Applies to all riders	Yes
Applies to all engine types	Yes
Exception to the legislation	No
Helmet standards mandated	No
Enforcement[a]	0 1 **2** 3 4 5 6 7 8 9 10
Seat-belt law	Yes
Applies to front-seat occupants	Yes
Applies to rear-seat occupants	No
Enforcement applied to:	front-seat occupants only
Enforcement[a]	0 1 2 3 4 5 **6** 7 8 9 10
Law requiring child restraints in cars	No
Enforcement[a]	NA

[a] The enforcement score represents a consensus based on the professional opinion of respondents on a scale of 0 to 10, where 0 is not effective and 10 is highly effective.

Road safety audits

Formal audits required for major new road construction projects	Yes
Regular audits of existing road infrastructure	Yes

Vehicle standards

No car manufacturers

Promoting transport alternatives to cars

National policies to promote walking or cycling	No
Investment in bicycle lanes	NA
Investment in foot paths	NA
Traffic-calming measures	NA
Investment for increasing cycling	NA
Disincentives for private car use	NA
National policies to promote public transport	No
Subsidized pricing of public transport	NA
Improving the frequency and coverage of public transport	NA
Disincentives for private car use	NA

Vehicle regulations

Compulsory insurance for vehicles	Yes
Periodic vehicle inspection for:	
cars	Yes
motorized 2- or 3-wheeled vehicles	Yes
minibuses and vans	Yes
lorries	Yes
buses	Yes

Registered motor vehicles

Total (2007)	259 421
Cars	86%
Motorized 2- and 3-wheelers	2%
Lorries	8%
Buses	1%
Other	3%

Source: Ministry of Interior, Sector for Information Technology

Care after road crashes

Formal, publicly available prehospital care system	Yes
National universal access telephone number	Yes (194)

Acknowledgements

Authority approving the data for publication: Ministry of Health
National data coordinator: Fimka Tozija, Republic Institute for Health Protection
Respondents: Spase Jovkovski, Representative of The Automobila Union of the Republic of Macedonia (AMSM); Boris Murgoski, Police Academy; Cane Kostvski, Ministry of Interior; Marjan Kopevski, Ministry of Transport and Communications; Elena Eftimovska, Macedonian Red Cross; Ljubica Damceska, State Statistical Office

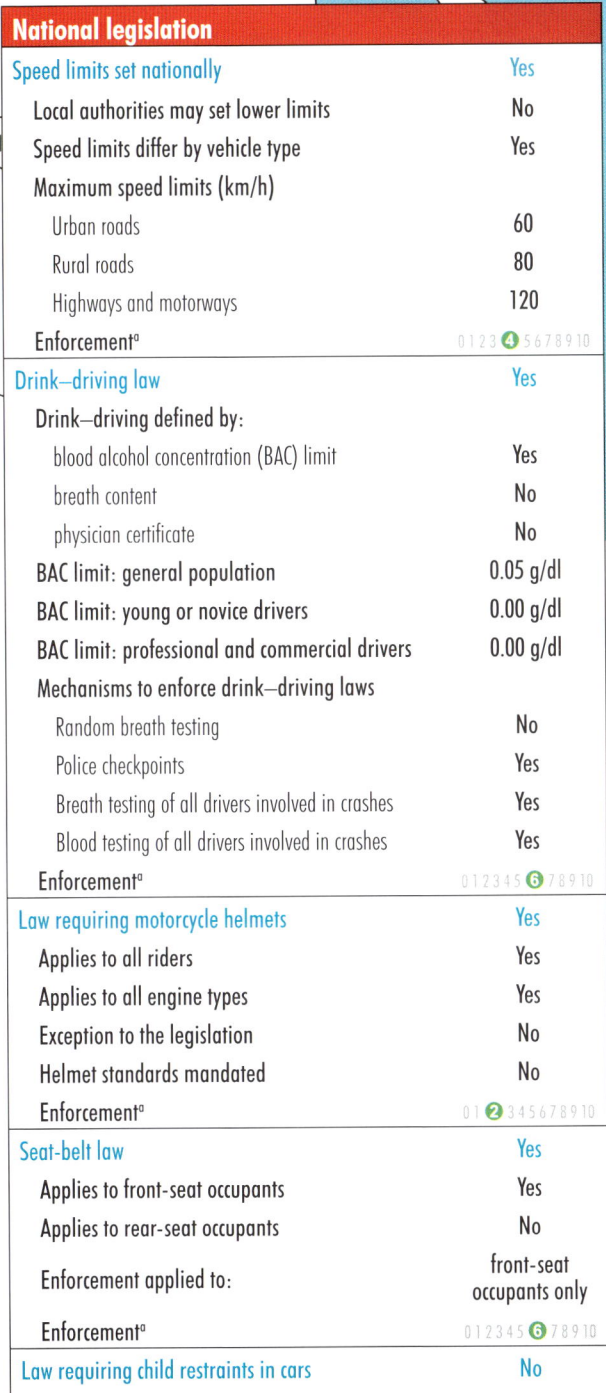

Turkey

Population: **74.88 million (2007)**

Median age: **27** years

Life expectancy at birth: **73** years

Income group:[a] **middle**

Gross national income per person: **US$ 8020** Rank: **30** of 49[b]

Human Development Index:[c] **0.798** Rank: **40** of 49[b]

Private car ownership per 1000 population:[d] **87.1**

CO_2 emissions (tonnes) per person per year:[a] **3.2**

[a] World Bank data.
[b] Rank among the 49 countries in the WHO European Region participating in the survey.
[c] United Nations Development Programme data.
[d] WHO European Region average: 339.

Institutional framework for road safety

Lead agency: Board of Road Traffic Safety	
Status of the agency	Interministerial
Funded in national budget	Yes
National road safety strategy	**Multiple strategies**
Measurable targets	NA
Implementation funded	NA
Money allocated (in € (year))	NA

Key data

Reported number of road traffic deaths (2006)	4633[a] (77% males, 23% females)
Reported number of non-fatal road traffic injuries (2007)	169 080[b]
Road traffic deaths involving alcohol	2.0%[c]
Wearing motorcycle helmets	12% Drivers[c]
Using seat-belts in cars	
Overall	70%[d]
Front-seat occupants	No information
Rear-seat occupants	No information
Costing study available	**Yes**
Annual estimated costs (in € (2002))	8.92 billion
Study included deaths, injuries or both	Both deaths and injuries
Methods used	No information

[a] Turkish Statistical Institute data, defined as died at crash scene.
[b] Turkish Statistical Institute data.
[c] 2005–2007, Security Directorate.
[d] 2007, Security Directorate, data apply to rural roads only (20% in city centres roads).

NA: not applicable

Trends in road traffic deaths

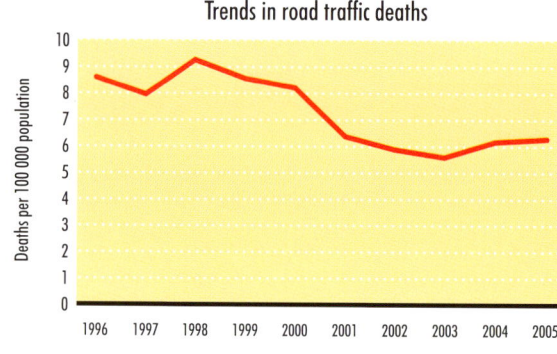

Source: *Traffic Accident Statistics (Road) 2007*, Turkish Statistical Institute

Age-specific mortality rates from road traffic injuries

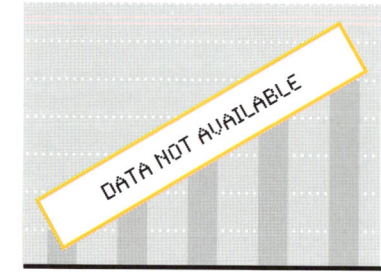

Deaths by road user category

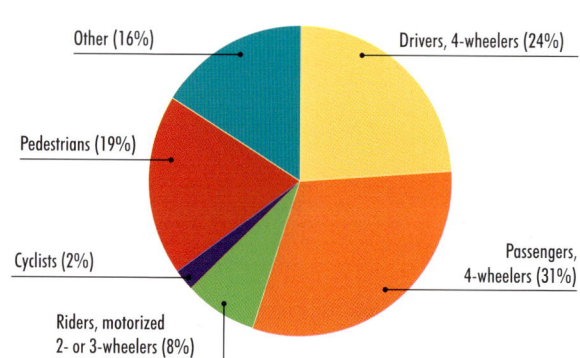

Source: 2006, Security General Directorate

126 EUROPEAN STATUS REPORT ON ROAD SAFETY

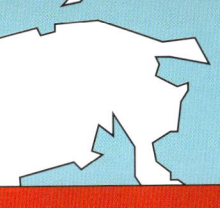

National legislation

Speed limits set nationally	Yes
Local authorities may set lower limits	Yes
Speed limits differ by vehicle type	Yes
Maximum speed limits (km/h)	
Urban roads	50
Rural roads	90
Highways and motorways	120
Enforcement[a]	0 1 2 3 4 5 6 7 **8** 9 10
Drink–driving law	Yes
Drink–driving defined by:	
blood alcohol concentration (BAC) limit	Yes
breath content	Yes
physician certificate	No
BAC limit: general population	0.05 g/dl
BAC limit: young or novice drivers	0.05 g/dl
BAC limit: professional and commercial drivers	0.00 g/dl
Mechanisms to enforce drink–driving laws	
Random breath testing	Yes
Police checkpoints	Yes
Breath testing of all drivers involved in crashes	Yes
Blood testing of all drivers involved in crashes	Yes
Enforcement[a]	0 1 2 3 4 5 6 7 8 **9** 10
Law requiring motorcycle helmets	Yes
Applies to all riders	Yes
Applies to all engine types	Yes
Exception to the legislation	No
Helmet standards mandated	Yes
Enforcement[a]	0 1 2 3 4 **5** 6 7 8 9 10
Seat-belt law	Yes
Applies to front-seat occupants	Yes
Applies to rear-seat occupants	Yes
Enforcement applied to:	front- and rear-seat occupants
Enforcement[a]	0 1 2 3 4 5 6 7 **8** 9 10
Law requiring child restraints in cars	Yes
Enforcement[a]	0 1 2 3 4 5 6 **7** 8 9 10

[a] The enforcement score represents a consensus based on the professional opinion of respondents on a scale of 0 to 10, where 0 is not effective and 10 is highly effective.

Road safety audits

Formal audits required for major new road construction projects	Yes
Regular audits of existing road infrastructure	Yes

Vehicle standards

Car manufacturers required to adhere to standards on	
Fuel consumption	Yes
Seat-belt installation for all seats	Yes

Promoting transport alternatives to cars

National policies to promote walking or cycling	No (subnational)
Investment in bicycle lanes	NA
Investment in foot paths	NA
Traffic-calming measures	NA
Investment for increasing cycling	NA
Disincentives for private car use	NA
National policies to promote public transport	Yes
Subsidized pricing of public transport	No
Improving the frequency and coverage of public transport	Yes
Disincentives for private car use	Yes

Vehicle regulations

Compulsory insurance for vehicles	Yes
Periodic vehicle inspection for:	
cars	Yes
motorized 2- or 3-wheeled vehicles	Yes
minibuses and vans	Yes
lorries	Yes
buses	Yes

Registered motor vehicles

Total (2008)	13 311 000
Cars	50%
Motorized 2- and 3-wheelers	15%
Minibuses, vans, etc. (seating <20 people)	18%
Lorries	6%
Buses	2%
Non-motorized vehicles	1%
Other	9%

Source: Turkstat through Security Directorate

Care after road crashes

Formal, publicly available prehospital care system	Yes
National universal access telephone number	Yes (112)

Acknowledgements

Authority approving the data for publication: Ministry of Health
National data coordinator: Huseyin Fazil Inan, Ministry of Health
Respondents: Bora Kayser, Ministry of Health; Senturk Demiral, Security General Directorate; Ismet Temel, Turkish Statistical Institute (Turkstat); Veysel Akkus, Highways General Directorate; Erpulat Ozis, Ufuk University; A. Haki Turkdemir, Ankara Province Health Directorate; Y. Mehmet Kontas, WHO Country Office Turkey

Turkmenistan

Population: **5.0 million (2007)**

Median age: **24 years**

Life expectancy at birth: **63 years**

Income group:[a] **middle**

Gross national income per person: **US$ 1234**   Rank: **46 of 49**[b]

Human Development Index:[c] **0.728**   Rank: **44 of 49**[b]

Private car ownership per 1000 population:[d] **80.9**

CO_2 emissions (tonnes) per person per year:[a] **8.7**

[a] World Bank data.
[b] Rank among the 49 countries in the WHO European Region participating in the survey.
[c] United Nations Development Programme data.
[d] WHO European Region average: 339.

Institutional framework for road safety	
Lead agency:	No
Status of the agency	NA
Funded in national budget	NA
National road safety strategy	Multiple strategies
Measurable targets	NA
Implementation funded	NA
Money allocated (in € (year))	NA

Key data	
Reported number of road traffic deaths (2006)	650[a]
Reported number of non-fatal road traffic injuries (2006)	1606[b]
Road traffic deaths involving alcohol	7.4%[c]
Wearing motorcycle helmets	No information
Using seat-belts in cars	
Overall	No information
Front-seat occupants	No information
Rear-seat occupants	No information
Costing study available	No
Annual estimated costs (in € (year))	NA
Study included deaths, injuries or both	NA
Methods used	NA

[a] Department of Police Road Supervision of the Ministry of Internal Affairs data, defined as died within 7 days of the crash.
[b] Department of Police Road Supervision of the Ministry of Internal Affairs data.
[c] 2008, Department of Road Police Supervision of the Ministry of Internal Affairs.

NA: not applicable

Trends in road traffic deaths

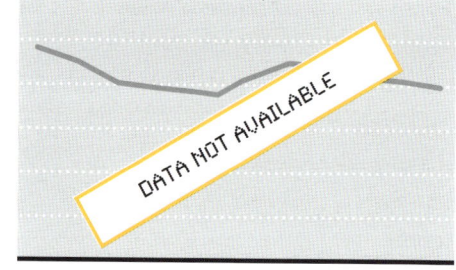

Age-specific mortality rates from road traffic injuries

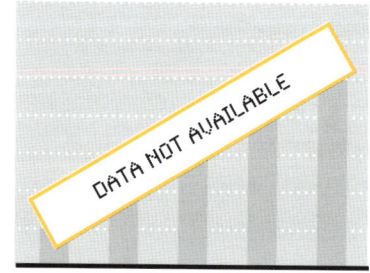

Deaths by road user category

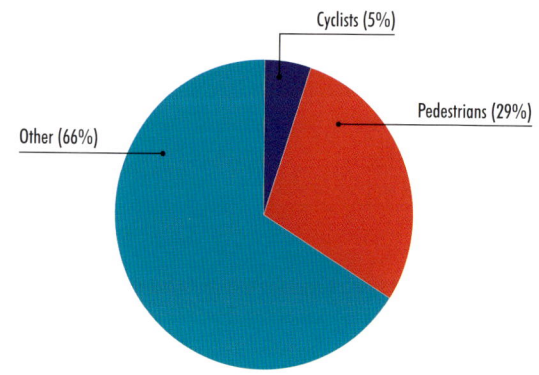

Source: Department of Police Road Supervision of the Ministry of Internal Affairs

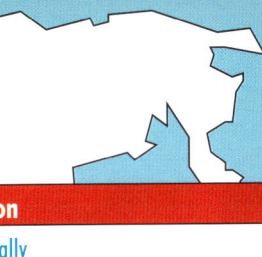

National legislation	
Speed limits set nationally	Yes
Local authorities may set lower limits	No
Speed limits differ by vehicle type	No
Maximum speed limits (km/h)	
Urban roads	60
Rural roads	90
Highways and motorways	110
Enforcement[a]	9/10
Drink–driving law	Yes
Drink–driving defined by:	
blood alcohol concentration (BAC) limit	Yes
breath content	Yes
physician certificate	Yes
BAC limit: general population	0.05 g/dl
BAC limit: young or novice drivers	0.05 g/dl
BAC limit: professional and commercial drivers	0.05 g/dl
Mechanisms to enforce drink–driving laws	
Random breath testing	Yes
Police checkpoints	Yes
Breath testing of all drivers involved in crashes	Yes
Blood testing of all drivers involved in crashes	Yes
Enforcement[a]	10/10
Law requiring motorcycle helmets	Yes
Applies to all riders	Yes
Applies to all engine types	No
Exception to the legislation	No
Helmet standards mandated	No
Enforcement[a]	8/10
Seat-belt law	Yes
Applies to front-seat occupants	Yes
Applies to rear-seat occupants	No
Enforcement applied to:	front-seat occupants only
Enforcement[a]	7/10
Law requiring child restraints in cars	No
Enforcement[a]	NA

[a] The enforcement score represents a consensus based on the professional opinion of respondents on a scale of 0 to 10, where 0 is not effective and 10 is highly effective.

Road safety audits	
Formal audits required for major new road construction projects	Yes
Regular audits of existing road infrastructure	Yes

Vehicle standards	
No car manufacturers	

Promoting transport alternatives to cars	
National policies to promote walking or cycling	No information
Investment in bicycle lanes	NA
Investment in foot paths	NA
Traffic-calming measures	NA
Investment for increasing cycling	NA
Disincentives for private car use	NA
National policies to promote public transport	Yes
Subsidized pricing of public transport	Yes
Improving the frequency and coverage of public transport	Yes
Disincentives for private car use	No

Vehicle regulations	
Compulsory insurance for vehicles	Yes
Periodic vehicle inspection for:	
cars	Yes
motorized 2- or 3-wheeled vehicles	Yes
minibuses and vans	Yes
lorries	Yes
buses	Yes

Registered motor vehicles	
Total (2008)	651 564
Cars	62%
Motorized 2- and 3-wheelers	18%
Lorries	16%
Buses	4%

Source: Department of Road Police Supervision of the Ministry of Internal Affairs

Care after road crashes	
Formal, publicly available prehospital care system	Yes
National universal access telephone number	Yes (03)

Acknowledgements

Authority approving the data for publication: Ministry of Foreign Affairs
National data coordinator: Begklich Ovezklichev, Ministry of Public Health and Medical Industry of Turkmenistan
Respondents: Gurbanmurad Shihmuradov, National Concern "Turkmenavtoellary"; Mekan Gaipov, Department of Police Road Supervision of the Ministry of Internal Affairs of Turkmenistan; Maral Kakisheva, Ashgabat Town Center of Traumatology and Urgent Surgery; Nataliya Levaya, National Society of the Turkmenistan Red Crescent; Irina Kivandova, Ashgabat Town Center of Drug Prevention, Alcohol and Psycologic Diseases to the Ministry of Public Health and Medical Industry of Turkmenistan; Maral Kakabaeva, Governmental Statistics Committee of Turkmenistan; Dovran Ovezov, Emergency centre to the Ministry of Public Health and Medical Industry of Turkmenistan; Ata Boppiev, Information Centre; Mamedov Meylis, Ministry of Road Transport of Turkmenistan

Ukraine

Population: 46.21 million (2007)
Median age: 39 years
Life expectancy at birth: 67 years
Income group:[a] middle
Gross national income per person: US$ 2550   **Rank:** 43 of 49[b]
Human Development Index:[c] 0.800   **Rank:** 39 of 49[b]
Private car ownership per 1000 population:[d] No information
CO_2 emissions (tonnes) per person per year:[a] 6.9

[a] World Bank data.
[b] Rank among the 49 countries in the WHO European Region participating in the survey.
[c] United Nations Development Programme data.
[d] WHO European Region average: 339.

Institutional framework for road safety

Lead agency: Ministry of Public Health	
Status of the agency	Government
Funded in national budget	Yes
National road safety strategy	Multiple strategies
Measurable targets	NA
Implementation funded	NA
Money allocated (in € (year))	NA

Key data

Reported number of road traffic deaths (2007)	9921[a] (76% males, 24% females)
Reported number of non-fatal road traffic injuries (2007)	40 887[b]
Road traffic deaths involving alcohol	No information
Wearing motorcycle helmets	No information
Using seat-belts in cars	
Overall	No information
Front-seat occupants	No information
Rear-seat occupants	No information
Costing study available	No
Annual estimated costs (in € (year))	NA
Study included deaths, injuries or both	NA
Methods used	NA

[a] Health data, defined as died within 30 days of the crash.
[b] Data source not specified.

NA: not applicable

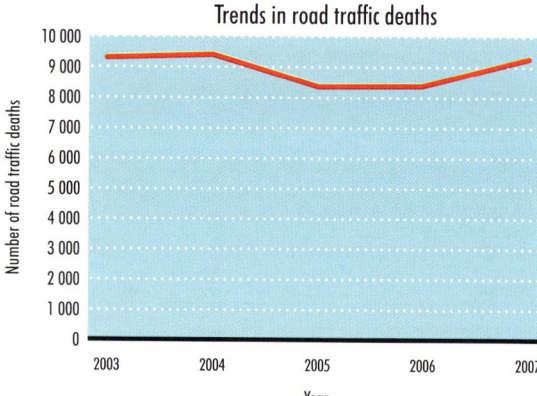

Trends in road traffic deaths

Source: State Medical Statistics Centre

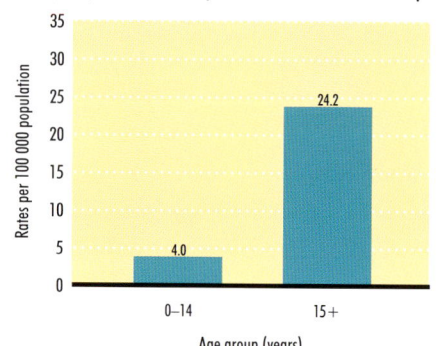

Age-specific mortality rates from road traffic injuries

Source: 2006, Department of Statistics of Transportation and Communication of National Statistical Service

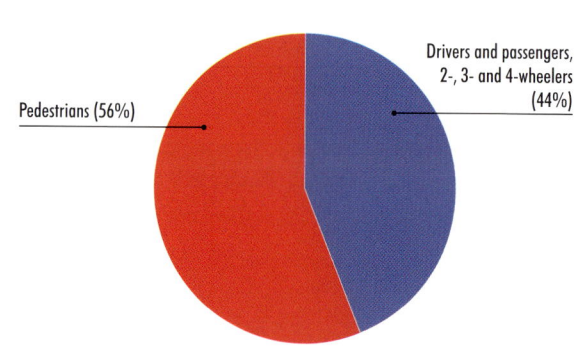

Deaths by road user category

Pedestrians (56%)
Drivers and passengers, 2-, 3- and 4-wheelers (44%)

Source: State Medical Statistics Centre

National legislation	
Speed limits set nationally	Yes
Local authorities may set lower limits	No
Speed limits differ by vehicle type	No
Maximum speed limits (km/h)	
Urban roads	60
Rural roads	40
Highways and motorways	90
Enforcement[a]	No consensus
Drink–driving law	Yes
Drink–driving defined by:	
blood alcohol concentration (BAC) limit	Yes
breath content	Yes
physician certificate	No
BAC limit: general population	0.00 g/dl
BAC limit: young or novice drivers	0.00 g/dl
BAC limit: professional and commercial drivers	0.00 g/dl
Mechanisms to enforce drink–driving laws	
Random breath testing	Yes
Police checkpoints	No
Breath testing of all drivers involved in crashes	Yes
Blood testing of all drivers involved in crashes	Yes
Enforcement[a]	No consensus
Law requiring motorcycle helmets	No
Applies to all riders	NA
Applies to all engine types	NA
Exception to the legislation	NA
Helmet standards mandated	NA
Enforcement[a]	NA
Seat-belt law	Yes
Applies to front-seat occupants	Yes
Applies to rear-seat occupants	No
Enforcement applied to:	front-seat occupants only
Enforcement[a]	No consensus
Law requiring child restraints in cars	No
Enforcement[a]	NA

[a] The enforcement score represents a consensus based on the professional opinion of respondents on a scale of 0 to 10, where 0 is not effective and 10 is highly effective.

Promoting transport alternatives to cars	
National policies to promote walking or cycling	No
Investment in bicycle lanes	NA
Investment in foot paths	NA
Traffic-calming measures	NA
Investment for increasing cycling	NA
Disincentives for private car use	NA
National policies to promote public transport	No (subnational)
Subsidized pricing of public transport	NA
Improving the frequency and coverage of public transport	NA
Disincentives for private car use	NA

Vehicle regulations	
Compulsory insurance for vehicles	Yes
Periodic vehicle inspection for:	
cars	Yes
motorized 2- or 3-wheeled vehicles	Yes
minibuses and vans	Yes
lorries	Yes
buses	Yes

Registered motor vehicles	
Total, year:	No information

Care after road crashes	
Formal, publicly available prehospital care system	Yes
National universal access telephone number	Yes (03)

Road safety audits	
Formal audits required for major new road construction projects	Yes
Regular audits of existing road infrastructure	No

Vehicle standards	
Car manufacturers required to adhere to standards on	
Fuel consumption	No
Seat-belt installation for all seats	No

Acknowledgements

Authority approving the data for publication: Data were not cleared by the government of Ukraine in time for publication of this report.
National data coordinator: Irina Fedenko, Ministry of Public Health
Respondents: Mikhail Golubchikov, Ministry of Public Health of Ukraine; Svetlana Sinelnik, Ministry of Public Health of Ukraine

United Kingdom

Population: **60.77 million (2007)**

Median age: **39** years

Life expectancy at birth: **79** years

Income group:[a] **high**

Gross national income per person: **US$ 42 740**   Rank: **8** of 49[b]

Human Development Index:[c] **0.942**   Rank: **14** of 49[b]

Private car ownership per 1000 population:[d] **476.5**

CO_2 emissions (tonnes) per person per year:[a] **9.8**

[a] World Bank data.
[b] Rank among the 49 countries in the WHO European Region participating in the survey.
[c] United Nations Development Programme data.
[d] WHO European Region average: 339.

Institutional framework for road safety	
Lead agency:	No
Status of the agency	NA
Funded in national budget	NA
National road safety strategy	Yes
Measurable targets	Yes
Implementation funded	Yes
Money allocated (in € (year))	No information

Key data	
Reported number of road traffic deaths (2006)	3298[a] (76% males, 24% females)
Reported number of non-fatal road traffic injuries (2006)	264 288[b]
Road traffic deaths involving alcohol	17.0%[c]
Wearing motorcycle helmets	98%[d]
Using seat-belts in cars	
Overall	No information
Front-seat occupants	91%[e]
Rear-seat occupants	84–90%[e]
Costing study available	Yes
Annual estimated costs (in € (2006))	19.49 billion
Study included deaths, injuries or both	Both deaths and injuries
Methods used	Willingness to pay

[a] Police data, defined as died within 30 days of the crash.
[b] Police data.
[c] 2006, Road Casualties Great Britain: 2006 Annual Report, Department for Transport
[d] 2006, Department for Transport estimation.
[e] 2006–2007, Department for Transport, observational studies.

NA: not applicable

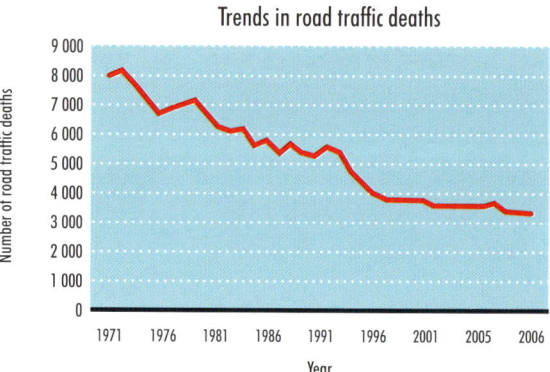

Trends in road traffic deaths

Source: Road Casualties Great Britain: 2006 Annual Report, Department for Transport, Road Traffic Collision Statistics Annual Report 2006, Police Service of Northern Ireland

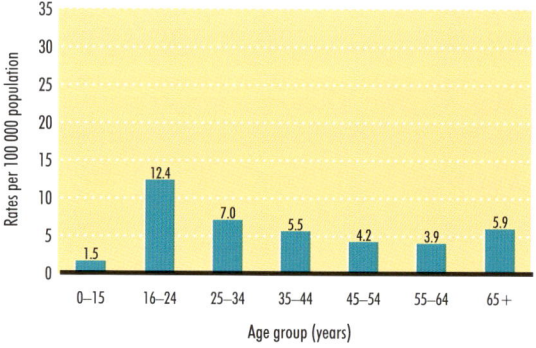

Age-specific mortality rates from road traffic injuries

Source: 2006, Road Casualties Great Britain: 2006 Annual Report, Department for Transport, Road Traffic Collision Statistics Annual Report 2006, Police Service of Northern Ireland

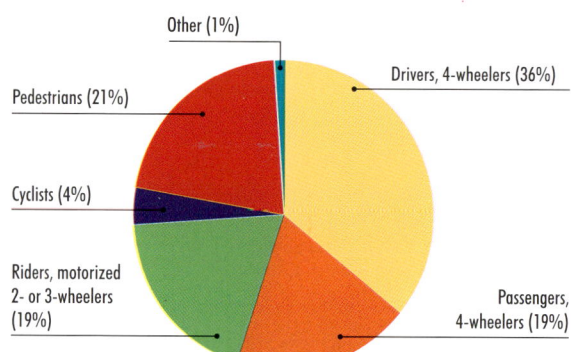

Deaths by road user category

- Drivers, 4-wheelers (36%)
- Passengers, 4-wheelers (19%)
- Riders, motorized 2- or 3-wheelers (19%)
- Cyclists (4%)
- Pedestrians (21%)
- Other (1%)

Source: 2006, Road Casualties Great Britain: 2006 Annual Report, Department for Transport, Road Traffic Collision Statistics Annual Report 2006, Police Service of Northern Ireland

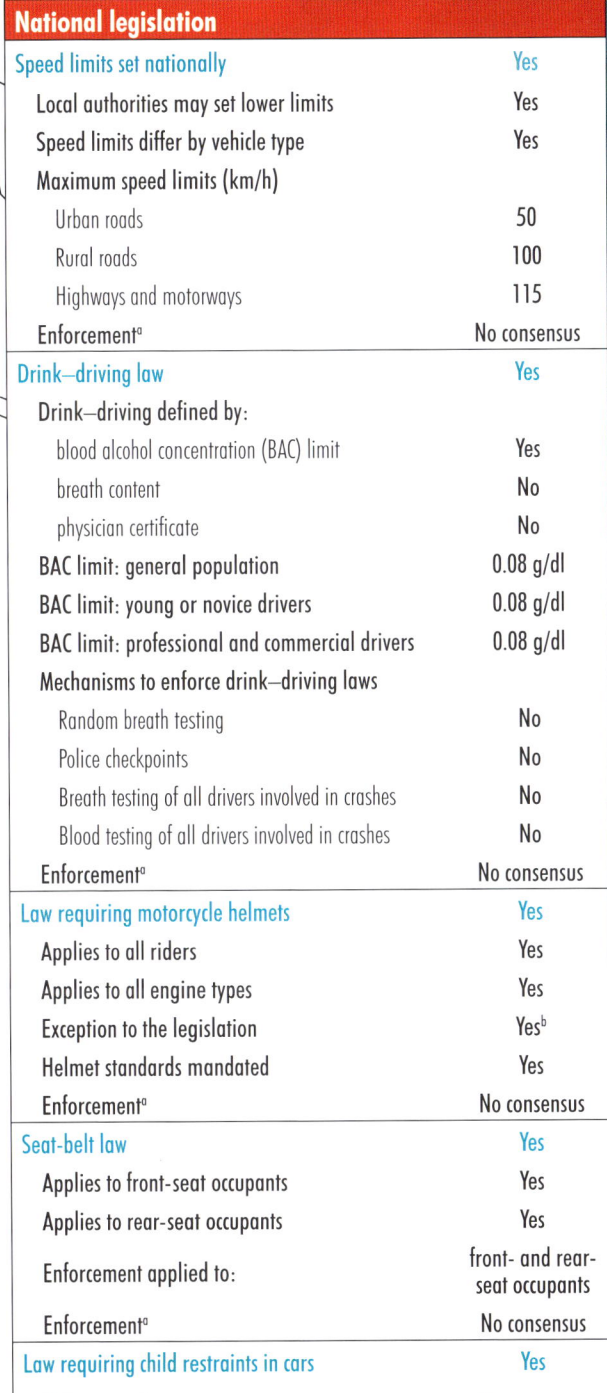

National legislation

Speed limits set nationally	Yes
Local authorities may set lower limits	Yes
Speed limits differ by vehicle type	Yes
Maximum speed limits (km/h)	
Urban roads	50
Rural roads	100
Highways and motorways	115
Enforcement[a]	No consensus
Drink–driving law	Yes
Drink–driving defined by:	
blood alcohol concentration (BAC) limit	Yes
breath content	No
physician certificate	No
BAC limit: general population	0.08 g/dl
BAC limit: young or novice drivers	0.08 g/dl
BAC limit: professional and commercial drivers	0.08 g/dl
Mechanisms to enforce drink–driving laws	
Random breath testing	No
Police checkpoints	No
Breath testing of all drivers involved in crashes	No
Blood testing of all drivers involved in crashes	No
Enforcement[a]	No consensus
Law requiring motorcycle helmets	Yes
Applies to all riders	Yes
Applies to all engine types	Yes
Exception to the legislation	Yes[b]
Helmet standards mandated	Yes
Enforcement[a]	No consensus
Seat-belt law	Yes
Applies to front-seat occupants	Yes
Applies to rear-seat occupants	Yes
Enforcement applied to:	front- and rear-seat occupants
Enforcement[a]	No consensus
Law requiring child restraints in cars	Yes
Enforcement[a]	No consensus

[a] The enforcement score represents a consensus based on the professional opinion of respondents on a scale of 0 to 10, where 0 is not effective and 10 is highly effective.
[b] Exceptions: Sikhs while they are wearing a turban.

Road safety audits

Formal audits required for major new road construction projects	Yes
Regular audits of existing road infrastructure	Yes

Vehicle standards

Car manufacturers required to adhere to standards on	
Fuel consumption	Yes
Seat-belt installation for all seats	Yes

Promoting transport alternatives to cars

National policies to promote walking or cycling	Yes[a]
Investment in bicycle lanes	Yes
Investment in foot paths	Yes
Traffic-calming measures	Yes
Investment for increasing cycling	No
Disincentives for private car use	No
National policies to promote public transport	Yes
Subsidized pricing of public transport	Yes
Improving the frequency and coverage of public transport	Yes
Disincentives for private car use	No

[a] Other policies are implemented in addition to those listed.

Vehicle regulations

Compulsory insurance for vehicles	Yes
Periodic vehicle inspection for:	
cars	Yes
motorized 2- or 3-wheeled vehicles	Yes
minibuses and vans	Yes
lorries	Yes
buses	Yes

Registered motor vehicles

Total (2006)	34 327 520
Cars	84%
Motorized 2- and 3-wheelers	4%
Minibuses, vans, etc. (seating <20 people)	9%
Lorries	1%
Buses	1%
Other	1%

Source: Vehicle Licensing Statistics: 2006, Department for Transport, *Northern Ireland Transport Statistics 2006*, Department for Regional Development

Care after road crashes

Formal, publicly available prehospital care system	Yes
National universal access telephone number	Yes (999)

Acknowledgements

Authority approving the data for publication: Department for Transport
National data coordinator: Mark Bellis, Centre for Public Health, Liverpool John Moores University; Sara Hughes, Centre for Public Health, Liverpool John Moores University
Respondents: Andrew Colski, Department for Transport; Pat Kilbey, Department for Transport; Harry Green, Department of the Environment; Carol Ann Munn, Scottish Government; Paul Taylor, Association of Chief Police Officers; Sue Maisey, Department of Health; Meryl James, Welsh Assembly Government

Uzbekistan

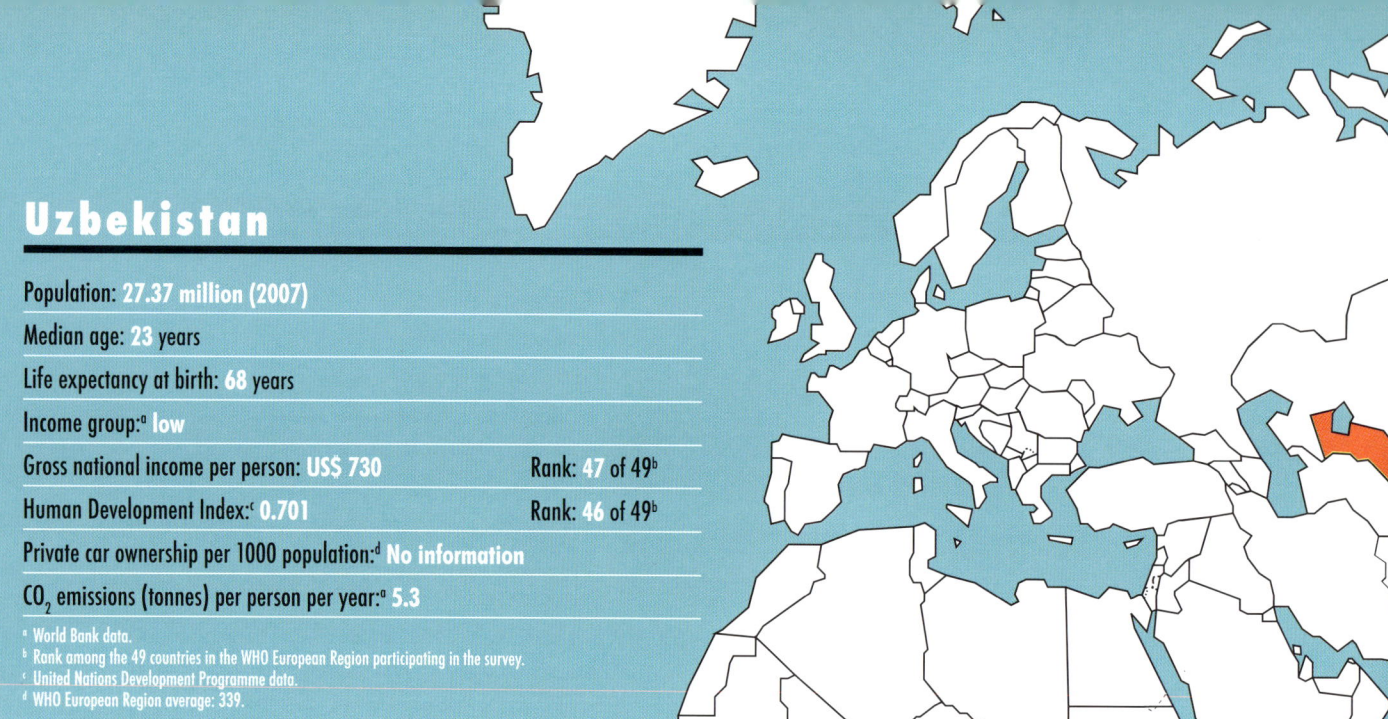

Population: 27.37 million (2007)
Median age: 23 years
Life expectancy at birth: 68 years
Income group:[a] low
Gross national income per person: US$ 730   Rank: 47 of 49[b]
Human Development Index:[c] 0.701   Rank: 46 of 49[b]
Private car ownership per 1000 population:[d] No information
CO_2 emissions (tonnes) per person per year:[a] 5.3

[a] World Bank data.
[b] Rank among the 49 countries in the WHO European Region participating in the survey.
[c] United Nations Development Programme data.
[d] WHO European Region average: 339.

Institutional framework for road safety	
Lead agency: The State Motor-Vehicle Inspectorate, Ministry of Internal Affairs	
Status of the agency	Government
Funded in national budget	Yes
National road safety strategy	Yes
Measurable targets	Yes
Implementation funded	No information
Money allocated (in € (year))	NA

Key data	
Reported number of road traffic deaths (2006)	2034[a]
Reported number of non-fatal road traffic injuries (year)	No information
Road traffic deaths involving alcohol	No information
Wearing motorcycle helmets	No information
Using seat-belts in cars	
Overall	No information
Front-seat occupants	No information
Rear-seat occupants	No information
Costing study available	No
Annual estimated costs (in € (year))	NA
Study included deaths, injuries or both	NA
Methods used	NA

[a] Ministry of Internal Affairs data, defined as died at the crash scene.

NA: not applicable

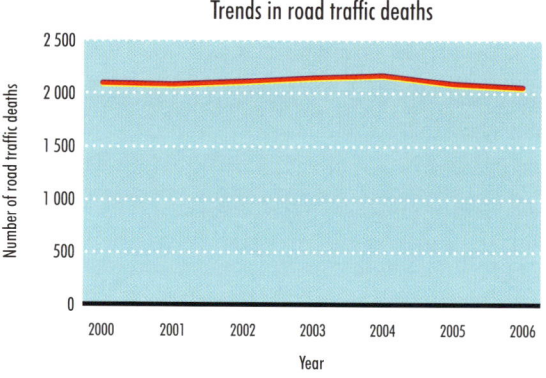

Trends in road traffic deaths

Source: Ministry of Internal Affairs

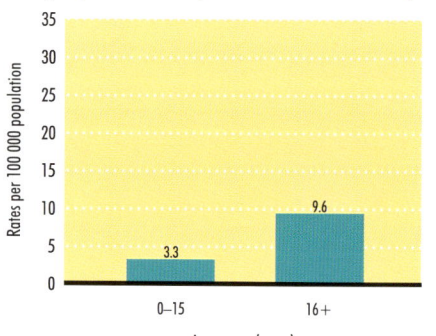

Age-specific mortality rates from road traffic injuries

Source: 2006, The State Motor-Vehicle Inspectorate, Ministry of Internal Affairs

Deaths by road user category

DATA NOT AVAILABLE

National legislation	
Speed limits set nationally	Yes
Local authorities may set lower limits	No
Speed limits differ by vehicle type	Yes
Maximum speed limits (km/h)	
Urban roads	70
Rural roads	70
Highways and motorways	90
Enforcement[a]	0 1 2 3 4 5 6 **7** 8 9 10
Drink–driving law	Yes
Drink–driving defined by:	
blood alcohol concentration (BAC) limit	Yes
breath content	Yes
physician certificate	Yes
BAC limit: general population	None
BAC limit: young or novice drivers	None
BAC limit: professional and commercial drivers	None
Mechanisms to enforce drink–driving laws	
Random breath testing	Yes
Police checkpoints	No
Breath testing of all drivers involved in crashes	Yes
Blood testing of all drivers involved in crashes	Yes
Enforcement[a]	0 1 2 3 4 5 6 7 8 **9** 10
Law requiring motorcycle helmets	Yes
Applies to all riders	Yes
Applies to all engine types	Yes
Exception to the legislation	No
Helmet standards mandated	No
Enforcement[a]	0 1 2 3 4 5 6 7 8 **9** 10
Seat-belt law	Yes
Applies to front-seat occupants	Yes
Applies to rear-seat occupants	Yes
Enforcement applied to:	front- and rear-seat occupants
Enforcement[a]	0 1 2 3 4 5 6 7 8 9 **10**
Law requiring child restraints in cars	No information
Enforcement[a]	NA

[a] The enforcement score represents a consensus based on the professional opinion of respondents on a scale of 0 to 10, where 0 is not effective and 10 is highly effective.

Road safety audits	
Formal audits required for major new road construction projects	Yes
Regular audits of existing road infrastructure	Yes

Vehicle standards	
Car manufacturers required to adhere to standards on	
Fuel consumption	Yes
Seat-belt installation for all seats	Yes

Promoting transport alternatives to cars	
National policies to promote walking or cycling	No information
Investment in bicycle lanes	NA
Investment in foot paths	NA
Traffic-calming measures	NA
Investment for increasing cycling	NA
Disincentives for private car use	NA
National policies to promote public transport	No information
Subsidized pricing of public transport	NA
Improving the frequency and coverage of public transport	NA
Disincentives for private car use	NA

Vehicle regulations	
Compulsory insurance for vehicles	Yes
Periodic vehicle inspection for:	
cars	Yes
motorized 2- or 3-wheeled vehicles	Yes
minibuses and vans	Yes
lorries	Yes
buses	Yes

Registered motor vehicles	
Total, year:	No information

Care after road crashes	
Formal, publicly available prehospital care system	Yes
National universal access telephone number	Yes (03)

Acknowledgements

Authority approving the data for publication: Ministry of Health
National data coordinator: Mirhakim Azizov, Research Institute of Traumatology and Orthopedy to the Ministry of Health of the Republic of Uzbekistan; Gulnora Kasimova, Scientific Research Institute of Traumatology and Orthopedy, Tashkent
Respondents: NA

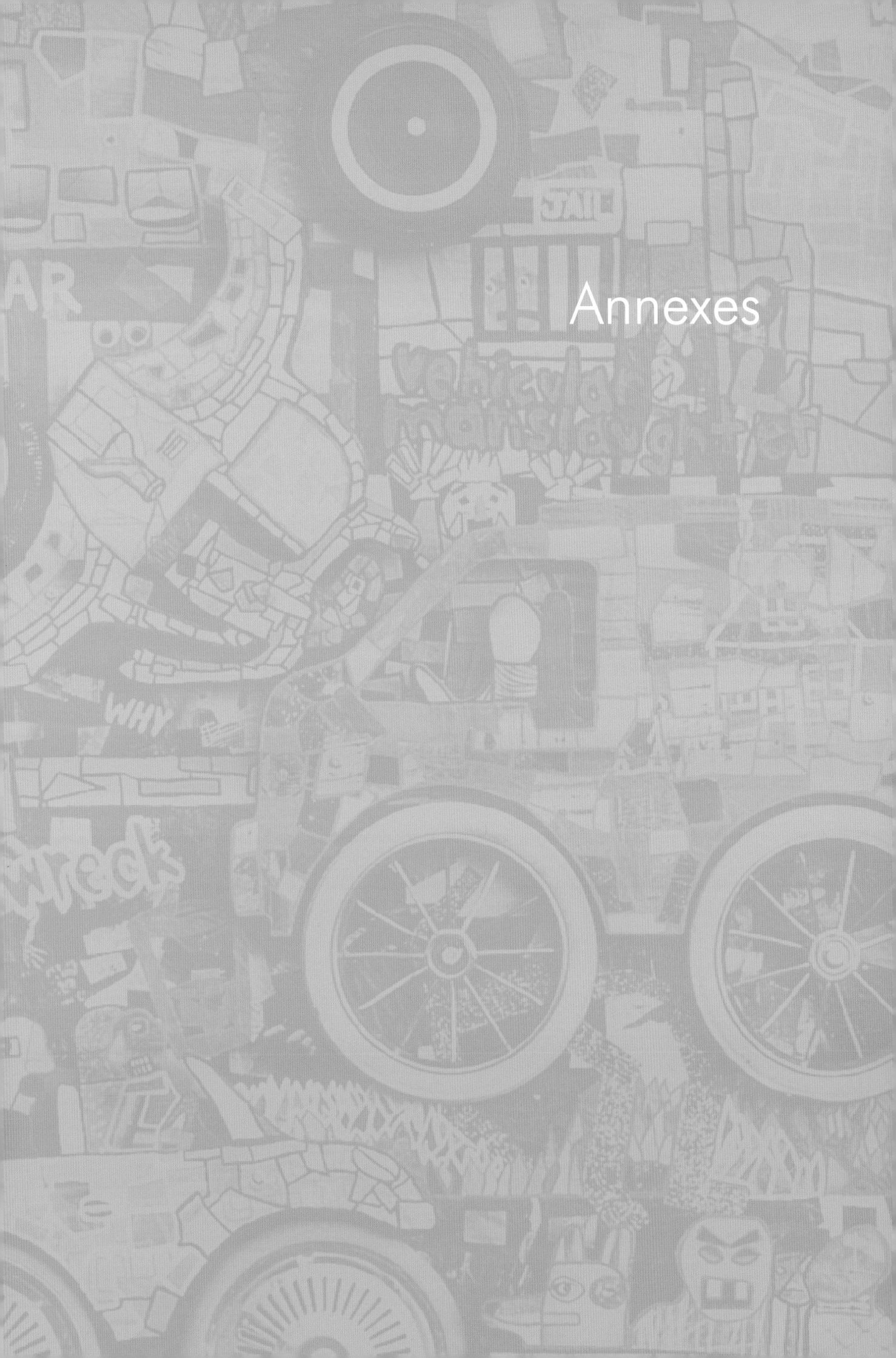

Annexes

Annex 1. Explanatory notes for Annexes 2–13

Background

The data presented in Annexes 2–13 were obtained through a self-administered questionnaire implemented in the 49 countries of the WHO European Region that participated in the first Global Survey on Road Safety in 2008. The survey focused on the recommendations of the *World report on road traffic injury prevention (1)* as the basis for its structure and content. Most countries used the same methods for data collection, as outlined in a survey protocol developed for the study. In 92% of the countries, a national data coordinator identified by the country coordinated the implementation of the survey, and teams of 6–8 key respondents including the national data coordinator completed the survey. The national data coordinators were trained in the methods and coordinated the collection, validation and clearance of data, as well as the data entry. The survey instrument, protocol and accompanying guidelines and training materials were available in the six official WHO languages. Where needed, national data coordinators coordinated the translation of these documents into the local language and then back-translated them for the data entry, which was done in English. More details on the methods used for data collection can be found at: www.who.int/violence_injury_prevention/road_traffic/road_safety_status/2009.

The following sections contain country-by-country data obtained from the survey.
- **Annex 2** includes the list of indicators explored in the survey.
- **Annex 3** provides detailed data on the 30-day adjusted number and rates per population of road traffic deaths and on the proportion of road users by country. The table includes modelled road traffic death numbers that have been generated. The process is briefly described below. Annex 3 also presents some general information on the countries, number of vehicles and rate of private car ownership and number and rates of injuries due to road crashes.
- **Annex 4** includes a graph presenting the mortality rates for road crashes by gross national income per person.
- **Annex 5** includes a list of objectives retrieved from the national strategies for the countries that reported a national strategy or a summary of it in English.
- **Annex 6** presents the estimated economic costs of one death in countries for which this was available.
- **Annexes 7–10** provide information on the status of laws, the enforcement of laws and the coverage and wearing rates relating to five road traffic risk factors: alcohol, seat-belts, child restraints, speed and helmets.
- **Annex 11** contains data on policy-related responses.
- **Annex 12** includes information related to the availability of prehospital care.
- **Annex 13** includes a list of national data coordinators and respondents who, in collaboration with national authorities, played a key part in conducting the survey.

Data processing

The data processing involved completing the survey instrument and entering data at the country level and validation at the regional level. WHO headquarters cleaned and modelled the data, and the WHO Country Office in the Russian Federation and the European Centre for Environment and Health, Rome Office, WHO Regional Office for Europe performed analysis and wrote the report.

Reporting of country-level data

National data coordinators entered the final country responses into an online database specially prepared by WHO for this project. National data coordinators also uploaded supporting documents where applicable and available. Data were then validated at the regional level. Once finalized and approved by regional data coordinators, the data were then exported into Microsoft Excel for cleaning. At this stage, each country's data were examined for accuracy, consistency and validity on a question-by-question basis. Where necessary, national data coordinators were contacted and additional supporting documents were requested to clarify inconsistencies. The survey instrument and study protocol are available at: http://www.who.int/violence_injury_prevention/road_traffic/road_safety_status/2009.

Types of data used

This report uses three types of data:
- data from countries and secondary sources;
- data adjusted for the 30-day definition of a road traffic death to facilitate comparability; and
- modelled numbers.

In addition to the data obtained directly from countries, secondary data sources were used:
- to classify countries into income categories; and
- to generate road safety indicators such as the adjusted road traffic deaths and modelled road traffic death rates (with a 90% confidence interval) as reported in Annex 3.

Population and income data from the United Nations Population Division *(2)* and the World Bank *(3)* were used for this analysis.

Annex 3 reports population estimates for 2007. If no estimate was available for a country for that year, published data for the latest year were used. Population estimates corresponding to the year of reporting were used for the modelling process.

Annex 3 uses World Bank (Atlas method) gross national income per capita for 2007 *(4)* (or latest available year) to categorize countries into:
- low-income = US$ 935 or less;
- middle-income = US$ 936 to US$ 11 455;
- high-income = US$ 11 456 or more *(3)*.

The modelling process used more detailed subgroups.

Adjusted data

Underreporting has been acknowledged for many years as an important reason for the difficulty in comparing road crash data between countries. Further, the lack of harmonized definitions for road traffic deaths, the use of different data sources and the quality of the reporting system have also been documented. Consequently, several mechanisms were used to address these issues and make data more comparable. The Global Survey used the following two methods:
- the European Conference of Ministers of Transport standardized 30-day road crash fatality factors *(5)* to adjust all reported country data; and
- a model using negative binomial regression (*Global status report on road safety*. Geneva, World Health Organization, 2009:231–234).

The "reported" data in Annex 3 have been adjusted to this 30-day definition (see Table 1 for adjustment factors). Data for Albania, Portugal, Slovakia, Turkey and Uzbekistan were adjusted by a factor of 1.30 to correct for deaths defined as died on the scene or within 24 hours. Data for Azerbaijan, Kazakhstan, the Russian Federation and Turkmenistan were adjusted by a factor of 1.08 to correct for road traffic deaths defined as died within 7 days of the crash. Data for Kyrgyzstan and the Republic of Moldova were adjusted by a factor of 0.97 to correct for deaths defined as died within 1 year of the crash.

The new adjusted numbers were therefore used in the corresponding model.

Table 1. European Conference of Ministers of Transport standardized 30-day factors for adjusting road crash fatalities

	30-day total	Adjustment factor
On the scene or 1 day	77%	1.30
3 days	87%	1.15
6 days	92%	1.09
7 days	93%	1.08
30 days	100%	1.00
365 days	103%	0.97

Modelled data

The model developed for estimating mortality rates used data obtained from all 178 countries participating in the Global Survey. The *Global status report on road safety* provides detailed information on the variables included in the model and how the estimates were achieved on pages 231–234.

Once data from all the countries participating in the survey had been adjusted for definition, countries were divided into two groups based on the completeness of vital registration data. Data from countries with good vital registration data and a population of more than 100 000 were used as a reference in constructing the negative binomial model. The model considered independent variables that are directly related to the outcome variable (road traffic deaths): gross national income per person, income level per person according to the World Bank classification of low, medium or high, population, vehicle density, road density, existence of a national helmet law, national speed limits on urban roads, national speed limits on rural roads, national policies that encourage walking and/or cycling, national policies that support investment in public transport, alcohol consumption and the strength of the health system. Estimates of the number of deaths with 90% confidence intervals were calculated using the model developed. The methods and formulas for the modelling process are fully described in the *Global status report on road safety (6)* on pages 231–234 and at the following web site: http://www.who.int/violence_injury_prevention/road_safety_status/2009.

Only six countries in the Region had incomplete vital registration data of less than 85% or external causes of death of undetermined intent greater than 30% *(7,8)*. Data on road traffic injury deaths from Albania, Armenia, Azerbaijan, Tajikistan, Turkey and Turkmenistan required modelling. Annex 3 presents results with 90% confidence intervals derived from the model. These results were also used to calculate mortality rates per 100 000 population, as shown in Fig. 3 in the main text.

References

1. Peden M et al., eds. *World report on road traffic injury prevention*. Geneva, World Health Organization, 2004 (http://www.who.int/violence_injury_prevention/publications/road_traffic/world_report/en/index.html, accessed 23 July 2009).
2. *World population prospects: the 2006 revision. Highlights.* New York, United Nations Population Division, 2007.
3. *World development indicators.* Washington, DC, World Bank, 2007.
4. *GNI per capita 2007: Atlas method and PPP.* Washington, DC, World Bank, 2007 (http://siteresources.worldbank.org/DATASTATISTICS/Resources/GNIPC.pdf, accessed 23 July 2009).

5. Jacobs G, Aeron-Thomas A, Astrop A. *Estimating global road fatalities*. Crowthorne, Transport Research Laboratory, 2000 (TRL Report 445; http://www.transport-links.org/transport_links/filearea/publications/1_329_TRL445.pdf, accessed 23 July 2009).
6. *Global status report on road safety*. Geneva, World Health Organization, 2009 (http://www.who.int/violence_injury_prevention/road_safety-status/2009/en/index.html, accessed 23 July 2009).
7. *The global burden of disease: 2004 update*. Geneva, World Health Organization, 2008 (http://www.who.int/healthinfo/global_burden_disease/GBD_report_2004update/en/index.html, accessed 23 July 2009).
8. Mathers CD et al. Counting the dead and what they died from: an assessment of the global status of cause of death data. *Bulletin of the World Health Organization,* 2005, 83:171–177.

Annex 2. **Indicators explored in the questionnaire developed for the** *Global status report on road safety*

1. Institutional framework, strategy and financial investment

Lead agency or coordinating body
    Existence of a lead agency
    Status of the lead agency
    Budget for the lead agency

Strategy: existence of a national road strategy or action plan
    Existence of a national strategy
    Measurable targets set
    Budget for the national strategy

2. Data

Fatalities
    Definition of road traffic death
    Number of official deaths and the agency collecting fatality data
    Fatalities by sex, age group, trend data and road user categories

Nonfatal injuries
    Number of injured subjects and agency collecting nonfatality data

Economic costs
    Existence of studies on the economic costs of road traffic crashes
    Estimated costs
    Methods used for estimating costs

3. Interventions

Exposure to risk
    Number of registered vehicles and distribution by vehicle category
    Existence of a policy that encourages walking and/or cycling
    Existence of policies that support investment in public transport
    Requirements for getting a driving licence

Infrastructure and vehicle standards
    Road safety audits on new and existing roads
    Car manufacturers required to adhere to safety standards
    Compulsoriness of insurance for all motorized vehicles
    Periodic vehicle inspection by vehicle types

Legislation
    Speed: limits set, difference of speed limits by vehicle type, by road types, local authorities entitled to change speed limits and perception of enforcement

Drink–driving: existence of a national law on drink–driving, blood alcohol concentration limit, mechanism of enforcement, perception of enforcement and estimation of the number of deaths attributable to drink–driving

Motorcycle helmet use: existence of legislation on helmet use, whether the law differentiates by road type or road user, existence of helmet standards, helmet use prevalence and perception of enforcement

Seat-belt and child restraints: existence of national legislation on restraint measures, compulsoriness by vehicle occupant position, seat-belt use prevalence and perception of enforcement

4. Post-crash care

Emergency health services

Availability of a prehospital care system
Availability of a universal access phone number

Annex 3. General information, vehicles, road traffic deaths and proportions of road user deaths by type and road traffic injuries for countries in the WHO European Region

Country	Population[a] for 2007	Gross national income per capita[b] for 2007 in US dollars	Income level[c]	Number of vehicles	Private car ownership per 1000 persons	Reported number of road traffic deaths[d]	Death defined in the country[e]	Estimated number of road traffic deaths[e] Point estimate	90% confidence interval	Estimated road traffic death rate per 100 000 population[f]
Albania	3 190 012	3 290	Middle	349 646	74.5	499	On the scene	445	366–522	13.9
Armenia	3 002 271	2 640	Middle	366 836	95.9	371	No time frame	417	352–489	13.9
Austria	8 360 746	42 700	High	5 796 973	507.5	691	Within 30 days	691	—	8.3
Azerbaijan	8 467 167	2 550	Middle	784 018	71.7	1 195	Within 7 days	1 099	900–1 319	13.0
Belarus	9 688 795	4 220	Middle	3 147 625	241.7	1 517	Within 30 days	1 517	—	15.7
Belgium	10 457 343	40 710	High	6 362 161	482.8	1 067	Within 30 days	1 067	—	10.2
Bosnia and Herzegovina	3 934 816	3 790	Middle	675 063	145.8	428[h]	Within 30 days	428	—	10.9
Bulgaria	7 638 831	4 590	Middle	2 628 680	258.2	1 006	Within 30 days	1 006	—	13.2
Croatia	4 555 398	10 460	Middle	1 949 936	327.5	619	Within 30 days	619	—	13.6
Cyprus	854 671	24 940	High	592 480	480.4	89	Within 30 days	89	—	10.4
Czech Republic	10 186 330	14 450	High	5 455 110	403.2	1 222	Within 30 days	1 222	—	12.0
Estonia	1 335 333	13 200	High	708 794	394.2	196	Within 30 days	196	—	14.7
Finland	5 276 892	44 400	High	4 656 370	540.0	380	Within 30 days	380	—	7.2
France	61 647 375	38 500	High	39 926 000	498.0	4 620	Within 30 days	4 620	—	7.5
Georgia	4 395 420	2 120	Middle	567 900	107.6	737	Within 20 days	737	—	16.8
Germany	82 599 471	38 860	High	55 511 374	564.5	4 949	Within 30 days	4 949	—	6.0
Greece	11 146 918	29 630	High	7 212 236	455.0	1 657	Within 30 days	1 657	—	14.9
Hungary	10 029 683	11 570	High	3 625 386	300.4	1 232	Within 30 days	1 232	—	12.3
Iceland	301 006	54 100	High	293 299	688.9	30	Within 30 days	30	—	10.0
Ireland	4 300 902	48 140	High	2 444 159	440.6	365	Within 30 days	365	—	8.5
Israel	6 927 677	21 900	High	2 283 634	257.1	398	Within 30 days	398	—	5.7
Italy	58 876 834	33 540	High	43 262 992	610.1	5 669	Within 30 days	5 669	—	9.6
Kazakhstan	15 421 861	5 060	Middle	3 105 954	157.2	4 714	Within 7 days	4 714	—	30.6
Kyrgyzstan	5 316 543	590	Low	318 581	—	1 214	Within 1 year	1 214	—	22.8
Latvia	2 277 040	9 930	Middle	1 062 935	358.9	407	Within 30 days	407	—	17.9
Lithuania	3 389 937	9 920	Middle	1 781 686	467.4	759	Within 30 days	759	—	22.4
Malta	406 582	14 575[g]	High	346 118	647.0	14	Within 30 days	14	—	3.4
Montenegro	597 983	5 180	Middle	199 014	298.5	122	Within 30 days	122	—	20.4
Netherlands	16 418 824	45 820	High	8 862 935	440.5	791	Within 30 days	791	—	4.8
Norway	4 698 097	76 450	High	2 599 712	442.7	233	Within 30 days	233	—	5.0
Poland	38 081 971	9 840	Middle	18 035 047	354.6	5 583	Within 30 days	5 583	—	14.7
Portugal	10 623 031	18 950	High	5 948 269	496.5	1 110	On the scene	1 110	—	10.4
Republic of Moldova	3 793 604	1 260	Middle	448 202	87.3	571	Within 1 year	571	—	15.1
Romania	21 437 887	6 150	Middle	4 611 362	170.1	2 712	Within 30 days	2 712	—	12.7
Russian Federation	142 498 532	7 560	Middle	38 695 996	195.5	35 972	Within 7 days	35 972	—	25.2
San Marino	30 926	41 044[g]	High	51 590	—	1	Within 30 days	1	—	3.2
Serbia	9 858 424	4 730	Middle	2 235 389	154.0	962	Within 30 days	962	—	9.8
Slovakia	5 390 035	11 730	High	2 039 745	272.1	815	Within 24 hrs	815	—	15.1
Slovenia	2 001 506	20 960	High	1 286 903	509.9	293	Within 30 days	293	—	14.6
Spain	44 279 180	29 450	High	31 441 152	480.0	4 104	Within 30 days	4 104	—	9.3
Sweden	9 118 955	46 060	High	5 500 000	464.4	471	Within 30 days	471	—	5.2
Switzerland	7 483 973	59 880	High	5 356 000	515.3	370	Within 30 days	370	—	4.9
Tajikistan	6 735 996	460	Low	268 018	28.8	464	Within 30 days	951	767–1 196	14.1
The former Yugoslav Republic of Macedonia	2 038 464	3 460	Middle	259 421	109.9	140	Within 30 days	140	—	6.9
Turkey	74 876 695	8 020	Middle	13 311 000	87.1	6 022	On the scene	10 066	8 394–11 839	13.4
Turkmenistan	4 965 278	1 234[g]	Middle	651 564	80.9	702	Within 7 days	926	694–1 343	18.6
Ukraine	46 205 382	2 550	Middle	—	—	9 921	Within 30 days	9 921	—	21.5
United Kingdom	60 768 946	42 740	High	34 327 520	476.5	3 298	Within 30 days	3 298	—	5.4
Uzbekistan	27 372 260	730	Low	—	—	2 644	On the scene	2 644	—	9.7

[a] Population Division of the Department of Economic and Social Affairs of the United Nations. *World population prospects: the 2006 revision, highlights.* New York, United Nations, 2007.
[b] Gross national income per capita is the value of a country's final income in a year divided by its population using the World Bank Atlas method. Data source: World Development Indicators database [online database]. Washington, DC, World Bank, 17 October 2008 (http://www.worldbank.org/data, accessed 10 June 2009).
[c] World Development Indicators database: low income is US$ 935 or less, middle income is US$ 936 to US$ 11 455 and high income is US$ 11 456 or more.
[d] Adjusted for 30-day definition of a road traffic death.
[e] Longest time frame applied in the country.
[f] Modelled using negative binomial regression (*Global status report on road safety*. Geneva, World Health Organization, 2009:231–234). Data from countries with good vital registration and countries with a population of less than 100 000 were not included in the model.

Country	Road user deaths (%)					Road traffic injuries		
	Drivers and passengers of four-wheeled vehicles	Drivers and passengers of motorized two-wheelers	Cyclists	Pedestrians	Other or unspecified users	Number of people injured	Injuries per 100 000 population	Ratio of injuries to deaths
Albania	45.3	9.0	5.7	40.0	—	1 344	42.1	3.0
Armenia	60.3	—	0.3	39.4	—	2 720	90.6	6.5
Austria	59.0	17.4	5.4	15.6	2.6	53 211	636.4	77.0
Azerbaijan	59.7	1.2	0.9	38.1	0.1	3 432	40.5	3.1
Belarus	47.3	3.8	9.1	39.8	—	7 991	82.5	5.3
Belgium	56.0	15.2	8.2	9.7	11.0	65 850	629.7	61.7
Bosnia and Herzegovina	61.0	4.7	5.8	23.7	4.8	11 647	296.0	27.2
Bulgaria	65.0	0.0	4.5	26.3	4.2	9 827	128.6	9.8
Croatia	49.9	18.8	4.5	20.0	6.8	25 092	550.8	40.5
Cyprus	50.6	28.1	3.4	18.0	—	2 119	247.9	23.8
Czech Republic	59.4	11.4	9.5	19.2	0.5	23 060	226.4	18.9
Estonia	66.0	6.0	9.0	19.0	—	3 270	244.9	16.7
Finland	70.3	10.8	5.8	12.6	0.5	8 446	160.1	22.2
France	59.2	25.0	3.1	12.1	0.6	77 007	124.9	16.7
Georgia	—	—	0.3	27.7	72.0	7 349	167.2	10.0
Germany	58.0	18.0	10.0	14.0	1.0	431 419	522.3	87.2
Greece	50.3	30.2	1.3	16.1	2.1	20 675	185.5	12.5
Hungary	54.4	10.1	11.7	22.7	1.1	27 452	273.7	22.3
Iceland	85.0	5.0	—	10.0	—	2 092	695.0	69.7
Ireland	61.9	7.9	2.5	20.0	7.7	8 575	199.4	23.5
Israel	57.6	9.3	1.5	31.6	—	2 079	30.0	5.2
Italy	49.0	26.0	5.5	13.4	6.1	332 995	565.6	58.7
Kazakhstan	—	—	—	16.2	83.8	32 988	213.9	7.0
Kyrgyzstan	55.0[i]	—	1.0	43.0	1.0	6 223	117.0	5.1
Latvia	50.4	4.2	8.1	37.3	—	5 404	237.3	13.3
Lithuania	53.7	4.5	6.9	31.9	3.0	8 254	243.5	10.9
Malta	35.7	28.6	—	35.7	—	1 195	293.9	85.4
Montenegro	75.4	4.1	—	20.5	0.1	2 796	467.6	22.9
Netherlands	46.0	18.0	24.0	12.0	—	16 750	102.0	21.2
Norway	67.0	17.0	3.0	10.0	3.0	11 755	250.2	50.5
Poland	51.0	5.0	9.0	35.0	—	63 224	166.0	11.3
Portugal	54.6	22.1	3.5	16.1	3.7	46 318	436.0	41.7
Republic of Moldova	57.3	4.1	2.4	34.3	1.9	2 985	78.7	5.2
Romania	74.5	8.0	6.8	10.8	—	29 832	139.2	11.0
Russian Federation	62.0	2.1	—	35.9	—	292 206	205.1	8.1
San Marino	60.0[j]	20.0[j]	—	20.0[j]	—	431	1463.1	431.0
Serbia	58.6	5.6	9.2	25.1	1.5	22 201	225.2	23.1
Slovakia	49.6	8.0	8.5	33.9	—	11 310	209.8	13.9
Slovenia	64.5[i]	18.1	5.8	11.3	0.3	16 449	821.8	56.1
Spain	62.0	19.0	2.0	15.0	1.0	143 450	324.0	35.0
Sweden	65.0	16.0	6.0	12.0	1.0	26 636	292.1	56.6
Switzerland	48.0	22.0	9.0	21.0	—	26 718	357.0	72.2
Tajikistan	48.7	1.1	6.0	43.6	0.7	2 048	30.4	2.2
The former Yugoslav Republic of Macedonia	41.4	10.7	3.6	34.3	10.0	6 133	300.9	43.8
Turkey	55.0	8.0	1.8	18.9	16.3	169 080	225.8	16.8
Turkmenistan	—	—	4.6	28.9	66.5	1 606	32.3	1.7
Ukraine	44.3[i]	—	—	55.7	—	40 887	88.5	4.1
United Kingdom	55.0	19.0	4.0	21.0	1.0	264 288	434.9	80.1
Uzbekistan	—	—	—	—	—	—	—	—

[g] 2007 data not available. Latest available used from: UN data [online database]. New York, United Nations, 2009 (http://data.un.org, accessed 10 June 2009).
[b] Death is defined as died at crash scene in the Federation of Bosnia and Herzegovina and as died within 30 days of the crash in the Republic of Srpska.
[i] Passengers and drivers of any motorized vehicle.
[j] Data apply to 5 deaths (2004-2007).
— Data not available.

Annex 4. Mortality rates for road traffic injuries per 100 000 population by gross national income per person in the WHO European Region, 2008[a]

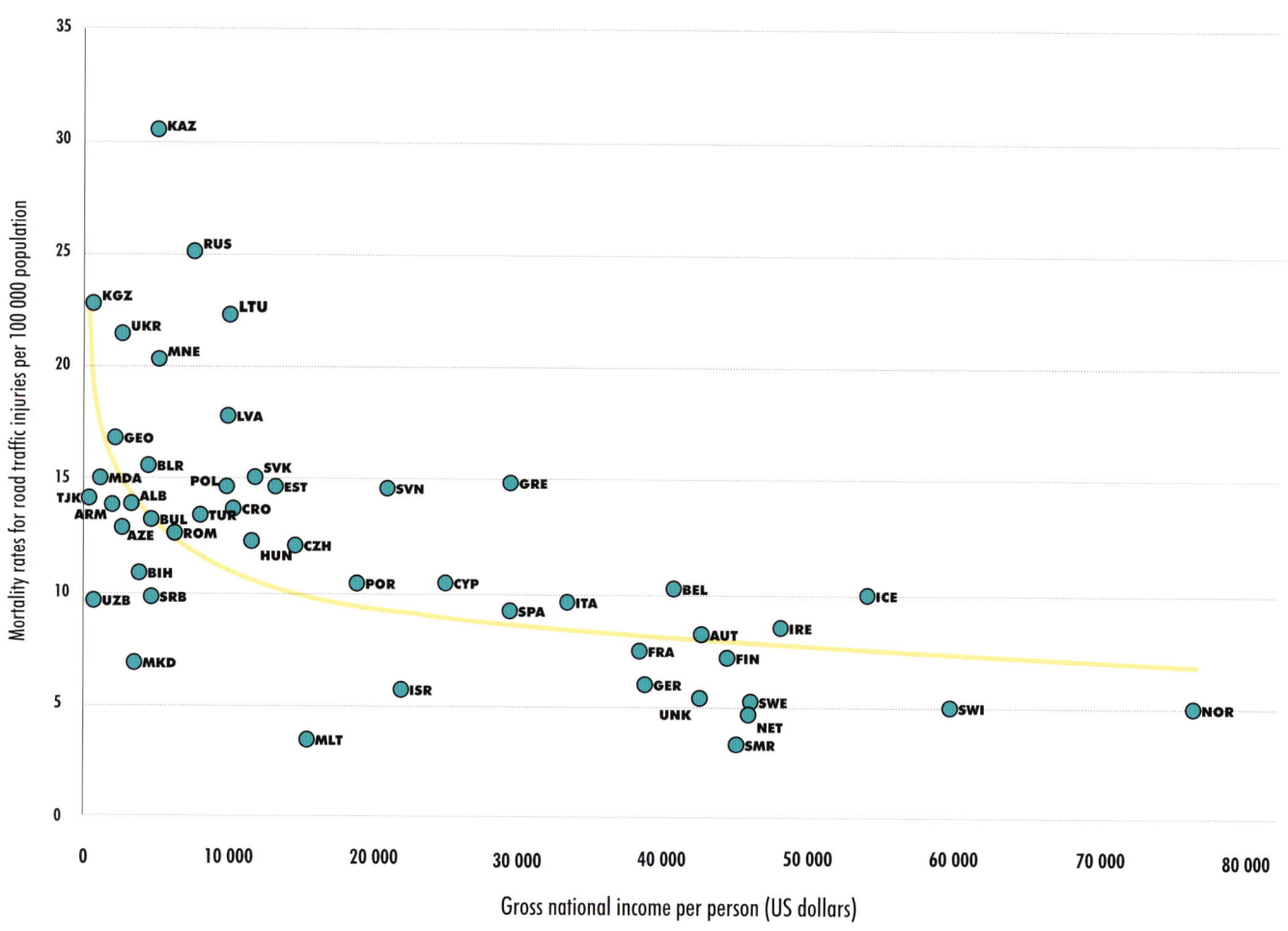

[a] The International Organization for Standardization acronyms are used in this figure: ALB: Albania; ARM: Armenia; AUT: Austria; AZE: Azerbaijan; BEL: Belgium; BIH: Bosnia and Herzegovina; BLR: Belarus; BUL: Bulgaria; CRO: Croatia; CYP: Cyprus; CZH: Czech Republic; DEU: Germany; EST: Estonia; FIN: Finland; FRA: France; GEO: Georgia; GRE: Greece; HUN: Hungary; ICE: Iceland; IRE: Ireland; ISR: Israel; ITA: Italy; KAZ: Kazakhstan; KGZ: Kyrgyzstan; LVA: Latvia; LTU: Lithuania; MDA: Republic of Moldova; MKD: The former Yugoslav Republic of Macedonia; MLT: Malta; MNE: Montenegro; NET: Netherlands; NOR: Norway; POL: Poland; POR: Portugal; ROM: Romania; RUS: Russian Federation; SMR: San Marino; SPA: Spain; SRB: Serbia; SVK: Slovakia; SVN: Slovenia; SWE: Sweden; SWI: Switzerland; TUR: Turkey; TJK: Tajikistan; UKR: Ukraine; UNK: United Kingdom; UZB: Uzbekistan.
Gross national income per person is from World Bank data for 2007.

Annex 5. **Sample objectives from national strategies implemented in countries in the WHO European Region**

Infrastructure

- Safety on rural and urban roads
- Tunnel safety
- Creating advisory committees for the road marking
- Creating "safety zones" on the roads
- Ensuring that walkways meet the standards for width and design
- Providing safe routes to schools
- Removing roadside hazards
- Improving curves
- Introducing centre-line rumble strips
- Improving road lighting
- Establishing safe crossing points for pedestrians and cyclists
- Proper equipment for winter conditions
- Routine road maintenance
- Installing road sign warnings on paths used by animals
- Constructing animal fences
- Black-spot treatment

Policy and enforcement

- Implementing stricter control of traffic rules (such as speed limits, use of safety equipment, valid driving licence and driving under the influence of alcohol or drugs)
- Routine road safety inspection
- Effectively controlling and sanctioning road offences
- Improving conditions of the examination of the driving licence
- Partnering with professional federations of road transport to develop road safety policies
- Imposing sanctions on the use of entertainment in driving situations
- Ensuring a decrease in the number of unlicensed drivers on the road
- Optimizing the operation of emergency care services and the rescue network
- Controlling rest regimes for professional drivers
- Conducting audits of road safety
- Improving the legal basis of road safety
- Conducting regular inspection of public transport, including school transport vehicles
- Enforcing regulations on transport operators for the carriage of goods and passengers, especially dangerous goods
- Enforcing safety regulations for parked cars
- Increasing roadside technical checks of heavy vehicles
- Enhancing tools and examinations used to assess driver competence
- Implementing automatic traffic surveillance
- Developing policies to curb the growth of the distance travelled by private vehicles
- Implementing awareness campaigns to educate the public about traffic dangers
- Positive reinforcement and penalty point system

Human behaviour

- Increasing the use of restraint systems, child safety seats and crash helmets (for motorcycle and moped drivers)
- Fighting the risks related to alcohol and drugs
- Ensuring that vehicles drive under speed limits
- Effective driver education and advanced driver training
- Elimination of driving fatigue
- Maintaining safe following distances
- Using daytime running lights
- Traffic education for children and adolescents (in schools)
- Black-spot treatment
- Providing advanced training for professional drivers
- Limiting the use of entertainment in driving situations
- Effective training and education for the employees of traffic control services
- Limiting the use of hand-held communication devices

Vehicles

- Lorry safety
- Equipping vehicles with child safety seats, if necessary
- Improving the visibility of heavyweight vehicles in the dark
- Improving the quality of vehicles through roadside vehicle testing
- Ensuring that vehicles are properly registered, inspected and licensed
- Encouraging the use of innovative technologies

Post-crash efforts

- Independent accident analysis
- First-aid training for drivers
- Promoting the use of roadside telematics
- Improving the efficiency of emergency care services
- Creating accident analysis groups

Research

- Accident analysis of the road network
- Conducting scientific studies intended for establishing a coordinating institution for road safety
- Conducting studies to assess the impact of transport on health by monitoring traffic volumes, environmental quality and proximity to urban areas

Annex 6. Estimated economic costs of one death in selected countries in the WHO European Region

Country	Costs per death in thousands of euros[a]	Method used	Year
Austria – including (excluding) human suffering	2676 (1399)	Willingness to pay	2006
Netherlands	2427	Gross output method; Willingness to pay	2003
United Kingdom	2137	Willingness to pay	2005
Finland	1752	Gross output method; Willingness to pay	2007
France	1194	Gross output method	2006
Germany	1162	Gross output method	2004
Hungary	769	Willingness to pay	2002
Estonia	767	Gross output method	2007
Cyprus	480	Gross output method	2008
Latvia	398	Gross output method	2006
Slovakia	287	Gross output method	2007

[a] Currencies were converted into euros using the appropriate mid-year exchange rate.

Annex 7. Drinking and driving laws, enforcement and road traffic deaths attributed to alcohol in countries in the WHO European Region, 2008

Country	National drink–driving law	How drink–driving is defined			Mechanisms to enforce bans on drink–driving			
		Blood alcohol concentration	Physician certificate	Breath content	Random breath testing	Police checkpoints	Breath testing of all drivers involved in crashes	Blood testing of all drivers involved in crashes
Albania	Yes	Yes	No	Yes	Yes	Yes	Yes	No
Armenia	Yes	Yes	No	Yes	Yes	No	Yes	Yes
Austria	Yes	Yes	No	Yes	Yes	Yes	Yes	Yes
Azerbaijan	Yes	Yes	Yes	Yes	Yes	Yes	Yes	Yes
Belarus	Yes	Yes	Yes	Yes	Yes	Yes	Yes	No
Belgium	Yes	Yes	No	Yes	Yes	Yes	Yes	Yes
Bosnia and Herzegovina	Yes	Yes	Yes	Yes	Yes	Yes	Yes	Yes
Bulgaria	Yes	Yes	Yes	Yes	Yes	Yes	Yes	Yes
Croatia	Yes	Yes	Yes	Yes	Yes	Yes	Yes	No
Cyprus	Yes	Yes	No	Yes	Yes	No	Yes	Yes
Czech Republic	Yes	Yes	No	No	Yes	No	Yes	Yes
Estonia	Yes	Yes	Yes	Yes	Yes	Yes	Yes	Yes
Finland	Yes	Yes	No	Yes	Yes	Yes	Yes	Yes
France	Yes	Yes	No	Yes	Yes	Yes	Yes	Yes
Georgia	Yes	Yes	Yes	Yes	No	No	Yes	Yes
Germany	Yes	Yes	No	Yes	No	Yes	Yes	Yes
Greece	Yes	Yes	No	Yes	Yes	Yes	Yes	Yes
Hungary	Yes	Yes	No	Yes	Yes	Yes	Yes	Yes
Iceland	Yes	Yes	No	Yes	Yes	Yes	No	No
Ireland	Yes	Yes	No	No	Yes	No	No	No
Israel	Yes	Yes	No	No	Yes	Yes	No	No
Italy	Yes	Yes	No	Yes	Yes	Yes	Yes	Yes
Kazakhstan	Yes	No	Yes	No	Yes	No	Yes	Yes
Kyrgyzstan	Yes	No	Yes	Yes	Yes	No	Yes	Yes
Latvia	Yes	Yes	No	No	Yes	No	Yes	Yes
Lithuania	Yes	Yes	No	No	Yes	Yes	No	No
Malta	Yes	Yes	No	Yes	No	No	No	No
Montenegro	Yes	Yes	Yes	Yes	Yes	No	Yes	Yes
Netherlands	Yes	Yes	No	Yes	Yes	No	No	No
Norway	Yes	Yes	No	Yes	Yes	Yes	No	No
Poland	Yes	Yes	No	Yes	Yes	Yes	Yes	Yes
Portugal	Yes	Yes	No	No	Yes	Yes	Yes	Yes
Republic of Moldova	Yes	Yes	Yes	Yes	Yes	Yes	Yes	Yes
Romania	Yes	Yes	Yes	Yes	Yes	Yes	Yes	Yes
Russian Federation	Yes	Yes	No	Yes	Yes	No	Yes	Yes
San Marino	Yes	Yes	No	No	No	Yes	No	Yes
Serbia	Yes	Yes	Yes	Yes	Yes	Yes	Yes	Yes
Slovakia	Yes	Yes	No	Yes	Yes	Yes	Yes	Yes
Slovenia	Yes	Yes	No	Yes	Yes	Yes	Yes	Yes
Spain	Yes	Yes	No	Yes	Yes	No	Yes	Yes
Sweden	Yes	Yes	No	Yes	Yes	Yes	No	No
Switzerland	Yes	Yes	No	No	Yes	Yes	Yes	Yes
Tajikistan	Yes	Yes	Yes	Yes	Yes	Yes	Yes	Yes
The former Yugoslav Republic of Macedonia	Yes	Yes	No	No	No	Yes	Yes	Yes
Turkey	Yes	Yes	No	Yes	Yes	Yes	Yes	Yes
Turkmenistan	Yes	Yes	Yes	Yes	Yes	Yes	Yes	Yes
Ukraine	Yes	Yes	No	Yes	Yes	No	Yes	Yes
United Kingdom	Yes	Yes	No	No	No	No	No	No
Uzbekistan	Yes	Yes	Yes	Yes	Yes	No	Yes	Yes

^a Drink–driving not defined by BAC limit.
— Data not available.
NA: not applicable.

Country	Effectiveness of overall enforcement (respondent consensus on a scale from 1 to 10, with 10 being the best)	National maximum legal blood alcohol concentration			Proportion (%) of road traffic deaths attributable to alcohol
		For the general population (g/dl)	For young or novice drivers (g/dl)	For professional or commercial driveres (g/dl)	
Albania	8	0.05	0.05	0.05	5.2
Armenia	5	0.08	0.08	0.08	6.1
Austria	9	0.05	0.01	0.01	8.1
Azerbaijan	9	0.00	0.00	0.00	2.7
Belarus	7	0.05	0.05	0.05	12.9
Belgium	3	0.05	0.05	0.05	—
Bosnia and Herzegovina	6	0.03	0.00	0.00	6.7
Bulgaria	7	0.05	0.05	0.05	4.7
Croatia	7	0.05	0.00	0.00	30.0
Cyprus	7	0.05	0.05	0.05	18.0
Czech Republic	9	0.00	0.00	0.00	3.4
Estonia	8	0.02	0.02	0.02	48.0
Finland	8	0.05	0.05	0.05	23.9
France	4	0.05	0.05	0.05	27.0
Georgia	9	0.02	0.02	0.02	37.0
Germany	NA	0.05	0.00	0.05	12.0
Greece	7	0.05	0.02	0.02	7.2
Hungary	5	0.00	0.00	0.00	12.0
Iceland	7	0.05	0.05	0.05	20.0
Ireland	No consensus	0.08	0.08	0.08	37.0
Israel	6	0.05	0.05	0.05	7.5
Italy	7	0.05	0.05	0.05	No consensus
Kazakhstan	10	None[a]	None[a]	None[a]	3.2
Kyrgyzstan	4	None[a]	None[a]	None[a]	—
Latvia	7	0.05	0.02	0.05	20.6
Lithuania	6	0.04	0.02	0.02	11.7
Malta	4	0.08	0.08	0.08	—
Montenegro	6	0.05	0.05	0.00	—
Netherlands	No consensus	0.05	0.02	0.05	25.0
Norway	4	0.02	0.02	0.02	20.0–30.0
Poland	7	0.02	0.02	0.02	14.0
Portugal	8	0.05	0.05	0.05	31.4
Republic of Moldova	2	0.05	0.05	0.05	17.0
Romania	8	0.00	0.00	0.00	1.5
Russian Federation	6	0.03	0.03	0.03	9.7
San Marino	6	0.05	0.05	0.05	—
Serbia	7	0.05	0.05	0.00	6.0
Slovakia	9	0.00	0.00	0.00	4.3
Slovenia	6	0.05	0.00	0.00	38.4
Spain	7	0.05	0.03	0.03	—
Sweden	6	0.02	0.02	0.02	20.0
Switzerland	6	0.05	0.05	0.05	16.0
Tajikistan	9	0.03	0.03	0.03	5.0
The former Yugoslav Republic of Macedonia	6	0.05	0.00	0.00	4.6
Turkey	9	0.05	0.05	0.00	2.0
Turkmenistan	10	0.05	0.05	0.05	7.4
Ukraine	NA	0.00	0.00	0.00	—
United Kingdom	No consensus	0.08	0.08	0.08	17.0
Uzbekistan	9	None	None	None	—

Annex 8. Seat-belt and child restraint laws, enforcement and wearing rates in countries in the WHO European Region, 2008

Country	Seat-belts				Using seat-belts in cars (%)			Child restraints	
	There is a national seat-belt law	The law applies to all occupants	Enforcement is applied to the following occupants	Effectiveness of seat-belt law enforcement (respondent consensus on a scale from 1 to 10)	Overall	Front-seat occupants	Rear-seat occupants	National law requiring child restraints	Effectiveness of enforcement of child restraint law (respondent consensus on a scale from 1 to 10)
Albania	Yes	Yes	All occupants	9	—	30	—	Yes	8
Armenia	Yes	Yes	All occupants	3	—	—	—	Yes	5
Austria	Yes	Yes	All occupants	7	88	89	49	Yes	9
Azerbaijan	Yes	Yes	All occupants	9	—	—	—	Yes	9
Belarus	Yes	Yes	—	7	—	—	—	Yes	6
Belgium	Yes	Yes	All occupants	3	—	79	46	Yes	6
Bosnia and Herzegovina	Yes	Yes	All occupants	7	—	—	—	Yes	5
Bulgaria	Yes	Yes	All occupants	8	—	—	—	Yes	4
Croatia	Yes	Yes	All occupants	7	45	—	—	Yes	5
Cyprus	Yes	Yes	All occupants	7	—	81	9	Yes	3
Czech Republic	Yes	Yes	All occupants	8	85	90	80	Yes	7
Estonia	Yes	Yes	All occupants	7	88	90	68	Yes	8
Finland	Yes	Yes	All occupants	7	—	89	80	Yes	7
France	Yes	Yes	All occupants	8	—	98	83	Yes	5
Georgia	Yes	No	Front-seat occupants only	8	—	—	—	Yes	7
Germany	Yes	Yes	All occupants	NA	95	95 (drivers); 96 (passengers)	88	Yes	NA
Greece	Yes	Yes	All occupants	7	—	75	42	Yes	6
Hungary	Yes	Yes	All occupants	4	69	71	40	Yes	4
Iceland	Yes	Yes	All occupants	8	80	88	68	Yes	8
Ireland	Yes	Yes	All occupants	No consensus	—	86	63	Yes	No consensus
Israel	Yes	Yes	All occupants	8	—	94 (drivers); 88 (passengers)	45	Yes	5
Italy	Yes	Yes	All occupants	7	—	65	10	Yes	7
Kazakhstan	Yes	Yes	Driver only	7	—	—	—	Yes	7
Kyrgyzstan	Yes	No	Front-seat occupants only	5	—	—	—	No	NA
Latvia	Yes	Yes	All occupants	7	—	77	32	Yes	6
Lithuania	Yes	Yes	All occupants	6	—	—	—	Yes	5
Malta	Yes	Yes	All occupants	8	—	96	21	Yes	6
Montenegro	Yes	Yes	All occupants	6	—	—	—	No	NA
Netherlands	Yes	Yes	All occupants	No consensus	92	94	73	Yes	No consensus
Norway	Yes	Yes	All occupants	6	88	93	85	Yes	9
Poland	Yes	Yes	All occupants	7	65	74	45	Yes	6
Portugal	Yes	Yes	All occupants	9	—	86 (urban roads); 93 (motorways)	28 (urban roads); 64 (motorways)	Yes	8
Republic of Moldova	Yes	Yes	All occupants	No consensus	—	—	—	No	NA
Romania	Yes	Yes	All occupants	5	50	80	20	Yes	3
Russian Federation	Yes	Yes	All occupants	7	—	33	—	Yes	8
San Marino	Yes	Yes	All occupants	6	—	—	—	Yes	6
Serbia	Yes	Yes	Front-seat occupants only	4	40–50	50–60	4-5	Subnational	NA
Slovakia	Yes	Yes	All occupants	8	—	—	—	Yes	9
Slovenia	Yes	Yes	All occupants	7	80	85	51	Yes	6
Spain	Yes	Yes	All occupants	8	84	89	69	Yes	7
Sweden	Yes	Yes	All occupants	3	94	96	90	Yes	2
Switzerland	Yes	Yes	All occupants	7	—	86	61	Yes	8
Tajikistan	Yes	Yes	All occupants	3	—	—	—	Yes	1
The former Yugoslav Republic of Macedonia	Yes	No	Front-seat occupants only	6	16	—	—	No	NA
Turkey	Yes	Yes	All occupants	8	70 (rural roads); 20 (city centres)	—	—	Yes	7
Turkmenistan	Yes	No	Front-seat occupants only	7	—	—	—	No	NA
Ukraine	Yes	No	Front-seat occupants only	NA	—	—	—	No	NA
United Kingdom	Yes	Yes	All occupants	No consensus	—	91	84 (Great Britain); 90 (Northern Ireland)	Yes	No consensus
Uzbekistan	Yes	Yes	All occupants	10	—	—	—	—	—

— Data not available.
NA: not applicable.

Annex 9. Speed limit laws and enforcement in countries in the WHO European Region, 2008

Country	Speed limits set at the national level	Speed limits modifiable at the local level	Legislation differs by vehicle type	Maximum speed			Effectiveness of overall enforcement (respondent consensus on a scale from 1 to 10)
				On urban roads (km/h)	On rural roads (km/h)	Intercity roads and highways	
Albania	Yes	Yes	Yes	40	80	90–110	9
Armenia	Yes	Yes	Yes	60	60	90–110	5
Austria	Yes	Yes	Yes	50	100	100	7
Azerbaijan	Yes	Yes	Yes	60	90	110	9
Belarus	Yes	No	Yes	60	—	90	6
Belgium	Yes	Yes	Yes	50	90	120	5
Bosnia and Herzegovina	Yes	Yes	Yes	60	—	130	6
Bulgaria	Yes	Yes	Yes	50	90	90–130	6
Croatia	Yes	Yes	Yes	50	90	130	6
Cyprus	Yes	Yes	No	50	80	100	6
Czech Republic	Yes	Yes	Yes	50	90	130	5
Estonia	Yes	Yes	No	50	90	90	6
Finland	Yes	Yes	Yes	50	80	80–100	7
France	Yes	Yes	Yes	50	90	130	7
Georgia	Yes	Yes	Yes	60	60	90–110	8
Germany	Yes	No	Yes	50	100	130[a]	NA
Greece	Yes	Yes	Yes	50	90	130	6
Hungary	Yes	Yes	Yes	50	90	130	4
Iceland	Yes	Yes	Yes	50	80–90	NA	7
Ireland	Yes	Yes	Yes	50	80	100	No consensus
Israel	Yes	Yes	Yes	50	80–90	90–110	5
Italy	Yes	Yes	Yes	50	90	110–130	7
Kazakhstan	Yes	No	No	60	60	120	5
Kyrgyzstan	Yes	Yes	—	60	60	100	7
Latvia	Yes	Yes	Yes	50	90	110	7
Lithuania	Yes	Yes	Yes	50	90	130	6
Malta	Yes	No	Yes	50	80	NA	5
Montenegro	Yes	Yes	Yes	50	80	100	6
Netherlands	Yes	Yes	Yes	50	80	120	No consensus
Norway	Yes	Yes	Yes	50	80	80	6
Poland	Yes	Yes	Yes	50	90	130	5
Portugal	Yes	Yes	Yes	50	90	90–100	8
Republic of Moldova	Yes	No	Yes	60	60	90	No consensus
Romania	Yes	Yes	Yes	50	50	90	5
Russian Federation	Yes	Yes	Yes	60	90[b]	110[c]	6
San Marino	Yes	No	Yes	50	70	70	5
Serbia	Yes	Yes	Yes	60	80	120	4
Slovakia	Yes	Yes	Yes	60	90	130	7
Slovenia	Yes	Yes	Yes	50	90	130	7
Spain	Yes	Yes	Yes	50	90	100	8
Sweden	Yes	Yes	Yes	50	70	90	5
Switzerland	Yes	Yes	Yes	50	80	120	7
Tajikistan	Yes	Yes	Yes	60	90	110	8
The former Yugoslav Republic of Macedonia	Yes	No	Yes	60	80	120	4
Turkey	Yes	Yes	Yes	50	90	120	8
Turkmenistan	Yes	No	No	60	90	110	9
Ukraine	Yes	No	No	60	40	90	NA
United Kingdom	Yes	Yes	Yes	50	100	115	No consensus
Uzbekistan	Yes	No	Yes	70	70	90	7

[a] Recommended speed limit.
[b] On roads out of populated regions and sites.
[c] On roads marked by special symbols.
— Data not available.
NA: not applicable.

Annex 10. Helmet laws, enforcement and wearing rates in countries in the WHO European Region, 2008

Country	National helmet law	Law applies to the following road users			Exceptions to the law		
		Drivers	Adult passenger	Child passengers	Exceptions to the helmet law	Helmet law applies to all road types	Helmet law applies to all engine types
Albania	Yes	Yes	Yes	Yes	—	Yes	Yes
Armenia	Yes	Yes	Yes	Yes	No	Yes	Yes
Austria	Yes	Yes	Yes	Yes	Yes	Yes	Yes
Azerbaijan	Yes	Yes	Yes	Yes	No	Yes	Yes
Belarus	Yes	Yes	Yes	Yes	No	Yes	No
Belgium	Yes	Yes	Yes	Yes	Yes	Yes	Yes
Bosnia and Herzegovina	Yes	Yes	Yes	Yes	No	Yes	Yes
Bulgaria	Yes	Yes	Yes	Yes	No	Yes	Yes
Croatia	Yes	Yes	Yes	Yes	No	Yes	Yes
Cyprus	Yes	Yes	Yes	Yes	Yes	Yes	Yes
Czech Republic	Yes	Yes	Yes	Yes	No	Yes	Yes
Estonia	Yes	Yes	Yes	Yes	No	Yes	Yes
Finland	Yes	Yes	Yes	Yes	Yes	Yes	Yes
France	Yes	Yes	Yes	Yes	Yes	Yes	Yes
Georgia	Yes	Yes	Yes	Yes	No	Yes	Yes
Germany	Yes	Yes	Yes	Yes	No	Yes	Yes
Greece	Yes	Yes	Yes	Yes	Yes	Yes	Yes
Hungary	Yes	Yes	Yes	Yes	No	Yes	Yes
Iceland	Yes	Yes	Yes	Yes	No	Yes	Yes
Ireland	Yes	Yes	Yes	Yes	No	Yes	Yes
Israel	Yes	Yes	Yes	Yes	No	Yes	Yes
Italy	Yes	Yes	Yes	Yes	Yes	Yes	Yes
Kazakhstan	Yes	Yes	Yes	Yes	—	Yes	No
Kyrgyzstan	Yes	Yes	Yes	Yes	No	Yes	Yes
Latvia	Yes	Yes	Yes	Yes	No	Yes	Yes
Lithuania	Yes	Yes	Yes	Yes	No	Yes	Yes
Malta	Yes	Yes	Yes	Yes	No	Yes	Yes
Montenegro	Yes	Yes	Yes	Yes	No	Yes	Yes
Netherlands	Yes	Yes	Yes	Yes	Yes	Yes	No
Norway	Yes	Yes	Yes	Yes	No	Yes	Yes
Poland	Yes	Yes	Yes	Yes	Yes	Yes	Yes
Portugal	Yes	Yes	Yes	Yes	No	Yes	Yes
Republic of Moldova	Yes	Yes	Yes	Yes	No	Yes	No
Romania	Yes	Yes	Yes	Yes	No	Yes	Yes
Russian Federation	Yes	Yes	Yes	Yes	No	Yes	Yes
San Marino	Yes	Yes	Yes	Yes	No	Yes	Yes
Serbia	Yes	Yes	Yes	Yes	No	Yes	Yes
Slovakia	Yes	Yes	Yes	Yes	No	Yes	Yes
Slovenia	Yes	Yes	Yes	Yes	No	Yes	No
Spain	Yes	Yes	Yes	Yes	Yes	Yes	Yes
Sweden	Yes	Yes	Yes	Yes	Yes	Yes	Yes
Switzerland	Yes	Yes	Yes	Yes	Yes	Yes	Yes
Tajikistan	Yes	Yes	Yes	Yes	No	Yes	No
The former Yugoslav Republic of Macedonia	Yes	Yes	Yes	Yes	No	Yes	Yes
Turkey	Yes	Yes	Yes	Yes	No	Yes	Yes
Turkmenistan	Yes	Yes	Yes	Yes	No	Yes	No
Ukraine	No	NA	NA	NA	NA	NA	NA
United Kingdom	Yes	Yes	Yes	Yes	Yes	Yes	Yes
Uzbekistan	Yes	Yes	Yes	Yes	No	Yes	Yes

— Data not available.
NA: not applicable.

Country	Effectiveness of overall enforcement (respondent consensus on a scale from 1 to 10)	Helmet standards	Estimated national helmet-wearing rate (%)
Albania	10	Yes	—
Armenia	5	No	—
Austria	9	Yes	95
Azerbaijan	9	No	—
Belarus	9	Yes	—
Belgium	8	Yes	—
Bosnia and Herzegovina	6	No	—
Bulgaria	7	Yes	—
Croatia	6	No	—
Cyprus	5	Yes	68 (drivers); 56 (passengers)
Czech Republic	9	Yes	97 (drivers); 85 (passengers)
Estonia	9	Yes	—
Finland	9	Yes	95 (drivers)
France	7	Yes	95
Georgia	6	No	—
Germany	NA	Yes	97 (drivers); 96 (passengers)
Greece	7	Yes	58 (drivers); 32 (passengers)
Hungary	9	Yes	95
Iceland	8	No	95
Ireland	No consensus	—	—
Israel	9	No	95
Italy	7	Yes	60
Kazakhstan	5	No	—
Kyrgyzstan	7	No	—
Latvia	6	No	93 (drivers)
Lithuania	6	No	—
Malta	9	No	—
Montenegro	6	No	—
Netherlands	No consensus	Yes	92 (drivers); 72 (passengers)
Norway	9	Yes	100
Poland	8	Yes	—
Portugal	9	Yes	—
Republic of Moldova	1	No	—
Romania	6	Yes	90 (drivers); 65 (passengers)
Russian Federation	6	Yes	—
San Marino	9	Yes	—
Serbia	3	No	—
Slovakia	8	Yes	—
Slovenia	7	Yes	—
Spain	8	Yes	98 (drivers); 92 (passengers)
Sweden	1	Yes	95
Switzerland	9	Yes	100
Tajikistan	6	No	—
The former Yugoslav Republic of Macedonia	2	No	1
Turkey	5	Yes	12 (drivers)
Turkmenistan	8	No	—
Ukraine	NA	NA	—
United Kingdom	No consensus	Yes	98
Uzbekistan	9	No	—

Annex 11. Road safety management, strategies and policies in countries in the WHO European Region

Country	Lead agency			Strategies				
	A lead agency is present	Lead agency status	Lead agency is funded	National road safety strategy	Strategy includes measurable national targets	Strategy is funded	National strategy: amount of money allocated (in millions of euros[a])	Year of funding
Albania	Yes	Interministerial	No	No	NA	NA	NA	NA
Armenia	Yes	Other	Yes	No	NA	NA	NA	NA
Austria	Yes	Government	Yes	Yes	Yes	No	NA	NA
Azerbaijan	Yes	Government	Yes	Yes	Yes	Yes	3.16	2007
Belarus	Yes	Interministerial	No	Yes	Yes	Yes	—	—
Belgium	Yes	Interministerial	Yes	Yes	Yes	Yes	94.00	2008
Bosnia and Herzegovina	Yes	Government	Yes	Yes	Yes	Yes	0.026[b]	2008
Bulgaria	Yes	Interministerial	Yes	Yes	Yes	Yes	—	—
Croatia	Yes	Interministerial	Yes	Yes	Yes	Yes	2.08	2008
Cyprus	Yes	Interministerial	Yes	Yes	Yes	Yes	7.00	2008
Czech Republic	Yes	Government	Yes	Yes	Yes	No	NA	NA
Estonia	Yes	Interministerial	Yes	Yes	Yes	Yes	15.40	2008
Finland	Yes	Government	Yes	Yes	Yes	Yes	—	—
France	Yes	Interministerial	Yes	Yes	Yes	Yes	2 295.00	2007
Georgia	Yes	Other	NA	Yes	Yes	Yes	—	—
Germany	Yes	—	Yes	Yes	No	Yes	—	—
Greece	No	NA	NA	Yes	Yes	No	NA	NA
Hungary	Yes	Interministerial	Yes	Yes	Yes	Yes	13.03	2008
Iceland	Yes	Government	Yes	Yes	Yes	Yes	3.49	2007
Ireland	Yes	Other	Yes	Yes	Yes	—	NA	NA
Israel	Yes	Other	Yes	Yes	Yes	Yes	101.78	2008
Italy	Yes	Government	Yes	Yes	Yes	Yes	53.00	2008
Kazakhstan	Yes	Government	Yes	Yes	No	Yes	—	—
Kyrgyzstan	Yes	Interministerial	No	Multiple strategies	NA	NA	NA	NA
Latvia	Yes	Interministerial	Yes	Yes	Yes	Yes	7.33	2006
Lithuania	Yes	Interministerial	No	Yes	Yes	Yes	5.69	2007
Malta	Yes	Government	Yes	Multiple strategies	NA	NA	NA	NA
Montenegro	No	NA	NA	No	NA	NA	NA	NA
Netherlands	Yes	Government	Yes	Yes	Yes	Yes	80.00	2008
Norway	Yes	Government	Yes	Yes	Yes	Yes	103.42	2007
Poland	Yes	Government	Yes	Yes	Yes	Yes	1 871.58	2005–2007
Portugal	Yes	Government	Yes	Yes	Yes	Yes	—	—
Republic of Moldova	Yes	Interministerial	No	Yes	Yes	Yes	—	—
Romania	Yes	Interministerial	Yes	Yes[d]	NA	NA	NA	NA
Russian Federation	Yes	Interministerial	No	Yes	Yes	Yes	245.73	2007
San Marino	Yes	Interministerial	No	Multiple strategies	NA	NA	NA	NA
Serbia	No	NA	NA	Multiple strategies	NA	NA	NA	NA
Slovakia	Yes	Government	Yes	Yes	Yes	Yes	0.96	2008
Slovenia	Yes	Interministerial	Yes	Yes	Yes	Yes	2.20	2008
Spain	Yes	Government	Yes	Yes	Yes	Yes	881.03	2008
Sweden	Yes	Government	Yes	Yes	Yes	Yes	—	—
Switzerland	Yes	Government	Yes	Yes[d]	NA	NA	NA	NA
Tajikistan	Yes	Government	Yes	Multiple strategies	NA	NA	NA	NA
The former Yugoslav Republic of Macedonia	Yes	Other	Yes	No	NA	NA	NA	NA
Turkey	Yes	Interministerial	Yes	Multiple strategies	NA	NA	NA	NA
Turkmenistan	No	NA	NA	Multiple strategies	NA	NA	NA	NA
Ukraine	Yes	Government	Yes	Multiple strategies	NA	NA	NA	NA
United Kingdom	No	NA	NA	Yes	Yes	Yes	—	—
Uzbekistan	Yes	Government	Yes	Yes	Yes	—	—	—

[a] Currencies were converted into euros using the appropriate mid-year exchange rate.
[b] Funds for the development of the strategy in the Federation of Bosnia and Herzegovina only.
[c] Costs for one road traffic death only.
[d] Not formally endorsed by the government.
— Data not available.
NA: not applicable.

Country	Economic costs					Policies on walking and cycling	
	Studies on economic costs	Estimates refer to	Estimated total annual economic costs (in millions of euros^a)	Year of estimation	Method for estimation	Presence of policy	Increased investment in bicycle lanes
Albania	No	NA	NA	NA	NA	No	NA
Armenia	No	NA	NA	NA	NA	No	NA
Austria	Yes	Both deaths and injuries	9 922.00	2006	Willingness to pay	Yes	Yes
Azerbaijan	No	NA	NA	NA	NA	No	NA
Belarus	Yes	Both deaths and injuries	179.65	2003	Gross output method	Yes	Yes
Belgium	No	NA	NA	NA	NA	Yes	Yes
Bosnia and Herzegovina	No	NA	NA	NA	NA	No	NA
Bulgaria	No	NA	NA	NA	NA	Local	NA
Croatia	—	NA	NA	NA	NA	No	NA
Cyprus	Yes	Deaths only	38.15	2001	Gross output method	Yes	Yes
Czech Republic	Yes	Both deaths and injuries	1 900.86	2007	Gross output method	Yes	Yes
Estonia	Yes	Both deaths and injuries	150.32	2007	Gross output method	Yes	Yes
Finland	Yes	Both deaths and injuries	2 532.33	2007	Gross output method; Willingness to pay	Yes	No
France	Yes	Both deaths and injuries	11 600.00	2006	Gross output method	Local	NA
Georgia	No	NA	NA	NA	NA	No	NA
Germany	Yes	Both deaths and injuries	30 900.00	2004	Gross output method	Yes	Yes
Greece	No	NA	NA	NA	NA	Yes	No
Hungary	Yes	Deaths only	0.77^c	2002	Willingness to pay	Yes	Yes
Iceland	Yes	Both deaths and injuries	369.43	2005	Gross output method	Local	NA
Ireland	Yes	Both deaths and injuries	1 328.96	2006	—	No	NA
Israel	Yes	Both deaths and injuries	1328.00	2005	Gross output method	Local	NA
Italy	Yes	Both deaths and injuries	32 236.00	2006	Gross output method	Yes	Yes
Kazakhstan	—	NA	NA	NA	NA	Yes	No
Kyrgyzstan	No	NA	NA	NA	NA	No	NA
Latvia	Yes	Both deaths and injuries	191.78	2006	Gross output method	Local	NA
Lithuania	Yes	Both deaths and injuries	434.86	2006	—	Yes	Yes
Malta	No	NA	NA	NA	NA	No	NA
Montenegro	No	NA	NA	NA	NA	No	NA
Netherlands	Yes	Both deaths and injuries	12 300.00	2003	Gross output method; Willingness to pay	Yes	Yes
Norway	Yes	Both deaths and injuries	3 751.26	2008	Gross output method	Yes	Yes
Poland	Yes	Both deaths and injuries	4 319.65	2006	Gross output method	Yes	Yes
Portugal	No	NA	NA	NA	NA	Local	NA
Republic of Moldova	No	NA	NA	NA	NA	No	NA
Romania	Yes	Both deaths and injuries	1 200.08	2007	—	Yes	Yes
Russian Federation	Yes	Both deaths and injuries	8 033.09	2007	Direct costing	No	NA
San Marino	No	NA	NA	NA	NA	No	NA
Serbia	No	NA	NA	NA	NA	No	NA
Slovakia	Yes	Both deaths and injuries	297.96	2007	Gross output method	No	NA
Slovenia	No	NA	NA	NA	NA	Yes	Yes
Spain	Yes	Both deaths and injuries	6 280.36	1997	Gross output method; Willingness to pay	Local	NA
Sweden	Yes	Both deaths and injuries	3 252.59	2006	Willingness to pay	Yes	Yes
Switzerland	Yes	Both deaths and injuries	9 057.45	2003	Gross output method	Local	NA
Tajikistan	No	NA	NA	NA	NA	No	NA
The former Yugoslav Republic of Macedonia	Yes	Both deaths and injuries	28.25	2002	Gross output method	No	NA
Turkey	Yes	Both deaths and injuries	8 917.18	2002	—	Local	NA
Turkmenistan	No	NA	NA	NA	NA	—	NA
Ukraine	No	NA	NA	NA	NA	No	NA
United Kingdom	Yes	Both deaths and injuries	19 492.05	2006	Willingness to pay	Yes	Yes
Uzbekistan	No	NA	NA	NA	NA	—	NA

Annex 11. continued

Country	Policies on walking and cycling					Policies on public transport					Audits	
	Increased investment in foot paths	Traffic calming	Investment in increased cycling	Introduction of disincentives to private car use	Other	Presence of policy	Subsidized pricing	Improved frequency or coverage	Introduction of disincentives to private car use	Other	Formal audits on new roads	Regular audits on existing roads
Albania	NA	NA	NA	NA	NA	Yes	Yes	No	No	No	Yes	No
Armenia	NA	NA	NA	NA	NA	No	NA	NA	NA	NA	Yes	Yes
Austria	No	Yes	No	No	No	Yes	Yes	Yes	No	No	No	Yes
Azerbaijan	NA	NA	NA	NA	NA	Yes	Yes	Yes	No	No	Yes	Yes
Belarus	Yes	Yes	No	No	Yes	Yes	Yes	Yes	No	Yes	Yes	Yes
Belgium	Yes	Yes	Yes	No	Yes	Yes	Yes	Yes	No	Yes	No	No
Bosnia and Herzegovina	NA	NA	NA	NA	NA	No	NA	NA	NA	NA	Yes	Yes
Bulgaria	NA	NA	NA	NA	NA	Yes	No	No	No	Yes	Yes	Yes
Croatia	NA	NA	NA	NA	NA	No	NA	NA	NA	NA	Yes	Yes
Cyprus	Yes	Yes	No	No	No	Yes	Yes	No	No	No	No	Yes
Czech Republic	Yes	Yes	Yes	No	Yes	Local	NA	NA	NA	NA	No	No
Estonia	Yes	Yes	Yes	Yes	Yes	Yes	Yes	Yes	Yes	Yes	No	Yes
Finland	No	No	No	No	Yes	Yes	Yes	Yes	No	No	Yes	Yes
France	NA	NA	NA	NA	NA	Yes	Yes	No	No	No	Yes	No
Georgia	NA	NA	NA	NA	NA	Local	NA	NA	NA	NA	Yes	Yes
Germany	No	Yes	No	No	No	Yes	No	No	No	No	No	Yes
Greece	No	Yes	No	No	No	Yes	Yes	Yes	No	No	Yes	—
Hungary	No	Yes	No	No	No	Local	NA	NA	NA	NA	No	Yes
Iceland	NA	NA	NA	NA	NA	Local	NA	NA	NA	NA	Yes	No
Ireland	NA	NA	NA	NA	NA	Yes	Yes	No	No	Yes	Yes	Yes
Israel	NA	NA	NA	NA	NA	Yes	Yes	Yes	No	Yes	Yes	Yes
Italy	No	No	Yes	No	No	Yes	Yes	Yes	Yes	No	Yes	Yes
Kazakhstan	No	No	No	No	Yes	Yes	No	Yes	Yes	No	Yes	Yes
Kyrgyzstan	NA	NA	NA	NA	NA	Yes	Yes	No	No	No	Yes	Yes
Latvia	NA	NA	NA	NA	NA	Local	NA	NA	NA	NA	Yes	Yes
Lithuania	Yes	No	No	No	No	Local	NA	NA	NA	NA	Yes	Yes
Malta	NA	NA	NA	NA	NA	Yes	Yes	Yes	Yes	No	No	No
Montenegro	NA	NA	NA	NA	NA	No	NA	NA	NA	NA	Yes	Yes
Netherlands	No	Yes	Yes	No	Yes	Yes	Yes	No	Yes	No	No	No
Norway	Yes	Yes	No	No	No	Yes	Yes	Yes	No	No	Yes	Yes
Poland	Yes	Yes	No	No	No	Local	NA	NA	NA	NA	Yes	Yes
Portugal	NA	NA	NA	NA	NA	Yes	Yes	Yes	Yes	Yes	No	No
Republic of Moldova	NA	NA	NA	NA	NA	No	NA	NA	NA	NA	Yes	Yes
Romania	Yes	Yes	No	Yes	No	Yes	Yes	No	Yes	No	Yes	Yes
Russian Federation	NA	NA	NA	NA	NA	No	NA	NA	NA	NA	Yes	Yes
San Marino	NA	NA	NA	NA	NA	Yes	Subsidized	No	No	No	No	Yes
Serbia	NA	NA	NA	NA	NA	Yes	Yes	Yes	Yes	No	Yes	Yes
Slovakia	NA	NA	NA	NA	NA	No	NA	NA	NA	NA	Yes	Yes
Slovenia	Yes	Yes	Yes	No	No	Yes	Yes	Yes	No	Yes	No	No
Spain	NA	NA	NA	NA	NA	Yes	Yes	Yes	No	Yes	Yes	Yes
Sweden	Yes	Yes	No	Yes	No	Yes	Yes	Yes	Yes	No	No	No
Switzerland	NA	NA	NA	NA	NA	Yes	Yes	No	No	No	Yes	Yes
Tajikistan	NA	NA	NA	NA	NA	Local	NA	NA	NA	NA	Yes	Yes
The former Yugoslav Republic of Macedonia	NA	NA	NA	NA	NA	No	NA	NA	NA	NA	Yes	Yes
Turkey	NA	NA	NA	NA	NA	Yes	No	Yes	Yes	No	Yes	Yes
Turkmenistan	NA	NA	NA	NA	NA	Yes	Yes	Yes	No	No	Yes	Yes
Ukraine	NA	NA	NA	NA	NA	Local	NA	NA	NA	NA	Yes	No
United Kingdom	Yes	Yes	No	No	Yes	Yes	Yes	Yes	No	No	Yes	Yes
Uzbekistan	NA	NA	NA	NA	NA	NA	NA	NA	NA	NA	Yes	Yes

[a] Currencies were converted into euros using the appropriate mid-year exchange rate.
[b] Funds for the development of the strategy in the Federation of Bosnia and Herzegovina only.
[c] Costs for one road traffic death only.
[d] Not formally endorsed by the government.
— Data not available.
NA: not applicable.

Country	Driving tests			Compulsory vehicle insurance system	Vehicle inspections on					Car manufacturers	
	Written	Practical	Medical		Cars	Motorized 2- or 3-wheelers	Minibuses, vans	Lorries	Buses	Seat-belt installation (all seats)	Fuel consumption
Albania	Yes	Yes	No	Yes	Yes	Yes	Yes	Yes	Yes	NA	NA
Armenia	Yes	Yes	No	No	Yes	Yes	Yes	Yes	Yes	NA	NA
Austria	Yes	Yes	No	Yes	Yes	Yes	Yes	Yes	Yes	Yes	No
Azerbaijan	Yes	Yes	Yes	Yes	Yes	Yes	Yes	Yes	Yes	No	No
Belarus	Yes	Yes	No	Yes	Yes	Yes	Yes	Yes	Yes	Yes	Yes
Belgium	Yes	Yes	No	Yes	Yes	No	Yes	Yes	Yes	Yes	Yes
Bosnia and Herzegovina	Yes	Yes	No	Yes	Yes	Yes	Yes	Yes	Yes	Yes	Yes
Bulgaria	Yes	Yes	No	Yes	Yes	Yes	Yes	Yes	Yes	NA	NA
Croatia	Yes	Yes	Yes	Yes	Yes	Yes	Yes	Yes	Yes	NA	NA
Cyprus	Yes	Yes	No	Yes	Yes	No	Yes	Yes	Yes	NA	NA
Czech Republic	Yes	Yes	No	Yes	Yes	Yes	Yes	Yes	Yes	Yes	No
Estonia	Yes	Yes	No	Yes	Yes	Yes	Yes	Yes	Yes	NA	NA
Finland	Yes	Yes	Yes	Yes	Yes	No	Yes	Yes	Yes	Yes	Yes
France	Yes	Yes	No	Yes	Yes	No	Yes	Yes	Yes	Yes	No
Georgia	Yes	Yes	No	No	No	No	No	Yes	Yes	NA	NA
Germany	Yes	Yes	No	Yes	Yes	Yes	Yes	Yes	Yes	Yes	No
Greece	Yes	Yes	No	Yes	Yes	Yes	Yes	Yes	Yes	NA	NA
Hungary	Yes	Yes	No	Yes	Yes	Yes	Yes	Yes	Yes	Yes	No
Iceland	Yes	Yes	No	Yes	Yes	Yes	Yes	Yes	Yes	NA	NA
Ireland	Yes	Yes	No	Yes	Yes	No	Yes	Yes	Yes	NA	NA
Israel	Yes	Yes	No	Yes	Yes	Yes	Yes	Yes	Yes	NA	NA
Italy	Yes	Yes	No	Yes	Yes	Yes	Yes	Yes	Yes	Yes	Yes
Kazakhstan	Yes	Yes	No	Yes	Yes	Yes	Yes	Yes	Yes	NA	NA
Kyrgyzstan	Yes	Yes	No	No	Yes	Yes	Yes	Yes	Yes	NA	NA
Latvia	Yes	Yes	No	Yes	Yes	Yes	Yes	Yes	Yes	NA	NA
Lithuania	Yes	Yes	No	Yes	Yes	Yes	Yes	Yes	Yes	NA	NA
Malta	Yes	Yes	No	Yes	Yes	No	Yes	Yes	Yes	NA	NA
Montenegro	Yes	Yes	No	Yes	Yes	Yes	Yes	Yes	Yes	NA	NA
Netherlands	Yes	Yes	No	Yes	Yes	No	Yes	Yes	Yes	NA	NA
Norway	Yes	Yes	Yes	Yes	Yes	No	Yes	Yes	Yes	Yes	No
Poland	Yes	Yes	No	Yes	Yes	Yes	Yes	Yes	Yes	Yes	No
Portugal	Yes	Yes	No	Yes	Yes	No	Yes	Yes	Yes	Yes	No
Republic of Moldova	Yes	Yes	No	Yes	Yes	Yes	Yes	Yes	Yes	NA	NA
Romania	Yes	Yes	No	Yes	Yes	Yes	Yes	Yes	Yes	Yes	Yes
Russian Federation	Yes	Yes	No	Yes	Yes	Yes	Yes	Yes	Yes	Yes	Yes
San Marino	Yes	Yes	No	Yes	Yes	Yes	Yes	Yes	Yes	NA	NA
Serbia	Yes	Yes	No	Yes	Yes	Yes	Yes	Yes	Yes	Yes	No
Slovakia	Yes	Yes	No	Yes	Yes	Yes	Yes	Yes	Yes	Yes	Yes
Slovenia	Yes	Yes	No	Yes	Yes	Yes	Yes	Yes	Yes	Yes	No
Spain	Yes	Yes	No	Yes	Yes	Yes	Yes	Yes	Yes	Yes	Yes
Sweden	Yes	Yes	No	Yes	Yes	Yes	Yes	Yes	Yes	Yes	Yes
Switzerland	Yes	Yes	No	Yes	Yes	Yes	Yes	Yes	Yes	NA	NA
Tajikistan	Yes	Yes	No	Yes	Yes	Yes	Yes	Yes	Yes	NA	NA
The former Yugoslav Republic of Macedonia	Yes	Yes	Yes	Yes	Yes	Yes	Yes	Yes	Yes	NA	NA
Turkey	Yes	Yes	No	Yes	Yes	Yes	Yes	Yes	Yes	Yes	Yes
Turkmenistan	Yes	Yes	No	Yes	Yes	Yes	Yes	Yes	Yes	NA	NA
Ukraine	Yes	Yes	No	Yes	Yes	Yes	Yes	Yes	Yes	No	No
United Kingdom	Yes	Yes	No	Yes	Yes	Yes	Yes	Yes	Yes	Yes	Yes
Uzbekistan	Yes	Yes	No	Yes	Yes	Yes	Yes	Yes	Yes	Yes	Yes

Annex 12. Prehospital post-crash care systems in countries in the WHO European Region, 2008

Country	National prehospital care system	Universal access telephone number National	Universal access telephone number Regional	Telephone number(s)
Albania	Yes	No	Yes	2253364
Armenia	Yes	Yes	No	103
Austria	Yes	Yes	No	144
Azerbaijan	Yes	Yes	Yes	103
Belarus	Yes	Yes	No	103
Belgium	Yes	Yes	No	100
Bosnia and Herzegovina	Yes	Yes	Yes	124
Bulgaria	Yes	Yes	No	150
Croatia	Yes	Yes	No	112
Cyprus	Yes	Yes	Yes	199, 112
Czech Republic	Yes	Yes	No	112, 155
Estonia	Yes	Yes	No	112
Finland	Yes	Yes	No	112
France	Yes	Yes	No	112
Georgia	Yes	Yes	No	03
Germany	Yes	Yes	Yes	112
Greece	Yes	Yes	No	166
Hungary	Yes	Yes	No	112
Iceland	Yes	Yes	No	112
Ireland	Yes	Yes	No	999, 112
Israel	Yes	Yes	No	101
Italy	Yes	Yes	No	118
Kazakhstan	Yes	Yes	No	03
Kyrgyzstan	Yes	Yes	No	103
Latvia	Yes	Yes	No	112
Lithuania	Yes	Yes	No	112
Malta	Yes	Yes	No	112
Montenegro	Yes	Yes	No	124
Netherlands	Yes	Yes	No	112
Norway	Yes	Yes	No	113
Poland	Yes	Yes	No	112
Portugal	Yes	Yes	No	112
Republic of Moldova	Yes	Yes	No	903
Romania	Yes	Yes	No	112
Russian Federation	Yes	Yes	No	03
San Marino	Yes	Yes	No	118
Serbia	Yes	Yes	Yes	94
Slovakia	Yes	Yes	Yes	112
Slovenia	Yes	Yes	No	112
Spain	Yes	Yes	No	112
Sweden	Yes	Yes	No	112
Switzerland	Yes	Yes	No	144
Tajikistan	Yes	Yes	No	03
The former Yugoslav Republic of Macedonia	Yes	Yes	No	194
Turkey	Yes	Yes	No	112
Turkmenistan	Yes	Yes	No	03
Ukraine	Yes	Yes	No	03
United Kingdom	Yes	Yes	No	999
Uzbekistan	Yes	Yes	No	03

Annex 13. National data coordinators and survey respondents in countries in the WHO European Region

Country	National data coordinator(s)	Respondents
Albania	Maksim Bozo	Fatos Olldashi, Maksim Tasho, Demir Osmani, Luri Balla, Gentiana Qirjako
Armenia	Lilit Avetisyan	Ella Safaryan, Grigory Torosyan, Rubik Navoyan, Vardan Petrosyan, Vahe Petrosyan, Mariam Gukasyan
Austria	Rupert Kisser	Guenter Breyer, Martin Germ, Fritz Wagner, Martin Vergeiner, Thomas Fessl
Azerbaijan	Rustam Talishinskiy	Hikmet Ibishov, Ali Aliyarov, Anar Orujov, Rustam Humbetov, Mamed Jafarov, Arif Mirzoev
Belarus	Ivan Pikirenia	Pavel Bozhanov, Sergey Zarecky, Andrej Gusakov, Tatiana Goriainova, Anatoly Sushko
Belgium	Anne Meerkens	Leen Meulenbergs, Rudi Wagelmans, Miran Scheers, Jan Robben, Denis Hendrichs, Anneliese Heeren, Paul Deblaere
Bosnia and Herzegovina	Jasminka Kovacevic, Alen Seranic	Munira Zahiragic, Muhamed Ahmic, Pavo Boban, Irena Jokic, Natasa Kostic, Mira Bera, Zelimir Skrbic, Jelena Glamocika
Bulgaria	Irina Kovacheva	Valentin Panchev, Evelin Jordanova, Anton Antonov, George Petrishki, Diana Dimitrova
Croatia	Ivana Brkic Biloš	Tihomira Ivanda, Ivica Franić, Boris Orlović, Dinka Rajčić, Željko Remenar
Cyprus	Costas Antoniades, Olga Kalakouta	Soteris Koletias, Stavros Cleanthous, Andreas Kouppis, George Morfakis, Charilaos Evripidou
Czech Republic	Veronika Benesova	Sarka Kasalova Dankova, Josef Tesarik, Zuzana Ambrozova, Jaroslav Horin
Estonia	Ursel Kedars	Dago Antov, Erik Ernits, Jaak Kalda, Alo Kirsimäe, Toomas Ernits
Finland	Petri Jääskeläinen	Merja Söderholm, Leif Beilinson, Pasi Kemppainen, Marita Koivukoski
France	Bernard Laumon	Jean Chapelon, Mireille Chiron, Mouloud Haddak, Alexis Marsan, Yves Rauch
Georgia	Kakha Kheladze	Mamuka Vatsadze, Zaza Devdariani, Kakhaber Chikhradze, Eka Laliashvili, Aleqsandre Tudziladze
Germany[a]		Rosemarie Schleh
Greece	Dimitrios Efthymiadis	Spyros Panagopoulos, Vilelmini Paraschou, Vasiliki Mylona-Danelli, Georgios Kanellaidis, Maria Vaniotou, Konstantina Kosmidou
Hungary	Mária Bényi	Péter Holló, Ákos Probáld, Csaba Kiss, Kirisztina Tálas, Zsófia Szász
Iceland	Rósa Thorsteinsdóttir	Svanhildur Thorsteinsdóttir, Birna Hreiðarsdóttir, Kristján Ó Guðnason, Sigurður Helgason, Brynjólfur Mogensen
Ireland	Declan Hayes	Robbie Breen, Gerry O'Malley, Ann Cody, Harry Cullen, Michael Brosnan, Con O'Donohue
Israel	Kobi Peleg, Sarit Levi	Rinat Zaig, Orit Yalon-Shuqrun, Tsippy Lotan, Maya Siman-Tov, Vered Yeshouia, Zeev Shadmi
Italy	Maria Giuseppina Lecce	Vito Disanto, Giandomenico Protospataro, Raffaella Amato, Alba Rosa Bianchi, Alberto Valenti
Kazakhstan	Nurlan Batpenov	Galina Jaxybekova
Kyrgyzstan	Samatbek Toimatov	Viktor Kustov, Elvira Torobekova, Zoya Tulegenova, Ludmila Turgasheva, Imanali Sarkulov, Soolot Begaliev, Emil Omuraliev
Latvia	Jana Feldmane	Aldis Lama, Georgijs Sovetovs, Jolanta Skrule, Maija Gaide, Vida Lukasevica, Arnis Vilums, Anita Villerusa
Lithuania	Ramunė Meižienė	Gintaras Aliksandravičius, Marius Vitėnas, Jelena Selivonec, Aušra Želvienė, Aida Laukaitienė
Malta	Neville Calleja, Audrey Galea	Joseph Galea, Therese Ciantar, Josie Brincat, Maryanne Massa, Kathleen England
Montenegro	Svetlana Stojanovic	Saša Stefanovic, Dijana Subotic, Nevenka Tomic, Klikovac Dragan, Sovjetka Veljic, Slobodan Tadic
Netherlands	Martijn Vis	Niels Bos, Peter Van Vilet, Harry Derriks, Loek Hesemans, B. Van Bruggen
Norway	Jakob Linhave, Signe Vind	Marthe Lillehagen, Finn Harald Amundsen, Jan Guttormsen, Kristin Øyen
Poland	Barbara Król	Jacek Zalewski, Robert Trajan vel Trojanowski, Andrzej Grzegorczyk, Ryszard Krystek, Maria Dabrowska-Loranc, Anna Zielinska
Portugal	Gregória Paixão von Amann	Ana Coroado, Victor Lourenço, Luís Filipe Branco, Angelina Afonso, José Lisboa Santos, Maria da Conceição Jorge Proença, Samuel Bonito Martins, Rodolfo Manuel Martins Soares
Republic of Moldova	Filip Gornea	Iurie Untilov, Petru Crudu, Nicolae Mihul, Gheorghe Ceban
Romania	Raed Arafat	Gino Theodor Bosman, Cristian Constantinescu
Russian Federation	Gennady Kipor	Boris Grebenuk, Aleksei Koldin, Leonid Borisenko, Aleksei Voitenkov, Andrei Fonski, Alexandr Gordienko
San Marino	Andrea Gualtieri	Eleonora Liberotti, Vladimiro Selva, Eva Guidi, Dennis Guerra, Federica Renzi, Marco Podeschi
Serbia	Milena Paunovic	Jovica Vasiljevic, Demir Hadzic, Krsto Lipovac, Ivana Radojicic, Svetlana Trtica
Slovakia	Martin Smrek	Adam Hochel, Katarina Halzlova, Alena Petrikova, Stefan Pristas, Hruskovic Samuel, Darina Sedlakova
Slovenia	Matej Košir	Vesna Marinko, Bojan Zlender, Bostjan Smolej, Mateja Rok-Simon, Robert Staba
Spain	Vicenta Lizarbe	Pilar Zori Bertolin, Catherine Pérez, María Seguí-Gómez, Teodoro Casillas Martin, María Librada Escribano, María Antonia Astorga
Sweden	Thomas Lekander	Bengt Svensson, Åsa Ersson, Ulf Björnstig, Johan Lindberg, Gunnar Ågren, Lars Darin
Switzerland	Bertrand Graz	Christoph Jahn, Lukas Matti, Brigitte Buhmann
Tajikistan	Abduvali Razzakov	Kurbonkhon Saidov, Nazarali Rahmatulloev, Hasan Nazarov, Shuhratjon Ziyoboev, Shodi Jamshedov
The former Yugoslav Republic of Macedonia	Fimka Tozija	Spase Jovkovski, Boris Murgoski, Cane Kostvski, Marjan Kopevski, Elena Eftimovska, Ljubica Damceska
Turkey	Huseyin Fazil Inan	Bora Kayser, Senturk Demiral, Ismet Temel, Veysel Akkus, Erpulat Ozis, A. Haki Turkdemir, Y. Mehmet Kontas
Turkmenistan	Begklich Ovezklichev	Gurbanmurad Shihmuradov, Mekan Gaipov, Maral Kakisheva, Nataliya Levaya, Irina Kivandova, Maral Kakabaeva, Dovran Ovezov, Ata Boppiev, Mamedov Meylis
Ukraine	Irina Fedenko	Mikhail Golubchikov, Svetlana Sinelnik
United Kingdom	Mark Bellis, Sara Hughes	Andrew Colski, Pat Kilbey, Harry Green, Carol Ann Munn, Paul Taylor, Sue Maisey, Meryl James
Uzbekistan	Mirhakim Azizov, Gulnora Kasimova	

[a] Questionnaire completed by the Federal Highway Research Institute (BASt).